In the Light
of the Self

In the Light of the Self

Adi Shankara and the Yoga of Non-dualism

by

ALISTAIR SHEARER

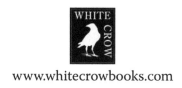

www.whitecrowbooks.com

BY THE SAME AUTHOR

Effortless Being (with photographs by Richard Lannoy)

The Upanishads (with Peter Russell & photographs by Richard Lannoy)

The Traveller's Key to Northern India

Thailand: The Lotus Kingdom

The Hindu Vision: Forms of the Formless

Buddha: The Intelligent Heart

Selections from the Upanishads

Islam through Art

Buddhism through Art

Hinduism through Art

The Spirit of Asia (with photographs by Michael Freeman)

India: Land of Living Traditions (with photographs by Michael Freeman)

The Yoga Sutras of Patanjali

Views from an Indian Bus

ABOUT THE AUTHOR

Alistair Shearer (www.alistairshearer.co.uk) has worked and travelled throughout the Land of the Veda over many years. He has taught courses on Indian art and architecture for several prestigious institutions, such as the *British Museum, The School of Oriental and African Studies* at *London University* and the auction houses *Sotheby's* and *Christie's*. A long-time teacher of meditation in the lineage of Shankara, he recently co-created an award-winning retreat hotel (www.neeleshwarhermitage.com) on the coast of Malabar, in the sage's homeland Kerala.

PRAISE FOR
ALISTAIR SHEARER'S BOOKS:

The Upanishads:

A lovely decanting of this very old wine into a sparkling new bottle
~ JOHN UPDIKE

This is the kind of text that one keeps close at hand like an old, wise and compassionate friend
~ RAM DASS

An elegant and valuable contribution to the growing corpus of Upanishadic texts in English
~ DR. KARAN SINGH

The Traveller's Key to Northern India:

This is quite simply the most informed and the most literate guide to the great Indian keynotes. It is the vade mecum for the intelligent student of the subcontinent
~ GEOFFREY MOORHOUSE

Superb. A well-written, vivid and informative guide
~ TRAVEL & LEISURE

By far the best guidebook on India I have ever seen
~ HUSTON SMITH

The Yoga Sutras of Patanjali:

> *A wonderful translation, full of contemporary insight yet luminous with eternal truth*
>
> ~ JACOB NEEDLEMAN

The Spirit of Asia:

> *An engaging and lively narrative of first hand experience ... one is touched not only by the deep mystery of these sacred places but by the devotion and sensitivity that the author brings to his task*
>
> ~ PARABOLA

'Just because something is not immediately visible does not mean it does not exist. Consider the case of light. In itself, it is imperceptible, yet it spreads through endless space. When all objects are removed, that light is not perceived anymore because all the objects that reflected it and made it visible have gone. But that does not mean that light itself, in its own pure nature, has vanished'.

ADI SHANKARA *(COMMENTARY ON THE BRAHMA SUTRA 1.1.4.)*

CONTENTS

INTRODUCTION

Few people outside India know the name Adi Shankara, though in his homeland this philosopher-saint is a hailed as a national treasure, even amongst secularists. Jawaharlal Nehru, the first leader of independent India and a westernised socialist with no time for religion, paid tribute to Shankara as 'a curious mixture of a philosopher and a scholar, an agnostic and a mystic, a poet and a saint, and in addition to all this, a practical reformer and able organiser'. The comprehensive nature of Shankara's genius is actually far more than that rather dismissive 'curious mixture', it is an astonishing phenomenon. As a champion of Vedic orthodoxy, he is celebrated for giving a coherent structure to many of the beliefs and practices that the West calls Hinduism and India *Sanatana Dharma* 'the Eternal Law'. That structure persists today. Gratefully remembered by the orthodox for purifying and re-invigorating disparate schools and sects to form a united bulwark against the challenges posed by Buddhism, he is also revered for establishing puissant centres of learning, each with its lineage of leaders, orders of monks and traditions of instruction, that continue to direct the religious instincts of millions. For intellectuals, his widest-reaching achievement is the extensive body of commentary he wrote on many major scriptures, the authority of which has never been surpassed. There were also many original compositions: both erudite metaphysical works and heartfelt hymns of popular devotion. All of these writings still uplift and inspire seekers after truth in both East and West.

So, if we were to recast Nehru's assessment and describe this prolific luminary in Christian terms, we could say he combined the metaphysical insight of a Meister Eckhart with the organising power of an Ignatius Loyola, and the exegetical authority of a St. Augustine with the devotional sensitivity of a Julian of Norwich. And all of these energetic talents were rolled together into one very short life; Adi Shankara died at the age of only thirty-two.

The life

What, then, do we know of Shankara the man? The answer is: almost nothing for certain. Tradition tells us he was born in a village called Kaladi near Cochin (modern Kochi) in Kerala, into a very high caste, the Nambudiri *brahmins* who, then as now, were the hereditary guardians of orthodox Vedic knowledge. The boy studied all the traditional disciplines incumbent on a male with his social status. He showed exceptional intellectual prowess from the start and renounced home and family at an early age, leaving his native place to find enlightenment. Travelling north towards the Himalayas in search of a Master, he finally found him in central India and spent time there serving his *guru* and studying sacred knowledge. All of this conforms to the idealised paradigm laid down for a refined *brahmin* youth in the Upanishads, sacred texts dating from perhaps 800 BC, that were to be the bedrock of Shankara's own message. After being initiated into the formal vow of renunciation (*sannyasa)* by his teacher and imbued with a quite extraordinary creative energy, the young monk then embarked on his teaching mission, spending much of his life travelling the length and breadth of the subcontinent. We do not know where he died; two of the most popular traditions cite places a good twelve hundred miles apart.[a]

Such are the bare bones of the life, but just when it took place continues to be a matter of fierce debate. On the one hand scholars and academics place Shankara sometime in the eighth century AD, citing in support of their view references from his own writings to places and people. Over the years academia has reached a consensus, first proposed over 100 years ago by the eminent German indologist Max Mueller, that he lived from 788 – 820 AD. On the other hand, a spectacularly different timeline is advanced by the holders of Shankara's lineage. Three of the five major monasteries he established hold records of an unbroken apostolic succession stretching back to their founding some twelve hundred years earlier than this date.[b] Their argument is that the scholars have long confused a later teacher of the same name or title with the original Master[c] and that Shankara was in fact born in 509 BC. If correct, this would mean he lived not long after the Buddha whose teachings, at least as they were being presented by the Buddhists he encountered, he often and vigorously refutes. An independent Jain text confirms this early date but, to add further confusion, the fourth of the principal monasteries he founded

supports a tradition that he was born later, in 44 BC.[d] Even by the no-
toriously imprecise chronology of early Indian history, such glaring
discrepancies are exceptional.

If we follow the scholars and place Shankara's birth in the last
quarter of the eighth century AD. we can at least gain some recognisable historical context. This would tell us that he was born at a time
the proselytising armies of Islam were energetically fanning out east
and west from the birthplace of their Prophet, who had died a hundred and fifty years earlier. Nearer home, the textual commentaries
of the 'Northern Saints' of Christianity – St. Cuthbert and the Venerable Bede – had been galvanising monastic communities in Britain for
over a century by the time that the south Indian sage embarked on
his own remarkable works of exegesis. We do know that the eighth
century was a period of great political and social instability in the
subcontinent; the surrounding disorder could well have been an added impetus to spur the young monk on to revive orthodox teachings
and instigate doctrinal, and thence social, reform. Despite his youth,
he himself alludes to the need for such a reform with all the nostal-
gia of a seasoned traditionalist:

> Whoever claims that the people of olden times were no more capable
> of directly communing with the gods than we are today might as
> well claim that because there is no one universal ruler alive now,
> none such existed in former times, or that the duties and obligations
> incumbent on the various different levels of society were always
> as casually disregarded as they are nowadays.[e]

The records

What little we do know of Shankara's life and travels comes from a
handful of biographies, none of which is older than the fourteenth
century AD. Even these are disputed. Sometimes overlapping, sometimes deviating in their details, they are devotional works, hagiographies rather than strictly historical records, full of the miraculous
happenings and supernatural interventions so dear to the Indian
imagination. The most generally recognised among them is the
Madhaviya Shankaradigvijaya, ('Shankara's Tour of Victory according to Madhav') authored by Madhava Vidyaranya, a fourteenth-cen-
tury abbot of one of the original five monasteries established by the

Master.[f] Added to these mythistorical works are numerous more recent accounts that retell the essential story in many of the Indian languages and also in English.

The central thread of all these narratives is the victorious journey – *digvijaya* – that the young renunciate made around the country: teaching, establishing monasteries, renovating and re-energising temples. This folkloric tradition is a body of living legend that connects him to holy places in all parts of the subcontinent. Indeed, there is hardly a temple or shrine that would not like to claim some connection with the youthful saint, so great is his reputation, and very many enthusiastically do so. It is not uncommon to find the same miraculous event attributed to places hundreds of miles apart, a fact which does nothing whatsoever to shake the faith of the believer. This present account mentions some of these events to add some spice to the narrative while aligning it to traditional sources, but it does not place undue emphasis on them. By the same token, I have not made great efforts to try to disentangle the exact sequence of his supposed travels; the several accounts are not consistent. And while many partisan biographies assume Shankara to be one who was born already perfect – what the Indians call an *avatar* ('direct descent') of Lord Shiva – my own intent is more prosaic: to present him as a young man, albeit an extraordinarily gifted one, whose spiritual understanding grew and matured over time. One implication of this more modest perspective is that the Truth he discovered, lived and taught is open and available to all of us.

In fact, it matters little that the verifiable facts we have about Shankara's life are so few. Traditionally, India has tended to treat history not as a precise and chronological record of the past but as an exemplary body of knowledge whose purpose is to inspire and uplift the present, offering guidelines for the living. This didactic purpose is perhaps even stronger in the case of saints and enlightened teachers. What is important in the lives of such great beings is not the minutiae of where they went, and when and what they did, or didn't do, but the degree to which they radiated the Divine at all times, in all places and in all their actions. To try to assess such a life by the details that comprised it is like trying to gauge the status of a mighty ocean by painstakingly cataloguing the waves that rise and fall on its surface. The persisting import of Shankara's own life was his realisation of the Absolute behind all lives and its purpose was to manifest that level of Being wherever he went and whatever he did. In this he shared the mission of every truly great teacher: which is continuously to remind us of who we essentially are, and thence what the world fundamentally is. The ultimate importance of Shankara's time on earth is the degree to which his message conveys this one indivisible Truth to those of us who come and go after him. In this sense, he is an archetypal, rather than a merely historical, figure.

The writings

A large part of the great reverence in which the young saint is held is due to his authoritative commentaries on several major religious and philosophical texts. In these he saw himself as a timely reformer motivated, as he tells us in his commentary to the Bhagavad Gita, by 'finding the texts being interpreted in all sorts of contradictory and conflicting ways'. His major commentaries, known collectively as the *Prastana Traya*, comprise: the ten 'major' *Upanishads* (so-called due to his having selected them to elucidate), the *Brahma Sutra* a highly abstract metaphysical work authored by Badaryana and the *Bhagavad Gita*, Hinduism's most popular scripture and a continuing inspiration of much religious devotion today. He also composed a number of original works, the best known of which are: 'The Crown Jewel of Discernment' *(Vivekachudamani)*, 'The Thousand Teachings' *(Upadeshasasahasri)*, 'Self-knowledge' *(Atmabodhi)* and 'Direct Self-realisation' *(Aparokshanubhuti)* as well as the devotional works: 'Just Praise God' *(Bhaja Govindam)*, 'The Wave of Shiva's Bliss' *(Shivanandalahari)*, A Hymn to Dakshinamurti – a form of Shiva *(Dakshinamurti stotra)*, A Hymn to Vishnu - He who Forgives all Sins *(Hari stotra)* and two hymns to the Great Goddess: 'The Wave of Beauty' *(Soundaryalahari)* and 'The Wave of Bliss' *(Anandalahari)*. Relatively recently, a work with a completely different feeling-tone from these hymns, the commentary on the classical *Yoga Sutra* of Patanjali, has also been attributed to the South Indian prodigy.

This is a conservative list; there are very many other works popularly believed to be his. In fact, the standard edition of the collected works in over twenty volumes contains more than 400 titles but considerable debate remains over which are genuinely Shankara's. Modern scholars deem about twenty-five of these to be authentic, at most. Once again, we are faced here with the huge difference between committed devotee and sceptical scholar that we have already encountered when considering the sage's dates.[g]

Whatever be the exact numbers, Shankara's work has earned him unparalleled respect as an author and exegetist. But it has left us with a severely one-dimensional picture of him. The commentaries, brilliant though they may be, remain for most people something left untouched on the dusty top shelf of the library, too far above normal life for all but the most dedicated to reach. By contrast, the saints that India really takes to her heart are not dry, remote academics but the full-blooded sons and daughters of her ancient soil, superhuman in some way perhaps, but also fully human in their characteristics and personal foibles. No matter how sublime their otherworldliness, as they sit surrounded by devotees in the intimacy of *darshan*, these saints are also beloved members of the family: earthy, humorous and grounded in familiar realities, their sanctified fingers firmly on the pulse of those around them. Adi Shankara, however, has nothing of this warmth.

To compound things further, alongside this apparent lack of endearing human qualities, Shankara's teaching is generally (though incorrectly) seen as a sterile life-denying philosophy based on the cardinal principle of *maya*: the doctrine that the world is 'an illusion'. That such a resolutely austere character with such an unprepossessing message should enjoy such a hallowed and enduring reputation is an extraordinary paradox, and surely one worth investigating. Accordingly, one of my aims in writing this book has been to add some warm flesh to the dusty academic bones and present what must have been a most unusual human being as not only a great scholar but a popular and compassionate teacher, always energetically and dispassionately available to help those who came to him. In this untiring and selflessly engaged role he must, no less than other great teachers we know of, have possessed endearing human qualities. These, along with his metaphysical brilliance, must have played their part in assisting his students to achieve, if not full liberation, at least a greater understanding of the source of their sufferings and a surer orientation on the path to transcend them.

The teaching

However remarkable his personality may have been, above and beyond Shankara the man lies his teaching. It is known as Advaita Vedanta, which translates as 'the Supreme Knowledge of Non-duality' and although rooted in the Vedic-Hindu context, it is by no means confined to that culture. In fact, Advaita ('non-duality') can lay claim to be the supreme expression of what is often called the Perennial Philosophy, a term coined by the German polymath Gottfried Leibniz at the end of the seventeenth century and popularised in the twentieth by the English writer Aldous Huxley.[h] As such, it is the knowledge of life itself, unbounded by time or place.

The essential tenets of this perennial wisdom of non-dualism can be reduced to four:

- There is an infinite and unchanging Absolute which underlies, informs and ultimately transcends the world of change;
- this absolute Reality is the essence of everything, including each one of us;
- the high purpose and evolutionary imperative of human life is to realize this divine Reality and live it in everyday life;
- the means to this realisation is the systematic purification and refinement of body, mind and heart.

The non-dualist outlook is sometimes erroneously described as 'pantheism', (a view which holds that the Divine and the universe are identical) and as such it is typically judged to be a less evolved spiritual understanding than Semitic 'monotheism', the doctrine of a personalised deity who stands over and against all the other, lesser, gods. But if we are to be accurate, Advaita is actually 'panentheism' – a term taken from the Greek meaning 'all-in-God' – which is the teaching that the absolute Divine principle not only informs, but simultaneously transcends, all its myriad manifestations. Crucial to this monism is an understanding of the relationship between the Divine and non-Divine and the ultimate significance of both. The varying degrees of this distinction have historically been the subject of much debate among the more metaphysically inclined of its adherents.

While such arcane topics may hold a fascination for those few of us inclined to the abstractions of philosophy, the teachings of Advaita also address a far more immediate and down-to-earth psychological need. We live in a time when the age-old question "Who am I?" is being asked with increasing urgency and frequency. All the traditional and certain markers that have hitherto defined our sense of who and what we are – be they definitions of race, genetics, nationality, family, social role, sexuality or even gender – are currently being scrutinised and re-formed. As our sense of identity becomes ever more fluid and tenuous, the commercial imperatives of the digital world render it ever more marketable and exploited. Yet despite all the choices on offer to determine that most basic need of knowing who we are, we are no nearer to answering the ancient and enduring question. A truly satisfying answer, one that binds us together as a human family in a world peopled by many different species, while simultaneously freeing us to celebrate our manifold differences, continues to be elusive.

On the contrary, as life becomes ever more uncertain and our day-to-day living increasingly mechanised, we can see on all sides a growing obsession with image and an increasingly desperate attempt to carve out for ourselves a lasting marriage of presentation and reality, substance and essence. On the one hand, this can take the form of a consoling retreat from confusion into a narrow and bounded sense of identity that inevitably brings us into conflict with others. The disastrous results of this are clear to see in political, religious and social spheres. Looking at the current position more positively, the desire for expansive self-knowledge has never been higher. More time, money and effort is spent on individual 'self-development' than ever before, while on the collective level, for all its dehumanising effects, globalisation has also fostered the intuitive recognition that the broader our sense of identity, the more we can comprehend, live alongside and perhaps even embrace the apparent 'other'.

Perhaps unexpectedly, Shankara is entirely relevant to this contemporary dilemma, as his prime concern is precisely this perennial question of selfhood. His perspective is both radical and uncompromising and it produces an answer that involves a complete reassessment not only of our individual identity but of our role, purpose and ultimate possibility both as members of the human family and as fellow participants in the wider cosmic drama. Shankara's Advaita is a constant and continuous celebration of the real Self which exists beyond any limiting form – spatial or material, conceptual or psychic – and which informs them all. This formless Self, infinite and unlimited, is our own non-dual nature, waiting to be discovered; it is the very root of ourselves as conscious beings. The teaching thus presents an all-inclusive paradigm of our human identity: we are both limited and universal at the one time, simultaneously individual and cosmic. This exalted vision is not just a subjective or philosophical luxury, it is something of far wider practical importance. For, as he himself says, if we do not know who we really are, then how can we claim to know anything profound about the world? Knowledge based on ignorance is no real knowledge at all.

Non-duality and religion

Since earliest times, the magnificently variegated edifice of human culture has been borne along the uneven road of history by the wheels of religion. The separate spokes of these wheels may be set far apart along the rim but the nearer they come to converging at the hub, the closer they are. This hub is an empty space that permits all to join it, no matter how divergent their starting point, and is thus a fitting symbol of the non-dual Absolute beyond all forms and divisions. The teaching that stems directly from this transcendental unity of religion is uncluttered by particular dogmas and superficial differences; it can accommodate any specific viewpoint, but is bound by none. From another angle, Advaita Vedanta is the apogee of *Yoga*, a word which means 'union'. Despite these days being so often reduced to a mildly esoteric regime of oriental gymnastics, *Yoga* is in fact the systematic procedure of uniting the individual mind with the cosmic intelligence. As such, it is at one with the heart of all the great mystical traditions of humankind.

The resolute absolutism of Advaita being all-inclusive, it does not preclude more conventional religious practices if they serve the cause of liberation. Of these, devotion to some form of God and the practice of prescribed ritual are both considered a valid, and for most people necessary, help in achieving the ultimate spiritual goal of 'supreme knowledge'. If the highest evolutionary state is the unbroken experience of the non-dual Absolute that transcends all forms, it is typically achieved only gradually and by stages and at each stage a different means may be useful.

The legitimacy and utility of self-transcending devotion on the path to this enlightenment is clear both from Shankara's own life and writings and from the activities of the Vedic-Hindu tradition that energetically continues to spread his message today. Theistic worship, carried on within an overriding framework of non-dualism, follows a procedure that was laid down by the Master in his commentary on the *Bhagavad Gita* and is consistently credited to him by popular tradition: namely, a focus on the six main forms of God: Shiva, Vishnu, The Goddess, Surya, Ganapati and Ishvara, the supreme Lord. This last is a non-sectarian deity and perhaps comes closest to what the West would typically understand by the idea of an all-powerful creator God, though it is by no means synonymous with it. The worship of these different aspects of the one Divine continues to be the backbone of orthodox (*smarta*) Hinduism today.

In addition, tradition has the young sage instituting in each of the five major *maths* both a female deity and a crystal *lingam* – the symbol of Lord Shiva – brought from the sacred Mount Kailash in Tibet. The worship resulting from these ancient installations is still in full swing today.[i] Moreover, even ascetics from the orders he established have consistently worshipped personal gods. From another angle, the devotion of the student to his *guru* also plays a central role in the practice of Advaita. Shankara's own spiritual apprenticeship as well as that of many teachers in his lineage provide stellar examples of this praxis.

In its inclusivity, the living tradition of Advaita is revealed to be a spiritual path that addresses the entire range of existence. This comprises various relative realms – the gross level of form perceptible to the senses, the many subtle realms with their assorted, discarnate intelligences – and ultimately the transcendent, absolute field that lies beyond all manifestation. In whatever way they may be envisioned or symbolised, these nested layers of life, when taken together as one indivisible whole, are known in Shankara's teaching as 'the Totality' (*brahman*).

The method

Although he is usually considered such, Shankara is not a philosopher in the conventional sense of that word. His intellectual acuity notwithstanding, he is not just a professional thinker who painstakingly and sequentially weaves conceptual threads together to create his own particular tapestry of truth. The Advaitin perspective of non-dualism derives instead from a settled state of mature, radical and spiritual insight technically known as *jnana* and usually trans-lated rather misleadingly as 'knowledge'. This direct insight stems not from simply thinking about life but from going within and plumb-ing the depths of our being from which our very life springs forth. It is this clear cognition into the very heart of what constitutes the self, rather than simply a consistently maintained conceptual posi-tion, that characterises all Shankara's work and teaching. Nonethe-less, when he wishes to, the master Advaitin can employ relentless reasoning to defend or advance this radical cognitive insight and he frequently enjoys doing so. But his methodology can sometimes be difficult for the modern mind to accept. The Master's logic – some-times quite brilliant, sometimes playful and impish – can be elusive. Take for example his assertion that:

> It is not possible to deny the Self, for it is always the very Self of the one who would deny it![j]

Such circularity is impossible to counter and may be criticised as sophistry, but the wider point here is that the Truth is not proven by any argument. Indeed, for Truth to dawn, our most cherished tool – the thinking mind – must itself be transcended. Here Shankara is in complete accord with his inherited tradition of the Upanishads, and with mystics the world over, in asserting that what is needed is an immediate, irrefutable and liberating perception, whereby the fact of the matter becomes as obvious as 'a gooseberry fruit lying in the palm of one's hand' as Indian texts quaintly put it. To help those whose minds are too dull to enjoy this direct apprehension, the compassion-ate teacher will employ logic, dialectic, provisional truth, humour, outrage or whatever other means are deemed necessary to precipi-tate such an insight, while remaining always mindful that the Truth lies prior to all such strategies. They will be employed only so long as they continue to be a 'useful means' (*upaya*).

One of these means that the modern reader may find sometimes unconvincing is the use of analogy, a device that occurs very fre-quently in all Indian systems of wisdom. Analogy, like symbolism, is a wonderful way to render concrete and comprehensible something that is abstract and unfamiliar, but to the Westernised intellect, ha-bituated to discern differences, the comparison between two appar-ently quite unrelated things may have a poetic charm but it does not *prove* anything. On the other hand, to the awareness that realises everything to be a modification of an underlying unity, analogy is a peculiarly apt device because it accurately reflects the fact that behind all observed differences lie deep causal principles that silently unify life's surface diversities whilst at the same time, paradoxically, maintaining them.

Whatever form they may take, all such pedagogic strategies are examples of what the Indian traditions call 'using a thorn to remove a thorn' – in other words, employing familiar mental categories only in order radically to transcend them. The aim is always to effect a turn-around in the student's awareness, propelling him or her towards the abstract reality that is their own Self. As this consciousness lies patiently beyond any thought, feeling, imagination or archetype, such transcendence is almost impossible to achieve through mere discussion or discursive reasoning. Our minds are too habituated to concretised experience and binding concepts, too unfamiliar with more abstract, emptier modes of functioning. This is precisely why the methodology of silencing the mind through deep meditation is an indispensable part of the journey to Self-realisation. Whenever that journey may be completed, the practical thing is to make a start. As the master Vedantin himself disarmingly confides:

> 'First let me set them on the right path, then in time I will gradually be able to bring them round to the final Truth'.[k]

The form

Many of Shankara's commentaries are structured as a type of Socratic dialogue, a dialectical debate between himself, usually referred to as 'the Vedantin', and one or more others typically called 'the Opponent'. This format of juxtaposition allows the subject in question to be approached from many different angles successively, until all possible wrong views have been put forward and eliminated, allowing the truth of the situation to stand forth, alone and clear. I have followed this method in my storytelling as it remains faithful to the original while at the same time providing some human and dramatic context to what are often highly abstract topics.

The path

Advaita Vedanta, then, derives its meaning and validation from the practitioner's direct experience. Such an opening in consciousness is typically nurtured by meditation and may involve appropriate religious observance. Ultimately, what is called 'direct knowledge of the Totality' (*brahmavidya*) has nothing to do with either intellectual concepts or religious ritual but is the result of consciously transcending all physical and psychic limitations. Rare though it may be, according to Advaita this intuitive vision of unicity is our natural state and as such it constitutes true 'knowledge'. Given this, the teaching has no hesitation in dismissing our habitually dualistic modes of perception – in other words, whatever we experience while waking or dreaming – as 'ignorance'(*avidya*). And although it is technically a state of non-experience, sleep is also contained in this category, if only because, like the other two, it is a transitory mode of mind and thus ineligible as a valid means though which to ascertain ultimate truth, which in all Indian systems of thought, is that which does not change.

Though it will turn our common-sense view of reality on its head, knowledge of the Self is based on profound human understandings. This is why, for all his intellectual persistence and respect for textual authority, Shankara frequently refers to the value of everyday or common-sense experience as the yardstick against which clever reasoning and scripture are to be measured. Indeed, he gives priority to such experience, insisting that truths initially derived from scripture or intellect must be internalised and experienced afresh in one's own case if they are to have any lasting value.

In sum

This book is not intended as a chronological or historically accurate account of Shankara's life. It seeks rather to serve as reader in his teaching that is compiled of many short sections, each of which stands alone and can be contemplated in its own time. In fact, these teachings are best taken in small, as it were, homeopathic, doses - one or two at a time. An overdose will lower their potency.

In assembling these sections I have utilised three sources. First and foremost is my own translation, interpretation and summary of excerpts from original sacred texts and, particularly, Shankara's commentaries on them. Prime among these are the *Bhagavad Gita*, the *Brahma Sutra* and some of the major *Upanishads*. Amongst these last, I have paid particular attention to the *Brihadaranyaka* and the *Chandogya* which are the two that Shankara himself seemed to prefer. They are the oldest and longest of that venerable corpus and they contain the greatest amount of purely Vedic material. My own translations have been backed up of course by several others; textual reference for the source of each teaching is provided in the Notes at the end of the book.

My second source of inspiration has been the example of some of the great beings who have lived and taught non-duality in recent times. One of these is the incomparable Anandamayi Ma; another is Sri Ramana Maharshi of Arunachala, perhaps the best-known modern exponent of classical Advaita. Ramana so revered Shankara that he referred to him simply as 'The Teacher' (*Acharya*) and he translated some of his writings. Maharishi Mahesh Yogi and his Master, Swami Brahmananda Saraswati, the former Jagadguru Shankaracharya of Jyotir Math, have both influenced my life and work profoundly over forty years or more, and continue to do so. Brahmanandji, as he is affectionately known in the Ganges lands, was once described by the first President of India, Dr. Rajendra Prasad, as 'Vedanta incarnate'. And then there is Swami Jayendra Saraswati, the current Jagadguru Shankaracharya of Kanchikamakoti Peetham who, in very difficult times, continues to radiate the spiritual effulgence of that extraordinary institution. Each of these great souls sings the same unending Song of Life, albeit in their differing accents. Over the years, I have been fortunate to spend a little time with some of them and it is with a sense of deep respect and gratitude that I salute them all.

Finally, I have included a few of the typical parables and stories with which the saints of the Land of the Veda have always spiced up their teaching. In doing so, they draw naturally and without effort from that fathomless well of folkloric wisdom that has nourished the Indian psyche for thousands of years, generation after generation. Long may it continue to do so.

Adi Shankara's work is an ongoing celebration of the Absolute that reconciles all apparent opposites while simultaneously transcending them. The realisation of this divine principle in the state of enlightenment is his unfailing context and constant interest. This beatitude – a state of plenitude beyond all boundaries – is universal. This being the case, it is perhaps fitting to end with some words from a time and place very far removed from Shankara's own. They come from a seventeenth century English poet who was also Dean of St Paul's Cathedral. Here John Donne speaks of attaining the celestial unity in words that the young South Indian *brahmin* who lived the enlightened life a thousand years earlier on the other side of the earth would instantly have recognised:

> 'And into that gate we shall enter, and in that house we shall dwell, where there shall be no cloud nor sun, no darkness nor dazzling, but one equal light; no noise nor silence, but one equal music; no fears nor hopes, but one equal possession; no foes nor friends, but one equal communion and identity; no ends nor beginnings, but one equal eternity'.[1]

Autumnal Equinox 2017
Laxfield,
Suffolk,
England.

PART ONE:

THE BOY

It was the hour of the cow-dust. To the east the clouds were dark and full of thunder but shot with red and gold from the setting sun. Each was a different shape and carried a light of its own; they hung towering over the ancient hills, immense, and between them patches of sky shone blue and delicate aquamarine. Each hill had its own character: one was dark and sculpted, another seemed almost transparent, as if lit from within. In the valley below, along the winding river bank, men and women were coming back from the fields in little groups, some chanting or singing, others silent from the day's toil. Among them stepped the patient animals, they knew their way home and were in no hurry, stretching their tired limbs with care. Further along the river lay the village, where a hundred fires had already been lit for the evening meal. As far as the eye could see, flat ribbons of smoke drifted out across the ground, while high above them long graceful lines of geese straggled across the sky on their way to roost. From the grove of sacred *banyan* trees on top of the small hill above the village came the sound of temple bells, as tiny oil lamps were lit for the evening *puja* to goddess Bhagavati, She who protects the night. It was a beautiful scene, and, despite the noisy flocks of crows gathering in the trees, full of contentment and the dignified repose that follows honest labour.

The hills became deep blue and dreamy in their folds and as the light rapidly faded, the trees became still and dark. The boy loved this twilight time, when the world hung suspended as the energies of the day retired and those of the night emerged. Sitting under one of the old trees at the edge of the *banyan* grove he had a clear view of the village below. Its houses were almost encircled by the wide, lazily twisting river; beyond them lay neatly cultivated fields and then dense woods stretching into the distance. Watching the winding down of the day's activities gave him a feeling of great peace but it was tinged with a poignancy at the inevitable passing of time.

The trees where he sat were visited by many birds and animals. Beady-eyed mynahs hopped and pecked along the ground and green parakeets gathered in untidy chattering groups before suddenly taking

3

wing, screeching, to wheel as one across the soft pink sky. Squirrels darted up and down the gnarled trunks, while lines of ants hurried purposefully across the forest floor watched by flat-headed lizards, stationed motionless among the dry fallen leaves as they patiently awaited their next meal. Sometimes a deer would come and shyly stand near him or a white-throated fishing eagle circle overhead, its wings hardly moving. All around, the roots of the ancient trees hung down in tangled tresses, giving a feeling of protection and aloneness.

The boy felt at home with that aloneness. From the very beginning he had been a solitary child, different from the others in the village. It was not that they disliked him, or resented him in any way, but there was something about him that marked him out as unusual and his fellows instinctively recognised it. He did not share their robust solidity; an aura of silence enfolded him, setting him apart. Adults noticed it too and some found the directness of his gaze unsettling. It was perhaps as well that none of them knew the circumstances of his birth, for his parents had kept their secret to themselves, well aware how people fear what they do not understand and how ignorant gossip can poison.

The boy's father, Shivaguru, was a pious and learned *brahmin* who traced his ancestry from the 'three thousand pure ones' who, long ago, had brought the sacred scriptures down from the North. These bearers of light settled inland, far beyond the eastern spice hills that rose in slow soft-pelted folds up from the coast, and to this day their descendants still live there, serving the great god whose dance of bliss sustains the universe.[1] At the time of the great famine, the boy's grandparents had come westwards over the hills in search of a livelihood, eventually arriving at the village he knew as home. Nambudiri *brahmins*, they brought with them both status and money, so settled into their new surroundings with ease and speed. Soon, they had a son, who they called Shivaguru. He was their only offspring, and from the start seemed a reclusive child, precociously interested in asceticism and spiritual knowledge. His father, Vidyadhiraja, needed all his powers of persuasion to get the boy to agree to marry and enter the householder way of life. A girl called Aryamba, from another Nambudiri family well-known for its piety, was chosen as a suitable bride for the introverted little boy.

Shivaguru and his new wife lived happily together. But after several years of marriage, despite their unswerving performance of all the appropriate rites, no child had arrived. Fearing that fate had marked her out to remain an empty vessel, Aryamba decided the couple should make a pilgrimage to the Hill of Joy at Vrishachala[2] near her ancestral family home, to seek a boon from the god who lived there and was renowned for his power to bless unlucky couples with children. Once at the temple, Shivaguru and Aryamba devoted themselves to the customary worship. They visited all the main shrines and made offerings, paid special reverence to the great Shiva *lingam* that, higher than a man, stood surrounded by lamps and glistening with libations of clarified butter, and they bathed daily in the sacred river that ran alongside the temple complex. To add weight to their efforts they also offered prayers to Lord Ganapati the Remover of all Obstacles and to the beautiful blue god Krishna, Lord of Love and, for good measure, payed their respects to other shrines belonging to the local guardian deities. When not worshipping in the temple the couple wandered timidly together around the town, open-mouthed with wonder at its size, busyness and splendour. On the last night of their stay, Shivaguru had a dream. An old man appeared to him and offered him a choice: many sons, each of whom would be strong and long-lived but average, or just one, who would be quite exceptional but live only a few years. Overcome, Shivaguru asked for permission to consult his wife on the matter. On waking he was amazed to learn that Aryamba had also had an unusual dream, but in hers Lord Shiva himself had appeared in all his glory, riding the sacred white bull Nandi, 'the Joyous'. Shiva informed her that her son was destined to become a great spiritual teacher, perhaps the greatest. Confused and overawed, the couple prayed humbly to the Lord not to test them but to do as He wished.

The first night back in their home village, Aryamba had another dream. This time Shiva appeared again. He told her he was gratified by the sincerity she and her husband had shown and as a reward for their piety, He himself would be born as their son. But they must heed the warning that his sojourn on earth could not last long.

And so it happened that the next spring the boy was born. The women who attended the birth to sing comforting songs, hold Aryamba's hands and wipe the sweat from her brow were struck by two things. Firstly, the labour was unusually short – about ten minutes – and painless. Secondly, once he had slipped out, the baby did not cry at all; placed on his mother's breast he lay quite serenely, his skin brilliantly lustrous and his breath coming without hindrance. An overwhelming feeling of peace enveloped them all. As the women

5

cleaned the room and lit the lamps to celebrate a new life, Devaki, the oldest and wisest of them, announced that this new arrival was surely destined for great things.

Throughout the proceedings Shivaguru had been waiting outside the birth-room. His nerves were calmed when one of his wife's relatives opened the door and whispered the traditional 'shirasoday-am' – 'the head has appeared'. Shivaguru immediately sent word to Raghavan the astrologer, so that the time for the birth chart could be logged correctly. The following morning the old man was formally invited to the house to perform his scholarly task and, after completing the appropriate rituals at the family shrine, set to work with his papers. Before long he announced that the new arrival did indeed have a remarkably auspicious birth-chart and was destined to lead a life of quite extraordinary achievement, although no unusual longevity was presaged. Fee in hand, he happily departed, leaving behind him the two new parents, overjoyed with the arrival of their new son but not a little awed by the responsibility that lay ahead.

According to custom the boy was named by the syllables that denoted the time of his birth. As he grew, he was not only unusually self-sufficient and quite without fear, but possessed of such a sweet nature that everyone loved him immediately. Even when busy, people started to find an excuse to drop by Aryamba's house just to spend a few minutes with the child. Despite his age he seemed quite selfless, unmindful of his own needs but always obliging and ready to help anyone. Yet despite this natural conviviality, he also manifested a love of solitude, choosing whenever possible to be by himself rather than join in the noisy games enjoyed by the other children in the village.

The boy was always happiest when outdoors. Most of all, he loved to walk. He would walk all through and around the village, keenly aware of all he saw and noting how the light created varying shades and textures on the walls and roofs and fell differently on straw and brick. He walked each of the winding paths beyond the village houses, stretching up to pluck fruit from the branches that reached down to him, or kneeling down to rummage among the bushes and grasses for the wild berries waiting to be discovered. He followed the banks of the wide river, where the rise and fall of the water etched delicate patterns in the sand and the leaping fish spread ripples that reflected off each tree trunk, each overhanging leaf. He felt no separation from the scrubby thorn bushes and the waving grasses sprinkled with brilliant flowers. The thickets and the copses, the wide sweep of emerald paddy fields with their rich tang of dark, wet earth, the busy miniature worlds of the insects – all were his intimate friends and all seemed to him to exist generously for his pleasure. Trees he loved especially, and he would hug the strange, venerable beings with delight, chatting animatedly to them as his dear companions. The bamboos creaked and rustled as they vouchsafed their shady secrets, and the birds opened their velvet throats to sing to him as they dipped and dived and swooped above his head. His heart would leap to greet the animals, the tame ones that kindly sought him out and the timid ones that watched him from a distance with their soft eyes. Sometimes he would skip and sing and leap and jump along paths carpeted with scented herbs; sometimes he sat quietly to watch the tumbling play of the clouds or the subtle shades of dawn and dusk as they unfolded surreptitiously across the huge sky. Everywhere he went he learned to read the book of nature: smelling the changes of weather and reading the portents of the shifting seasons long before they arrived, and from the wind he heard strange whispered tales of far-away places.

At night, when his parents were asleep, the boy would often slip out of the house to sit at the bends of the river and watch the hunting crocodiles as they steered fish into the bank with their long spiky tails. Or he would wander through forest groves dappled silver with moonlight, opening his ears to the hidden sounds of darkness. Lying on his back in a clearing, he would gaze up at the night sky above him, and the longer he looked, the more the twinkling points of light increased, star behind star behind star, until he felt himself stretch out, expanding and expanding until he dissolved into the blackness.

There was another side to this carefree young life. As he grew older, the boy began to fall frequently into a trance-like state, losing all sense of bodily awareness. This could happen anywhere – on his solitary walks, in the middle of playing with the other children or even during meals. When the trance happened at home, Aryamba carried him to his bed and sat anxiously by him bathing his forehead until he regained awareness, which was usually after some minutes. When he was away from home and did not return at the expected time, she anxiously set out herself to find him. Later, when such absences had become part of the household's routine she was less worried, even sending one of the other children to find him. Sometimes he was discovered at one of his favourite places in a half-conscious state, at other times he could not be found anywhere and she just had to wait for his return. When he did eventually come back he was invariably serene, though disoriented and embarrassed at the consternation his absence had caused.

Little by little his parents grew used to this strange behaviour. At first they assumed it was evidence of some sort of physical weakness but old Damodaran who knew the secrets of herbs and health, pronounced the boy fit and well. Then there was gossip that some spirit was causing the family mischief by possessing the boy but as he seemed to suffer no permanent ill effects from the trances, and was otherwise developing well and healthily, his parents gradually lost their concern. Remembering the words of Lord Shiva, they accepted the trances as a sign of his destiny, which they knew lay beyond their understanding. All they could do was watch him carefully, do their best to look after him and wait.

The boy was particularly close to his father. Each morning just after sunrise he went with him to the hilltop shrine and helped in the preparation of the offerings to Goddess Bhagavati who lived there. It was a small building, with wooden walls and a roof made of thatched palm leaves, its sturdy door-pillars painted in blue and gold. His father would announce their arrival by ringing the old brass bell that hung from the ceiling of the porch, then the boy would follow him into the shrine, carefully carrying the fresh fruit and flowers across the threshold to set them down near the ancient image. He would watch his father make the preparations, always in the same order, always with the same unhurried sense of purpose. Chanting the different names of the Goddess, he first cleaned the small shrine, sweeping the floor with a twig brush and wiping the surfaces clean with a large orange cloth. He passed the brass and copper pots and trays to the boy to empty outside, for the villagers came and gave their offerings throughout the day and there was always a heap to clear away. Each day these vessels needed cleaning and he would sit and scrub them with a mixture of sand and ashes moistened with the juice of a lime.

The result was a fine sheen of innumerable tiny scratches that made the metal shine happily. Then the boy fetched fresh water from the spring behind the shrine while his father filled the smoke-blackened brass lamps with *ghee* and checked the cotton wicks were in good order. Sometimes the stubs need trimming off, sometimes new ones must be rolled from the soft white bundle kept under the altar. Next, his father took the scented block of black resinous incense, pulled off a sticky piece and rubbed it between his palms to create several lumpy, tapering cones. Once they were lit, heavy smoke with a thick, aromatic smell wafted through the shrine. Now all was ready to begin the *puja* that would bless the day ahead.

Throughout these measured preparations the boy felt dimly conscious of a long line of continuity, stretching back to the beginnings of time and passed on from father to son, generation after generation. He loved the safe and certain repetition of it all and his heart thrilled to the brilliant colour of the fresh flowers and vermilion paste offered to the image, the smell of powdered sandalwood and the warm, homely glow of the polished metal. Most of all he loved the majestic silence that entered the still scented room when the deity, who is always pleased by simple-hearted worship, descended to bestow her blessing.

From time to time there was a communal festival that brought the whole village together. The boy would long remember one in particular: a fire-offering that his father had sponsored to ensure a good harvest. As soon as old Raghavan, who knew about the movement of the stars and their effect on humans, had consulted his tattered cloth-bound books to find the correct time to begin the ritual, everyone caught the mood of excitement. Here, in their very own village, the gods who guarded the whole district from afar were coming to pay them a visit!

On the day of the ceremony the family rose even earlier than usual, well before sunrise. After a purifying bath, his father shaved his head and donned a special robe made of yellow silk before disappearing for meditation. As the boy and his mother took their breakfast of milk and fruits, a quiet sense of harmony enveloped them. Later, the three of them walked together with unhurried but purposeful steps down to the old temple ground down by the river, where many of the villagers were already sitting freshly bathed and in their best attire. In the dappled courtyard, under the huge and tranquil *banyan* tree that overlooked the water, a large square area had been fenced-off by bamboo poles and white cords, with a white awning stretched overhead. Within this area several smaller spaces had been marked off by poles painted with red powder; each contained a small shrine heaped with fruit and flowers. A number of brick pits of different sizes and shapes sat ready to carry the fires. Some were round, others square or semi-circular; they would be used to contact the invisible presences that watched over the village. The whole place was like a magical stage set, colourful and expectant.

Suddenly, a flurry announced the arrival of the priests. Belonging to the families that have guarded the precious jewels of language from the beginning of time, they knew the sacred sounds that connect mankind with the higher beings. As befitted their status, they exuded a natural authority, signalled by the sacred thread across their bare chests and their crisp white silk *lungis*. Each had his role: some would chant the *mantras* to drive away any lurking evil spirits and invite the deities, others would light and tend the fires, yet others would make the offerings. One group, that was responsible for a particularly difficult part of the ritual, had come from the far-off kingdom of the Tamils beyond the eastern mountains. Their language sounded strange to the villagers and they looked strange too. Some had their heads half-shaved at the front, others had glistening, freshly-oiled hair hanging heavy and loose or piled up in a bun fixed with an ornate silver pin. All had ear lobes stretched long and soft by the solid blocks of gold inserted in them.

The ground around the priests was soon cluttered with piles of objects: clay pots and vessels of bamboo to hold the sacred liquids of clarified butter, milk and curds; long-handled wooden ladles to convey offerings into the flames; boards and knives to chop the herbs, a pestle and mortar to grind them. And so many offerings! Piles of sacred *kusha* grass; rice cakes; mounds of barley, wheat and sesame seeds; cardamoms, saffron and many other grasses and leaves; papayas, water melons, bananas and other fruits, both fresh and dried; different types of pressed oil; clay pots of honey and crumbling blocks of raw sugar and sticky fistfuls of dark, resinous incense and myrrh. And everywhere you looked lay the mounds of tender young coconuts and best polished rice, piled up high on beds of plantain leaves stitched together by tiny wooden pins. Glittering discs of gold and silver lay heaped up too, while next to them were laid out the long bamboo pipes that the priests would use to blow the embers into life without polluting them with their breath, and the smooth black antelope horns they would use to scratch themselves when the evening midges started to bite. And all around were the hairy mounds of coconut husks that would keep the fires alive, hour after hour.

All day long the chanting droned on, like the soporific hum of a huge swarm of bees around the hive. The boy was entranced by its hypnotic textured patterns. Sometimes the sound was smooth and elongated, like the skeins of glossy silk stretched out to dry in front of the weavers' cottages; sometimes it rang out sharp and staccato, like an axe biting into new wood. It could bounce and bubble like a stream tumbling over boulders, or drift drowsily, heavy as temple incense, wafting the mind into a dreamy haze. These ancient chants sounded as if they came from the very beginning of time, before we humans appeared on earth, and they thrilled his little body with a tingling energy, leaving him exhilarated yet peaceful.

Within the whole dreamlike day, one particular incident would stand out in his memory: the arrival of the holy cow. One priest took some clarified butter in a ladle and put a piece of gold covered in sacred grass into it. Approaching the little creature, he gazed closely into her soft eyes, took the gold into his hand and meditated intently for some moments. Then as patrons of the event, the boy and his parents got up and followed him, walking behind the cow for a few paces. They bent to scoop up some of the earth she had trodden in and, sprinkling it with holy water, offered it to the flames. And always the chanting rumbled on, rising and falling like some primordial sea, while the measured and graceful gestures of the officiants fed the flames as they crackled and spat, rising hungrily to devour the offerings.

The ceremony lasted until the sun disappeared over the hills and the whole universe seemed held in its compass. For weeks afterwards a sense of deep contentment hung like a warm, scented haze over the village and people felt themselves to be part of some vast and communal being, returned to a natural harmony with the unseen rhythms that govern both heaven and earth.

Every so often fate would toss a pebble into the placid pond of village life. One of these was the arrival of visitors from the wider world. When any stranger turned up, the children were always first on the scene, materialising in an instant as if from nowhere to stand in curious groups scrutinising the intruders intently but from a safe distance. Then, drawn from their tasks by the excited shouts, little by little the adults would arrive, their initial suspicious frowns giving way to calls of recognition or shy smiles of welcome.

Exotic envoys from that huge, itinerant population that has always earned its living moving around the Land of the Veda, these visitors were a mixed bunch. Most numerous were the peddlers, weighed down with strange cloth bundles and oddly shaped packages that disgorged herbs, magic potions, animal claws and talismanic gemstones, along with dried berries, roots and good luck stones. Some of them could tell your fate from your face or hands or even from the shadow you cast; others had monkeys or parrots that picked out little chips of painted wood to indicate your fortune. There were the musicians, jugglers, puppet-masters and magicians, and the patient blind singers who were shuffling their slow way north to touch the feet of the great blue god who lived at Guruvayur.[3] Then there were the wild looking tribal folk, dry season travellers. Their trick was to carry tattered baskets into the centre of the village with exaggerated care and, after a lengthy, teasing preamble to gather the crowd, empty them out with a dramatic flourish to scatter writhing snakes and scuttling scorpions as shrieks of horror went up from the onlookers. The village sceptics claimed the creatures had been rendered harmless, but who knew for sure?

One of the best loved of these acts was the cow and bull trained to play the part of lovers. Decked out in bright cloths and coloured glass beads, they would be led into an open space nuzzling up together, then start to quarrel, stamping their hooves and turning their backs to each other with a dismissive toss of their painted heads. Finally, after many sulks and entreaties and backing to and fro, to squeals of delight from the audience they would at last make up again, with great wet licks. Sometimes too, shaggy bears red with dust would be led lumbering from house to house. They would dance to music and perform tricks, but they could also be hired to stick their blunt snouts into anthills and suck up the insects with their long rough tongues. Most of the villagers were delighted to give a few coins or some food to have such a persistent domestic nuisance removed so easily, but Mother Janaki who lived by the disused well and knew about these things would disapprove loudly, reminding everyone she came across that an anthill is the gateway to the underground kingdom of the serpent-gods and should be left well alone.

And then there were the *sadhus*. Alone or in groups of three or four, these strange, liminal figures would suddenly materialise as if from nowhere. Before any were seen, a firm and well-modulated voice would be heard at the edge of the village, sounding the traditional greeting that announced their presence: "*OM namo Narayana* – I bow down to the Lord of the universe!*"* Many of the children, and not a few of their parents, were frightened by the wild appearance and dubious reputation of such mendicants but whenever the boy heard their call he would immediately drop what he was doing and rush to greet them. By the time the women had arrived to offer food, he would be sitting chatting enthusiastically to the newcomers and telling them all about the village. He was completely at home with them, and found their strangeness curiously familiar.

These spiritual nomads, whose ceaseless travel reflected their abandonment of settled society, usually arrived early in the morning, just as the first smoke was rising from the fires before the men ate and left for the expectant fields, and their timing fitted nicely with the rule that the *sadhu* should only take cooked food when he is on the road. Those properly educated in mendicant etiquette took only a morsel from a number of different houses, thus spreading the burden of their alms bowl. The *sadhus* ate exactly what the villagers did, excepting anything very highly spiced or containing onions or garlic, foods considered too stimulating for the religious. On good days the bowl would overflow with a rich variety: fish, gourd, peas, pulses and fresh fruit. In the frequent lean times, like everyone else, they had to make do with rice or a single green vegetable. Those who fed a *sadhu*, even if they came from the most important families in the village, always thanked the half-clad visitor for the privilege, for do not the scriptures teach that giving purifies the giver? And although the curse of a holy man was greatly feared, it was not fear that prompted such generosity from people who often had little. They gave only because they received; nourished by his teaching, blessings and a glimpse of wider horizons, they were more than happy with the bargain. For the *sadhu* roamed freely through what was for them another and altogether unimaginable world, free of the numerous obligations that hedged in their daily existence, and the expanded vista he gave them opened a refreshing window on their sometimes airless lives.

13

With food secured in his bowl, the *sadhu* would retire to eat alone, while the news of his arrival flashed around the village, usually carried by the children who ran excitedly from house to house. By rights he should also have been alone for his chanting of the scriptures after the meal, but the boy always managed to sneak a vantage point from which he could observe the visitor. Then, as the others began to come, little by little a short informal audience would begin as guest and hosts politely sized each other up. Even the children, often carrying a younger brother or sister on their hips, were held quiet by the interaction. Later, they would run back and forwards carrying messages between the men and women who, sitting in their separate groups, were not supposed to communicate openly in such a sanctified environment. After some time, when the holy man lay down to take his rest, the villagers would remain sitting there, soaking up the mysterious power of his presence, his *darshan*.

Much later, with the cooling of the sun, a more formal session would begin. The men would be drifting in from the fields before too long, so the women took advantage of their absence to ask their own questions about those things no husband could understand. As the men arrived and joined the gathering, the *sadhu* would begin with some long-awaited news from the wide world beyond, describing what was happening in the villages he had recently visited, their ups and downs, highs and lows. Once this gossip was out of the way, one of the men, a *brahmin* or respected elder, would nervously clear his throat and initiate the formal audience with a question: "How are we to live in the world and still perform our religious duties?" or "What is the best way for householders such as we to worship God?" or "How can we escape misery and rebirth?" And so the teachings would unfurl. The boy had heard such questions countless times, and their answers, but he was always fascinated to follow the latest variant on what were well-established themes. His eyes never strayed from the *sadhu's* face, as he read the body language and unconscious movements, seeing how the words tallied with the man himself. His bright young attention was focussed like an animal sniffing out a new and intriguing scent; he missed nothing.

The more skilled *sadhus* spiced their teaching with drama and humour, holding the villagers spellbound, for they knew that a well-told story, however familiar, has never been heard before. Then, little by little the talk would shade off into more mundane topics and a more personal element began to creep in. A questioner would inadvertently let slip his own particular problem, others would follow suit, and soon the atmosphere had descended from the mountain heights of scripture to the warm, humorous and familial valley of common humanity. Illnesses of men and their beasts, disputes over land and water, unruly sons and stubborn daughters, barren wives and unproductive fields – all were legitimate topics for the *sadhu's* disinterested advice. Sometimes the visitor had healing powers. In this case, after the *darshan* was over, people would line up to see him privately and get special herbs and powerful amulets or the light touch of a magical hand.

While everyone enjoyed the visits of the *sadhus*, to the boy they were a life-line. As time went by, he felt increasingly distanced from what was going on around him. To his keen, fresh eye the villagers seemed so preoccupied with the narrow focus of their lives that they never really noticed the beauty and the blessings that surrounded them but lived as if imprisoned by their day-to-day concerns. And how quickly they aged! Wearied by toil, the men soon became drained by the demands of their women and families, the women in turn exhausted by child-bearing and the daily struggle to keep a family together. He saw how men sold their lives for wages and how rapidly they were rendered useless through illness or slavish through debt. He saw the mute, habitual struggle for power between the man and the wife, and his relatives and her relatives, on and on, from parents to children to grandchildren, generation after generation. He heard the continuing disputes over land and houses and cattle and money; quarrels over reputation, slights real or imagined. The prospect of such a life, bound fast into the closely woven fabric of the village community, left him feeling suffocated. At his core the boy knew that his way led elsewhere, and that he had no time for compromise. His path was different and, although he sensed its direction only dimly, he knew it was connected to the *sadhus*. And so his heart thrilled when he heard the ochre-robed figures quoting the classic lines from the Upanishads that applaud the seeker of spiritual knowledge, praising the one 'who abandons the desire for sons, for fame, for wealth and for the worlds, and devotes himself to seeking the Real, which is his own Self'.

This, he slowly came to realise, was what his life was for. This was the destiny he had been born to fulfil and nothing on earth would stop him.

In the boy's fifth spring his father died. It was quite unexpected. The passing was rapid and straightforward: sudden tiredness one afternoon, followed by fever with heavy sweating and shaking in the evening. Aryamba sat up all night, feeding her husband *margosa* water to calm the heat, but his breath came fast and shallow and he lost consciousness in the early hours. By the time dawn cracked the sky purple, he was gone.

In fact, for those with eyes to see, it had not been so unexpected. One night a few weeks earlier, Shivaguru had been sitting with a group of the men on his front veranda. They were talking softly about their ancestors and he had mentioned that many of the men on his father's side had died young. At that very moment, a dog howled on the path outside the house. Startled glances were exchanged; everyone knew the meaning of such a coincidence. The news of the bad omen spread rapidly all around the village, but it was another three full days before Aryamba managed surreptitiously to prise out of her good friend Radhika what lay behind those sympathetic and concerned looks she had been noticing from the other women.

Aryamba mentioned nothing to her husband of course, but waiting until he had left for his morning visit to the temple, she hurried to the house of Raghavan the astrologer. Although his body was bent with age, his gaze was as piercing as a bird's, and behind his back he was known as 'the man who has seen the beginning of the world'. In the opinion of the village, he had probably foreseen its end too. The ostensible tools of his trade were the ancient palm-leaf manuscripts heaped in untidy piles around his simple room, but most of his calculation was done in his head, and sometimes he gave a reading with hardly a glance at his tattered scripts. A quick consideration of Shivaguru's birth chart confirmed the worst: Shani,[4] the bringer of difficulty and loss, was very badly aspected for the next couple of months.

Aryamba kept her eyes open for any sign. One was not long in coming. Less than a week after the dog's bark, as she was sweeping the yard, she heard a loud and persistent chirruping from the southwest corner of the compound. It came from a large green lizard and, on seeing it, her heart sank; she knew that such a sign presaged loss of a family member. Worse still, the call was repeated on three separate occasions that same day. Sensing there was no time to lose, she made her plan. Telling Shivaguru that a relative living in a nearby village had suddenly been taken ill, she got him to agree to her spending a couple of days there. Surreptitiously, she took with her all the money she had saved, for her real motive for the trip was to visit the temple where Lord Shiva in his form as Vaidyanath, Lord of Healers, had been staying for many years. It was common knowledge that *pujas* performed to him could cure illness.

Once there she began her daily visits to the shrine, taking even more care than usual to find the most beautiful white flowers to offer. In the morning she chose only those that were pearled with dew and in the evening, those that had been shaded from direct sunlight and retained their freshness. She also gave the money she had brought with her to have a special *puja* performed to pacify Shani. Throughout the ceremony she prayed earnestly for Shivaguru's life to be saved but deep down she felt a terrible weight, as if some implacable destiny was moving against her wishes.

When her husband went, Aryamba felt as if her heart had been ripped out of her chest.

The boy was deeply shocked by his father's passing. About this time, possibly connected to his loss, a process began that was to last intermittently for several years. He called it 'the cleansing'. It started with the dreams – if dreams they really were – of violent images that tore him gasping out of sleep, heart pounding. With these images came memories of a long sequence of comings and goings, arrivals and departures, the painful procession of life after life. Each coming was a blind entering into a cramped, constricting mass, the memory of being forced into a tiny new house, unable to see anything in the darkness, feeling his way around as if each room was closed off and he had to stumble unseeing from door to door, room to room. Not knowing what or where he was, he was only dimly aware of trying to establish himself bit by bit in this fragile structure that was itself still struggling to function, with eyes that couldn't yet see, ears that couldn't yet hear, everything trying to find its rightful place to work. And then, after so long spent negotiating his new surroundings, which were all the time changing and growing too, after so many months hanging suspended in this cramped prison, suddenly he was violently wrenched and pushed out of it into the blinding glare of a new world, a new life of almost insufferable intensity.

And the leavings were no less painful. They involved an inverse kind of suffering: the heart-rending sadness of being torn away from a home which, over the long years, had become so familiar. So many precious rooms and precious objects, all so full of memories and comfort and familiarity, and each time nothing could go with him, no matter how dear it was – room after room with its knitted locks and well-closed doors was wrenched away. Even the breath which had filled his whole structure for so long had to withdraw; no force on earth could stop that awesome, unavoidable coldness creeping up from the feet, up through the legs and into the body. No force on earth could lighten that inevitable, crushing, flattening weight that bore down on him as the breath got shorter and shorter. And with the swamping discomfort the mind began to unravel, travelling quite beyond control through huge reaches of space, buffeted here and there by images, memories, flashes of coloured light and outlandish sounds in a vast unending blackness...

Another, less violent, aspect of 'the cleansing' were the night journeys. These were not dreams interrupting his sleep, nor were they memories of former lives and deaths, but travels out of his body that would often signal their onset by early evening. Suddenly overcome by a heavy lassitude, he felt as if all the life energy was withdrawing from his body. Weak and slightly nauseous he would retire early to his bed, where he lay stretched out on his back like an offering awaiting the knife. The breathing would become so shallow as to almost disappear while his awareness withdrew from the surroundings, thinning out into a slender thread centred in a steadily mounting pressure of heat in the chest or the forehead or the crown. Then deep in his body the shuddering would start, a steadily mounting vibration that seemed to shake some inner part of him loose from its outer covering. As the shuddering reached a certain point of intensity, his awareness would slip out of the body and rise above it. Sometimes he would be aware of flying high up over the house and the village and travelling far and wide. Moving with a wonderful and effortless buoyancy he would look down on roofs and settlements, rivers and hills, bright sunlit deserts and forested slopes. Usually, he recognised nothing, yet there was sometimes a sense of familiarity, as if at some distant time or place he had been there, or was there even now, somehow, in tandem to his present life.

Occasionally, before the flights took place, he would need to pass through a dreadful dark and murky realm, populated by many entities.

It was like a miasmic sea full of fish and he was the dangling bait. First the sounds came, whistling and buzzing, followed by disembodied voices calling his name and faces swimming towards him out of the darkness, with eyes shining with eager, hungry intent and lolling mouths. Then the beings would start to nibble and jostle him, biting and sucking, mocking and jeering. The more he resisted, the stronger and more unpleasant their attentions became, so he learned that the best way to navigate such seas was to abandon resistance and focus his attention beyond their inhabitants.

Sometimes Garuda, King of the Birds, would take him for a journey. He never saw the great one face to face but he knew it was he, as looking down he could see himself silhouetted on the ground below, surmounted by mighty wings spreading wide above, and he could feel the firm but gentle claws gripping him on the shoulder and around the ankles. The boy and the bird would travel together over strange and wonderful landscapes, full of curious sights and buildings and beings, many of whom seemed delighted by his arrival in their realm and approached to converse without words. There were scintillating bejewelled palaces bathed by soothing sounds and surrounded by brilliant water and flowered gardens filled with light and laughter and strange and beautiful creatures. At times the great bird took him to formless realms, and he would find himself floating immersed in a field of muted brilliance that shifted continuously through subtle hues of pure, exquisite feeling. With this came an indescribably sweet sense of having reached his true home, a realm of perfect harmony and belonging.

But Garuda also showed him other sights. They travelled over sunken pits filled with ghoulish, hairy creatures, their limbs ripped off with stumps and mutilated torsos dripping blood, who snarled and drooled and fought, or mounted each other in a frenzy, rutting with the blind, driven energy of bulls on heat. He saw beings with grotesquely swollen bellies and long thin necks, gorging on their own offspring yet forever unable to satisfy their hunger and others harnessed to heavy carts being driven and whipped like weeping beasts of burden. He saw some held in an agony of discomfort, standing up to the neck in pits of slowly undulating snakes surrounded by terrible hybrid creatures. But whatever he saw, no matter how terrible or beautiful, he knew its significance instantly. There was no need of instruction; in that state to see was to understand immediately, and when he lost consciousness and awoke later, he had little clear memory of what had happened.

At yet other times 'the cleansing' took the form of physical adjustment. It was if there were many hands working deep inside him, pulling, kneading and twisting the flesh, nerves and sinews, reshaping the very contours of his body and brain. The process was completely beyond his control as he lay there breathless, enduring its fiery benediction. The head might shake violently or the whole body be moved from side to side, but usually the pain was concentrated in the head or spine. It would come on steady and implacable, building to a crescendo so intense he could not even cry out, as his consciousness felt stretched to its very limit until he lost awareness. Sometimes the pain peaked then levelled out, receded and finally passed, leaving in its wake a feeling of such blessedness that had him lying without breath or movement in tears of gratitude and joy. And when he did eventually sleep after these episodes, he would wake feeling tired but exquisitely delicate, reborn as one enveloped by an unutterable sense of beatitude and purity.

There was another type of experience that usually occurred during the day and with eyes open. Suddenly, without warning, he would have the sensation of moving straight and easily into a pure light that grew in intensity with an inconceivable swiftness, taking his awareness not just beyond the horizon of his world, but beyond all forms and time itself, dissolving all sense of limitation into a naked sense of being. He would feel himself dissolve into a vast stillness that was without shadow or even the faintest movement. This stillness arose and covered everything – the trees, the fields, the people – and it was imbued with a limitless innocence and strength and naked purity, untouched by time and change and thought.

While all these happenings came and went, each different from the last, there was one vision that recurred frequently: the face. Bearded and with long hair like a *sadhu's*, its most remarkable feature were the eyes, whose gaze was of a startling directness. Brimming with love and compassion, at the same time those eyes offered a stark challenge. It was as if, able to see so deeply, they could locate something in him that he himself was unaware of. Gently and humorously, but with an adamantine insistence, they were goading him to find it.

The boy suffered all this meekly. He never questioned the meaning of what was happening to him nor did he tell anyone. He felt no need to put his experiences into words to make them more comprehensible to himself or to others, and anyway, who would understand? And even if they did, what difference would it make? He realised, obscurely, that he was in the hands of some force, some process that must have its way, and it would have its way no matter what, so there was no point in resisting it even if he could and he knew he could not. He had his path to tread, whatever it may entail, and he was not afraid to undergo what was being demanded of him.

One sultry and overcast morning many months after Shivaguru died, a *sadhu* arrived in the village. He wore an ochre loin-cloth and carried only two things: a gourd shell as a bowl and a long metal *trishula*, the trident of Lord Shiva. The newcomer was a bear of a man: well over six feet tall, handsome and fair-skinned, his serpentine locks matted with cow dung and falling almost to the ground. He moved like a king, with an imperious gait that had him swaying slightly from side to side as he walked, and he was the tallest person anyone in the village had ever seen. He was so tall that Padmavathi, the widow who lived at the edge of the old paddy field and knew about these things, informed people he was a time-traveller from the Golden Age of Righteousness when all men were giants and children were conceived by the power of thought alone.

That a *sadhu* had materialised out of nowhere to spend the rainy season retreat was not in itself so unusual, but his mode of arrival was. Entering the village from the east, he had walked purposefully through the lanes until he reached Aryamba's house, which lay amongst the other high-caste dwellings on the northern edge of the settlement. There he sat down at the gate of her compound and waited. While many villagers were keen to offer him hospitality, it was obvious fate had selected Shivaguru's widow for this honour. People were glad; she was someone who could afford to feed an extra mouth each day and anyway, he would provide a settling atmosphere for her in her grief and no doubt be a good influence on the young boy who had lost his father so early.

The evening of the *sadhu's* arrival, the rains began. For weeks banks of heavy clouds had covered the sun with an opaque silver tarnish and the village had borne the weight of a lethargy that tested even the most patient. That evening an eerie silence descended and for an hour or more the universe seemed to hang suspended, as if waiting. And then, suddenly, came the first large drops, splashing and slapping down noisily into the cracked and desiccated earth, raising little whirlwinds of dust. The drops rapidly became spears and the spears sheets and the sheets walls – solid walls of water, relentless and deafening. The villagers stayed inside their houses, peeking out at the deluge, torn between awe at this display of Indra's[5] power and concern that last year's repairs on the roof would hold good. The ferocity continued unabated for several hours, then eased off into a lighter, but still steady, downpour. The next morning, while it was still dark and the rain fell unabated, people began emerging from their houses into the streets, some laughing and dancing, others carrying containers to catch the precious liquid they had not seen for so many months. A feeling of relief and release coursed through the village like the water in the gutters.

But the rains did not bring universal joy. As the days and weeks went by and the downpours continued, flattened crops rotted and stank in foetid swamps, while many cattle were swept away in the brown frothing river that had overrun its banks and was twice its normal width. The air was full of biting insects and bodily discomfort. One afternoon, taking advantage of a break in the rain to walk along the edge of the swollen torrent, the boy came across a large group of vultures noisily hopping and prancing over a carcase. Their black wings rustled like heavy, new silk as they reluctantly shuffled aside to reveal a grotesquely swollen body, mottled and stiff-limbed, its bloodied eye-sockets skewed to the leaden sky.

The first thing the boy liked about the *sadhu* was the way he moved, particularly his hands. Despite his size, each of his gestures was deft and graceful, delineated with such an ease and lack of effort that his way of being in the world seemed just right. There was something perfect in such economy; it reminded the boy of how his father had conducted his *puja* each day: precise, unhurried and quietly authoritative.

This new visitor spread an atmosphere of quiet but palpable content wherever he went. Quite self-sufficient, he was happy to sit without fuss for what could be hours on end, yet he was always ready to engage with anyone who wished his company. Both people and animals seemed unusually relaxed in his presence. The daily stream of women visiting the widow Aryamba increased, but now it was not the usual need to unburden themselves of the latest village happenings that brought them, but their desire to see the *sadhu*. On entering the house, they would immediately notice how loudly they had been speaking, how caught up in their own little imaginings. The man had said or done nothing; somehow just his presence acted to cast a clear and objective light on the behaviour of those around him. So it was not long before a group would come quietly each morning to sit shyly before him, pausing at the yard gate to rearrange the bunch of freshly picked flowers or polish up the fruit they had brought, for they knew well that spiritual beings should never be visited empty-handed.[6] And the widow Aryamba was happy with all this, grateful for both his presence during these restricted months of rain, and the company of friends he brought her.

The boy quickly grew to love the *sadhu* and the *sadhu* him. They would spend much of the day together, beginning with the morning *puja* to Goddess Bhagavati. The boy showed him all the walks around the village and pointed out its special places: the ruined temples and abandoned wells with their many stories, the spots where the biggest clusters of wild bees could be found, those trees where the giant bats hung in their hundreds like living fruit, and those where the fierce red ants wove nests of leaves as big as three or four coconuts together. And he showed him the twists and turns of the river, and the places where the various spirits lived, recounting in detail all the mischief they had caused in the village over the years and to whom. But most importantly, he told him what he had never been able to tell anyone: his strange night-time journeys, the things he saw and the places he visited when he travelled out of the body, and the strange subtle intuitions that irrupted into in his waking life. It was an enormous relief. The *sadhu* listened intently to all he said on this, sometimes offering a comment or explanatory aside, sometimes just nodding encouragement and understanding. And when the boy spoke of his recurring image of the bearded, smiling face with the intense gaze, the *sadhu's* eyes filled with tears, but he said nothing.

For his part, the *sadhu* would describe the freedom of the life of *sannyasa* and all the adventures it brought. How it was to wake up each morning free of possessions, expectations and commitments, ready to take to the highway and see what Mother Nature had in store that day, bound only by the obligation to visit each and every shrine you passed. How it was never to know what you would eat or where you would spend the night; how it was to be able to treat all people equally as fellow players in this strange and wonderful dream of life, how it felt to bathe in the solitude that denies nothing. He described some of the strange people he had met on his travels, and seeing how the boy revelled in the natural world, he explained many things about it: the way the trees feel and react, which plants heal and which cause harm, how the crows carry messages from one holy man to another across the length and breadth of the Land of Veda and how, from their vantage point high above human activity, the birds can act as useful guides. His talk ranged far and wide, and the boy paid unswerving attention to everything, as if the words were food and drink. He taught the boy many things about life and the hidden energies that govern it, and he taught him also about the Being of all beings, the one for whom even the greatest of men are but food, and death is but the sauce.

The *sadhu* had a wonderful voice, deep and melodious, and he would often spontaneously break into song. One of the first things he taught the boy was a song they often sang together:

> There is no happiness for him who does not travel, Rohita! This is what we have heard. Living in the society of men, even the best becomes a sinner...so go wandering!
>
> Oh, the feet of the wanderer are like the flower, his soul is growing and reaping the fruit; and all his sins are destroyed by his moving on, so go wandering!
>
> The fortune of him who is sitting, sits; it rises when he rises; it sleeps when he sleeps; it moves on when he moves. So, go wandering, Rohita, go wandering![7]

As each day passed the boy felt more fired to follow his new friend's example and dedicate his life to the open road. So often were the incongruous pair seen together, the huge man and the small neat boy trotting happily along by his side, that they became known as 'Ganesha and his mouse'. And unwittingly the villagers were right, for Lord Ganesh is the God of Good Beginnings and the *sadhu* had been sent to quicken his little friend's destiny.

The time had come for the great initiation known as 'the second birth', the assumption of the sacred thread that enlivens the body of light lying dormant within the physical form. Unless this was done, although the boy was by birth a *brahmin*, he would remain as any other being born of flesh: unfit to study the scriptures or realise their inner meaning. The custom was to take the thread at the age of eight and the boy was now not much more than five, but bearing in mind his exceptional spiritual gifts and remembering Lord Shiva's promise, the widow Aryamba consulted Gangadharanji, the village *pandit* who knew about these things. He confirmed that for those destined to see the light of God, the ceremony could certainly be performed at such an early age. Raghavan the astrologer's consultation with the ancient texts revealed the auspicious time for the ceremony and one of Aryamba's relatives, a priest from the great temple in Vrishachala, agreed to come and perform the initiation.

Early on the appointed morning, after spending the night alone in a small straw hut that had been specially built behind their house, the boy sat with his mother to eat what was to be the last meal she would be allowed to cook for him. Aryamba could not hide her tears at losing this precious connection with the one person who gave her life meaning. Then, after taking a purifying bath and donning new clothes, they went out together into the soft sunlight of the compound where the priest was already waiting.

First he wrapped a soft cotton shawl around the young body and tied a girdle around his waist; then the small head was carefully shaved, leaving only a tuft of hair at the crown. Holding the sacred thread, made of nine strands of silk woven by one of the unmarried village girls, the priest took the boy's right hand and stretched out his four fingers. Explaining that the number four is what binds the world to God – the four Vedas, the four cosmic ages, the four castes, the four stages of life – he carefully wound the thread across the outstretched fingers, then knotted it to bind in the blessings of the departed ancestors. To the boy, it all seemed to take forever.

Finally, the thread was hung over his left shoulder and down across his chest: a strange new part of him had arrived. Cool drops of sacred water were sprinkled over him, sparkling in the sunlight, and *mantras* chanted. The priest motioned to him to rise and stand on a rock to symbolise his strength of purpose, and he was given a clay pot of curds to represent chastity, and the staff that would connect him with the higher beings that govern life. Then came the core of the initiation, the transference of the *gayatri* mantra, those sacred syllables through which the pious *brahmin* enlivens the divine intelligence within himself at the start of each new day. Covering them both with a white cloth, the priest whispered the *mantra* into the boy's right ear. The charge of the ancient sounds penetrate deep into his being and resonate there, quickening an energy in his solar plexus that rose and spread across his chest in waves of heat. His felt his awareness expand beyond his body and he seemed to be watching from a distance as the priest performed the final fire-ceremony inviting the gods to give their blessings.

And so the boy became a *brahmachari*,[8] one of those twice-born qualified to study the Veda and devote his life to realising and spreading its teachings. Turning to his mother, he uttered for the first time the words that would become his daily rite: "Honourable person, please give alms". Eyes downcast to avoid her gaze, he took the food she offered, then began his first alms round by walking to the houses of his female relatives who were waiting with their food ready.

The boy loved his new routine. Each morning and evening he would sit with the other *brahmacharis* in front of Gangadharanji's house, repeating, learning and reciting the sacred sounds of nature. The *pandit* was a man of few words and a fierce temper when needed, but the discipline he imposed was never unjust and his students soon grew to love him. Wearing robes died yellow to stimulate the intellect, the group of boys, through their intense studies, also innocently acted as a filter to cleanse and regenerate the environment. The hypnotic rhythms of their chanting wove a tapestry of vibrations that draped the surroundings like some protective being, warm and benign. And so the nodes of the day were marked, and the village linked to the wider cadences of nature. Animals would come and sit some yards behind the group; even the jungle crows would quieten down and perch on the backs of the cattle, their heads cocked attentively to one side. And everyone remarked that the flowers and plants around the *pandit's* house were the happiest in the village.

As all mankind benefits from the chanting of the Veda, the *brahmacharis* were supported without question by the village. Once they had taken the sacred thread they would no longer live off their parents but gather their own food from the houses each morning. The self-sufficiency this bred would serve them in good stead for the time when, householder's life done, they would set out on the life of a solitary mendicant. It was then that the knowledge they were storing now would really bear fruit. As the village had a high proportion of *brahmins* there was a fair number of *brahmachari* boys, and a system had been evolved whereby they took their handful of food from those families who could afford it, rather than burden the less well-off. Accordingly, the wealthier houses were divided between the group so each boy had a regular round, often composed of members of his own extended family and their friends. In this way everyone involved felt the bond of kinship in a display of practical generosity that served both the general good and their own *karma*. And of course over time, the women of each house would come to know their visiting *brahmachari* quite well, watching him carefully to see if he might be a suitable match for one of their daughters when the time for marriage came.

The boy was well aware that one of his mother's neighbours had a daughter she was lining up for him. He had caught the speculative glances and felt almost suffocated by the extra fuss she made of him whenever he called at their door with his alms bowl. It was not just that he felt embarrassed by the whole business. The prospect of marriage and embroilment in the duties of householder life had always filled him with dread and, at the thought of such a fate, his spirit sank like a bird faced with a cage.

One night he overheard Aryamba and her friends discussing the matter on the veranda outside his window when they thought he was asleep. His worst fears were confirmed. He awoke with a sense of deepening gloom, and when the time for the morning alms round came he decided to skip the girl's house and keep moving down the quiet shaded path to the neighbouring one. As it happened, the place belonged to a couple that everyone knew weren't worth a turmeric root. Their ungrateful children had left home long since and they were living out their declining years in poverty, alone and unaided. Each year, almost as soon as their meagre crops began to sprout, a flock of screeching green parrots would descend to nip each bud in the field with their razor-sharp bills, or a band of chattering monkeys would swing down from the high branches of the great *banyan* to take the unripe fruit from their few spindly papaya trees. Yet, despite their misfortunes, the couple were unfailingly pious and humble, and the villagers were dismayed that such good people should suffer this undeserved hardship. Once, after a rock fell inexplicably on their roof on the night of no moon, it was generally agreed that the old couple must be possessed by a *chatan*.[9] Several of the wealthier members of the village got together and decided to hire the services of an *ashtavaidya*[10] skilled in dealing with such spirits. He duly came all the way from Trichur, bringing with him a copper-bound clay pot containing ten-year-old *ghee*[11] fortified by herbs and empowered by mantras to the Goddess and Ganesh. He talked gently to the couple, recited sacred verses and tied the protective black thread round their wrists; he performed *puja* with special incense beneath the old *peepal* tree where the *chatan* was probably living. But it was all to no avail. Their crops continued to suffer and their fortunes to decline.

Knowing all this, the boy's initial reaction was to pass by the house and continue down to the next, but something drew him to the dilapidated door. The woman of the house answered his call and her face lit up to see the little *brahmachari* standing there, but her pleasure at being asked to donate to a bowl of such good repute turned rapidly to embarrassment. There was no food in the house. Explaining that her husband was at that moment foraging for some leaves in the forest, she went back inside to return a few minutes later with all that she had: a single shrivelled *amalaka* fruit.[12] Lowering her eyes in shame, she placed the fruit in the bowl and putting her thin hands together in salutation, bowed down.

The boy felt overwhelmed at such devotion. He closed his eyes and a silent prayer to Lakshmi, the Goddess of Abundance, rose up from his heart:

> Oh Mother Lakshmi, energy of the Divine, may your compassionate gaze become the clouds and your grace become the wind, and let them together pour down rain to extinguish the flames of this poor woman's *karmas*. May your celestial rain shower riches over this sorrowful little bird of yours![13]

No one knows just what happened next, but it is said the woman remembered everything around her dissolving into a brilliant light and an overwhelming sense of softness and delicacy, the very essence of femininity, sweeping over her. The light intensified, and then from the densest point at its centre appeared the form of the goddess Lakshmi. She was huge and radiant, with an expression of indescribable sweetness, and two of her hands held a lotus flower. From another of her hands a stream of gold came forth, bubbling and glittering. At this point the old woman lost consciousness. When she came to, both the Goddess and the boy had gone, but the ground around her was heaped with gold coins.

At first the woman and her husband told nobody about what had happened, but the change in their fortunes became obvious to everyone and the story soon came out. The village was polarised. Those who had always believed that the boy was some sort of divine being were delighted with this proof. But others, who had long felt threatened by his obvious difference from the other children, muttered amongst themselves that they had always known he was possessed by some shape-shifter, and this incident with the pauper lady only confirmed it.

After much thought, the widow Aryamba decided that the best way to deal with this new turn of events was for the boy to leave the village for a while. It was time anyway for him to take his study of the Veda further. He had already assimilated most of Gangadharanji's knowledge and there was no-one else in the village who could teach him anything. A neighbour had a contact at the *pandit* school attached to the great Vrishachala temple, and so it was arranged for the boy to be apprenticed there and begin the next stage of his education.

After three years the boy arrived back from the Vedic school. He was considerably taller and subtly changed. His teachers there had been astonished at his progress and the ease with which he learned even the most recondite texts. From his side, the boy felt that each lesson was not so much a meeting with the new, but more a means to jog his memory of something he was already familiar with. The knowledge was somehow lying quietly within, waiting to be uncovered, and so it was easily retrieved. Indeed, often it seemed to emerge fully formed by itself once the prompt had been given. The teacher would chant a phrase or a verse and the whole relevant passage would pass before the boy's inner eye and into his speech without any effort, spontaneously. He would witness himself learning verses and reciting them, watching as if from a distance, while feeling himself strangely free of the process and quite spared the effort that the other pupils had to put in.

As a result, the boy quickly became the most adept among them, overtaking even advanced students several years his senior. As his reputation grew, many of the scholars visiting the temple came to the school to observe him, curious to see for themselves this precocious lad from Kaladi. Another child of his age might well have felt overawed by this attention from such renowned intellectuals, but so great was the boy's self-possession that he was not upset by it at all; indeed, he greatly enjoyed his time with these wise elders, just as he had always sought out the company of the *sadhus* who visited his village. He would recite and discuss with them as one of their own, and they in turn began to realise that here was something special, a great being had come into their midst in the guise of a seven-year-old boy. Amongst themselves the *pandits* began calling him *Manusha Shiva* or 'Shiva in human form'.

Once home, the boy settled back into the soporific rhythm of village life: looking after his widowed mother, continuing his studies with the aid of texts he had brought back from the temple, reciting the scriptures, getting his food each day from door to door. And, of course, long periods of meditation. But his time away had only quickened the latent desire to leave home and find his *guru*, to devote himself full time to the life of a *sannyasi*, the homeless seeker after truth. Nothing else really interested him.

A tension began to smoulder between the boy and his mother. Now that he had finished the first part of his studies she was keen that they make efforts to find the girl he would marry, so that everything could be secured for the future. But however much he wanted her to feel secure for her old age, there was nothing the boy wanted less than to fit in with her plans. Yet he could not just leave her, especially without her blessing. The situation seemed quite stuck, and it gnawed at his heart like a rat at a sack of grain. Then, not long after his return to the village, two curious incidents occurred that were to resolve the matter once and for all.

It was late in the monsoon season, humid and unhealthy, and the widow Aryamba had come down with a debilitating fever that had confined her to bed for days. As a result, she was too weak to walk to the river that ran some distance from her house to take her customary bath each morning. Seeing her mounting distress, the boy sank into a meditative trance, softly praying to the river deity to help the pious woman. That night there was a torrential downpour for several hours, much heavier than usual. The next morning it was seen that the river had burst its banks, expanding its course to carve out a tributary that flowed to within a few yards of the widow's door. Now she could take her morning bath with ease! It is said that the river still flows in this stream today.

Since her illness, the boy had got into the habit of accompanying his mother on her morning trip to the river. One day, while she was bathing, he took his usual seat astride a thick branch that stretched out low over the water. It was a beautiful and tranquil scene, the early morning sun was not too warm and, after all the recent rain, the river was the colour of molten caramel as it flowed under the vivid greens of fresh new growth. The air was full of birdsong and the busy chirping of insects. As often happened in such pleasant natural surroundings, the boy felt the outside world receding as his attention slipped deep within. Lost in abstraction, he failed to notice that one of the logs floating nearby was in fact a crocodile basking lazily in the sun. Almost imperceptibly the creature drifted towards the seated figure, then, perfectly positioned, it opened its huge jaws and grabbed his dangling leg. Pulled into the water, the boy screamed to his mother – "Mother, help me, help me! Let me take *sannyasa* before I die – at least I can then return in my next life in the right way!" Horrified, the woman realised that there was nothing she could do to save him, and as an instinctive response, gave her permission. As the crocodile dragged him further out into the river, the boy loudly chanted the sacred *mantra* of renunciation, and suddenly, the grip of those terrible teeth relaxed and he was able to swim breathlessly back to the bank.

As he walked home, the boy remembered clearly the words of the great Vedic sage King Janaka that his *sadhu* friend had often repeated:

'On the day that he decides to renounce, on that very day let him set forth'.

He decided to leave home immediately and begin the wanderer's life. For her part, his mother was torn between relief at his escape from death and a deep sadness at his departure. Try as she may, she could not dissuade him. The boy consoled her that he would never want for company; from now on, every house would be his home, all the women who gave him alms would be his mother, the teachers who imparted him their knowledge would be his father and the whole world would be his family. Sad as she was, deep down Aryamba accepted that something inevitable was taking place; the momentum of the whole strange affair was unstoppable. She and Shivaguru had asked for an exceptional child and they had been granted one. The rest was God's will; she could hardly complain. But before the tearful parting she made her little son promise that, even if they were destined never to see each other again, he would at least return to Kaladi to carry out the proper funeral rites when her time came. Overcome with emotion he agreed, and, casting a last lingering look around the familiar surroundings, set out alone on his journey. He was eight years old.

Part Two:

THE MONK

The Narmada river flows broad and blue through the heart of the Land of the Veda, dividing the north from the south. Pilgrims walk her entire length from the Eastern *ghats* to the great sea of the West, stopping at each of the myriad temples and shrines that line her holy banks like jewels strung on a languorous necklace. Even the poorest will toss a featherweight coin and a prayer into her limpid waters; no other river commands such heartfelt devotion. She is the daughter of Lord Shiva, a goddess born from her father's throat to cleanse the world of evil. To this day there stands a temple that marks the spot of her first emergence on the vast mountain plateau of Amarkantak, a spot which is known as The King of Pilgrimages. Here she is worshipped in an image that is as black as infinity, holding in her outstretched hands the symbols of her father's power: the trident and the *lingam*.

Tumbling down from the great height of Amarkantak the Goddess descends with a ferocious joy through dramatic waterfalls and lush jungle, while elegant conifers line her royal processional route, swaying in respect as she passes. She continues onwards through leafy, gentler hills, now flowing broad and sometimes several hundred feet deep, while along her banks the monkey armies of Lord Hanumanji stop their chattering to watch her stately progress, and tribal people cast flower offerings into her waves from boats carved from a single log of teak. Everywhere she goes the Goddess brings bounty, spawning the most beautiful eggs of marble that glow a translucent pink or lilac or blue, countless glossy pebbles that are prized as her own magical *lingams,* each one an emblem of her mysterious divine power.

It was these pebbles that now held the boy fascinated, as he gazed at how they shimmered and danced in the light of the sparkling water. He bent and picked one up, turning it over in his hand. It was creamy white and veined with delicate violet streaks, beautifully smooth and no bigger than his thumb. He hesitated, was even this just another possession, a poisonous attachment to weigh down a wandering *brahmachari* such as himself? After a moment's thought, he decided to keep it – after all, surely the symbol of Lord Shiva could accompany him wherever he went?

Three years had passed since he left his home in the south, three long years on the road moving slowly north-east across the Land of the Veda towards the mighty mountains where, he had always felt sure, he would meet his *guru*. As he travelled, he had immersed himself gradually in the ancient, sacred geography of the land, learning to read its mountains, rivers, caves and rocks as others might read a venerated manuscript. He had walked along so many roads that now blurred into one, through village after village, town after town, passed by countless doorways and innumerable alleyways that vainly sought to lure him into the labyrinthine possibilities of daily life. He had trod ancient isolated paths resonant with the dreams of those who had walked that way before. This constant movement was an exhilarating adventure but a lonely one, his days deprived of even those little routines that are the companions of the solitary. So often he was tempted to stay in one place, make some human connections and join again the warm, animal bustle of normal life. But the search for his *guru* kept his mind resolutely focused on the goal and, even if sometimes reluctantly, the boy always moved on.

Over the long months he had met many who claimed to know and teach the truth. Some of those he encountered were undoubtedly advanced souls, surrendered to God and in service to the world, and he had profited greatly from the time he spent with such beings. Some displayed a remarkable degree of self-sufficiency and lack of interest in worldly matters, such as those *sadhus* so detached from human society that they would not even take alms from householders, but instead observed the feeding habits of the birds and animals, and followed them in gathering their food direct from nature. But for all the talk of renunciation, much of what he saw was misunderstanding that masqueraded as spiritual knowledge. He had met a yogi who after many years of penance could produce flames out of thin air but still had not conquered the fire of his own temper. Another had taken twenty-five years to perfect the *siddhi* of walking on water and was offering to teach the same power. The boy thanked him politely but replied he would rather save the time and take the ferry. He came across a yogi who showed off a pet lion he had trained never to touch meat, another who had stood on one leg for seven years and ate only grass in a vow to win the grace of his chosen deity, and yet others who bound their genitals with iron chains to prevent any squandering of the life-energy in sexual activity. He saw those who were so sunk in the recesses of their own minds that they had lost the power of speech and lay unmoving on the ground like stones, and those who had sat for years in the jungle while their nails curved into long yellowed talons, and wasted muscles hung off their bones like scraps of cloth. Some practised the black arts and dealt with spirits and ghosts they contacted through sacrificing to bloodthirsty goddesses, bludgeoning tiny soft heads on crude jungle altars in their attempt to win subtle powers. Once he travelled many days through the forests to find a spiritual teacher with a widespread reputation, but instead of a saint he found a man obsessed with saving the world at large while remaining quite indifferent to the sufferings of those sitting beside him. And everywhere along the way lay the apathetic dreamers dulled with hashish and opium, mistaking their self-absorbed visions for spiritual truth.

Such were the 'holy men'; the temples were little better. Well-intentioned believers were often hoodwinked by *pandits* who claimed to know the scriptures while their Sanskrit was perfunctory or their pronunciation awry. Bullying, venal priests took money from the poor, the simple and the credulous to perform sacred rituals incorrectly, or even not at all. Everywhere there was fear feeding exploitation, and domination starving hope; it was a vista of the human spirit suffocated by the dead weight of a once-noble tradition that seemed to have run its course.

As time went by, disillusion was setting in. Dejected, the boy began to wonder if he would have the perseverance to reach the mountains and find his teacher. And yet, despite all the disappointments, one thing kept him going: wherever he went he had also found the unsatiated hunger of seekers after truth. In each temple, after the gods had been worshipped and the priests been given their due, came the heartfelt questions: "What is the state of enlightenment?" "Who are the real teachers?" "How can we realise the truth of life and go beyond suffering?" And in all these discussions, one name came up again and again, a man who many had heard of but no one seemed to have met, a teacher who evidently rose far above the typical so-called spirituality being peddled in the market-place. His name was Govinda Yogi and he was known to be the closest disciple of Gaudapada the Great, one of the most esteemed of those masters of Vedanta who teach the unity of all life. So great was Govinda's reputation that he was also known as Yogindra, 'the King of Yogis'. People said he usually stayed somewhere close to the mighty Goddess Narmada, wishing to place himself under her divine protection. As the mighty river lay on the boy's route to the Himalaya, he had decided to travel her length with eyes and ears open for signs of this elusive teacher.

There is a celebrated temple set on an island where the Goddess Narmada meets her younger sister Kauveri, fondly embraces her and grants her permission to travel further south and bring life and hope to the Land of the Tamils.[14] It is known that Lord Shiva is particularly partial to this place because the island is naturally formed in the shape of his great mantra OM. On one bank opposite the shrine a town has long existed to cater for the pilgrims who come to take *darshan*, especially numerous at the great Shivaratri festival each Spring.[15] The boy decided to visit the temple to get the Lord's blessings for his quest.

It was outside the temple that it happened. As he was about to enter the precincts for the evening *puja* the boy heard the music and commotion of a procession behind him. At first he thought it was some aristocratic marriage party, or perhaps the local *raja* who had come to visit the deity. But as he stood aside to let the procession pass, he saw that in the middle of the crowd was a large group of shaven-headed monks accompanying an open palanquin carried shoulder-high, and decorated with saffron flags and hung with ropes of orange marigolds. It must be some holy man or other. Raising his folded palms to salute the palanquin, he saw an orange-robed figure inside, sitting with his back to him. But just as the palanquin drew level, the figure turned to look directly down at him and the boy saw again the lucent countenance from his dreams. The look from those eyes, perfectly unobstructed, opened his heart, and his pilgrim soul was captured.

The boy had arrived at the feet of his Master as a man dying of thirst arrives at a well. Since that brief glimpse of the face in the palanquin, he could think of nothing else but how to arrange a meeting with the orange-robed figure. He managed to get a meal a day and a floor to sleep on by helping out in the kitchen of a pilgrim rest-house in the town opposite the temple, and he soon learned that Govinda's ashram lay some miles downriver. But how could he get to meet the Master? He knew that the gatekeepers there would never allow him entrance; their job was to vet anyone desiring to approach their teacher and protect him from unwelcomed visitors. Every young boy in the area knew the weight of their bamboo canes. So there was nothing he could do but wait and watch until an opportunity presented itself.

It was not long in coming. One morning, while he was clearing the tables in the dining-hall, he overheard two pilgrims planning to take *darshan* of the great saint. They had heard he was due to make a rare trip out from his ashram to spend a few days at the house of a pious *brahmin* scholar, a long-time devotee of high repute who lived locally. Shyly, the boy approached them and told them that he had travelled up from the far south just to meet the saint. They were astonished by the precocious child but, being open-hearted people, they reluctantly agreed to let him accompany them, on the strict condition that once they were at the scholar's place, he was on his own and it would be as if they had never met him.

It was the night of the full moon. The three had travelled in a horse-drawn cart to reach a large house on the outskirts of the town late in the evening. A sizeable group of people was already gathered on the veranda, sitting quietly in silence. Surprised to see more visitors arriving at that hour, a couple of the men frowned and put their fingers to their lips; the newcomers did the same to show that they would not disturb the atmosphere. Every so often, a *brahmachari* would come down from the first floor and invite some of the assembled group to follow him upstairs. Before long, the boy's two adult companions were selected and disappeared up the stairs, leaving him standing uncertainly at the back of the veranda. All around was darkness; only an oil lamp burnt dimly in one corner. An hour or more went past and by now there were only half a dozen people left waiting. Summoning up his courage, the boy finally whispered to one of them who looked a little more sympathetic than the others. "Good sir, is it possible that I could have *darshan* with Swamiji? Just *darshan*, no talking, I won't disturb him." Surprised, the man responded gruffly: "Who told you to come here?" The boy whispered, "Please sir, this is not the time to go into all that, all I'm asking is if I may have *darshan*". Frowning, the man said nothing more but when the *brahmachari* next appeared, he whispered in his ear. The young monk looked at the boy and shook his head. "Not possible, you'd better leave and come back some other day". The boy stood there without answering him. After about ten minutes the monk returned and impatiently motioned him to sit down. A flame of hope flickered in the boy's heart.

After perhaps another hour, two or three people came down the staircase followed by the same *brahmachari*. He motioned the boy upstairs. "Go in and just stand in front of Maharaj-ji. Make your prostration and come straight out. No talking and no hanging around" he said sternly. His heart in his mouth, the boy began to climb the stairs; there was no light and every step brought him into a more intense darkness. Feeling his way onwards he emerged uncertainly onto the upper terrace. Out in the open again, it was not so dark but it was still difficult to see clearly. Just at that moment it happened that the moon came out from behind a cloud and a sudden flood of brightness illuminated Govinda's face with an ethereal radiance.

After that first night, the boy somehow managed to join the group of perhaps a couple of dozen who went to the scholar's house every evening and were granted audience with the Master. He befriended the horse-cart *wallah* who let him sit up front with him without paying and, once they had arrived at the house, he would slip deftly into the back of the *darshan* group, where he sat spellbound by the sight of the man he had finally found as his teacher. This pattern lasted for a few days. Then on the evening before Govinda was due to return to his ashram, as the boy was going down the stairs, the *brahmachari* from the first night stopped him. Evidently embarrassed at having to deliver a message to a mere boy, the novice assumed an air of superior nonchalance as he said offhandedly: "The Master told me to tell you that you can come to the ashram tomorrow, if you feel like it".

When he was first accepted as a member of the ashram, the boy had expected that something special would happen. Nothing did. On arrival that first morning he had been subjected to an interview with a fierce old monk who wanted to know all the details of his family and education. A novice briefly showed him around the complex and after that, it was as if he didn't exist. There was no sign, no word, no acknowledgement from Govinda. Nothing. He just joined the ashram community and its unwavering routine of an early rise, prayers, *puja*, work, more prayers and *puja*, punctuated by sparse communal meals taken in silence in the dining-hall. Then it was early to bed, which for him was a pile of gunny sacks in the corner of a provisions storeroom. After some time, he was given various humble tasks around the place: cleaning, sweeping out the rooms, working in the kitchens. Then, once he had shown that he was prepared to accept without question whatever he was given, he was finally allowed to help with the many visitors who came each day to see the Master. At first he was as if invisible but, as time went by, his tender years and obvious sincerity began to endear him to everyone, residents and outsiders alike, and he became affectionately known as *bal brahmachari* 'the little novice'. For his part the boy was happy and grateful to have settled after so long on the road, but he could not disguise his disappointment that there was no sign that Govinda had even noticed him. After all his seeking he had arrived at the goal, but what had changed? Absolutely nothing. Even his remarkable learning was of no avail, as no one here bothered to speak to him of the Veda or philosophy. All he had was the occasional glimpse of the Master, the occasional possibility to be in his presence for a few moments, quite by accident and totally unacknowledged. For many long months this had to be enough.

But then, imperceptibly, things began to change. The boy learnt to organise things so he could spend time in the corridor outside Govinda's rooms and gradually befriend the senior monks who were in attendance there. From them he started to pick up errands: running here and there with messages, summoning a particular monk the Master wished to see. Then he began to act as an unofficial doorman, organising the almost constant stream of visitors into an orderly and patient queue, bringing the waiting people water, making sure they kept silence and refrained from chewing betel or smoking. From this role he graduated to helping clean out the Master's rooms, sweeping them each morning, bringing fresh flowers and removing the old ones, tidying the bundles of texts that were always lying around by the end of the day. His skill at reading and writing, uncommon among the other ashramites, then got him the job of helping attend to the correspondence that poured into the ashram office: requests for *darshan*, invitations to preside over religious functions near and far, petitions for blessings, help and advice.

Day by day these humble tasks afforded him increasing chances to enjoy some proximity to the Master, and the more this increased, the more a strange and profound transformation began quietly to make itself felt. For all the while the boy was innocently being schooled in a great truth of the spiritual life: in the path to the Divine, the connection with the Master is the most important thing. If the seeker finds a good Master, things move quickly; if not, he has to keep on going slowly and gradually by his own efforts and there may be no end to it. In fact, finding the proper Master is all that an aspirant on the path of truth needs to do, for with the right guide, a channel is opened up that allows the thing to be accomplished almost by itself, naturally. There is no greater power in nature than this spiritual channel and so it is that through complete surrender the disciple evolves into the Master. Little by little, the influence of the greater seeps into the lesser, and the more wholehearted the obedience, the more powerfully the transforming influence can flow. Meditation, rituals, penances, good works – all these form one well-trodden path to ultimate freedom. But the path of surrender is another way. And once it is perfected, the work of the spiritual quest is done. Nothing more is needed. Little by little, the boy grew in this surrender. He learnt the art of foregoing his own preferences and attuning his mind to the mind of his Master. Whatever Govinda liked, the boy began to like. If Govinda wanted him to go one way, he went that way, whether he himself wanted to or not. And having gone halfway, if Govinda wanted the boy to turn, he turned; if he wanted him to change direction, he changed direction; if he wanted him to go another way, he went that way; if he wanted him to return, he returned. The boy never objected, never complained, never deviated from what he was asked to do, whether it seemed to make sense or not, and much of the time it didn't. His whole attention was to carry out what his *guru* had asked him to do, and so long that the work was not done, he had no rest, he had no sleep, he had no food. He had no interest in socialising with his fellow *brahmacharis*, he would not think of it or care for it. His one-pointed attention was to carry out the wishes of his *guru* and nothing else.

In this manner, his own will became pliant and gradually subsumed into Govinda's will until, eventually, nothing of his own volition remained, only the Master's wish existed. Throughout this subtle alchemy, it was not the specific task that was important, that was just a pretext. What mattered was keeping in harmony with the flow of the Master's attention, so that the likes and dislikes of the Master became the likes and dislikes of the disciple. Gradually, the two minds became attuned and with this attunement, Govinda's thoughts became the boy's thoughts, Govinda's feelings became the boy's feelings and the gap between *guru* and disciple was bridged. Disciple and Master were two bodies yet one existence, two minds and yet one mind, two hearts and yet one. Learning to adjust his limited mind to the unlimited mind of the Master, the boy grew daily, nurtured by the quickening power that existed in the very atmosphere around the *guru*, which was so full of joy, so full of life, so full of silence. And within the apparent restrictions of this complete obedience, freedom began to blossom. This is how the sacred drama of discipleship naturally unfolds, and it is the most binding love affair there is.

In this attunement, the boy began to taste the priceless nectar in which the saints lose themselves and forget everything during their deep meditations in silent places, but he experienced it with his eyes open and in a completely wakeful state, just by the proximity to his Master. An inner bliss arose in waves to express itself as the forms and feature of daily life; he was as if drowned in ecstasy. An inexpressible happiness, a feeling of huge elation, overwhelmed his heart and swelled outwards as if rising in powerful torrents to the surface from somewhere deep inside a limitless ocean. Then, diving back inside again, and having struck the deepest depths, it rose outwards again and again, to fall mutely at Govinda's feet in ripples that heaved and vibrated in ecstasy. The boy felt as if he would burst with the fullness of that ecstatic feeling; each tiny atom of his body was enveloped in bliss, melting into it as if into an indivisible and everlasting union with a pure and radiant love, untouched by any constraint. It was invincibility and freedom, eternal stability and deep happiness, all experienced on the surface of life. And all this derived from the *guru's* grace and presence.

It was the most blessed time for the boy. Unaware of when the sun rose and set, or what day it was, he lived his whole life in surrender. He had no feeling of himself existing, he only knew his Master existed. Such a surrendered state of life is all but impossible for the world to understand, and that is why those who have had such supreme good fortune keep the matter to themselves.

One morning Govinda summoned the boy and informed him the time had come for him to take the formal vow of renunciation. He began by emphasising the necessity of having a realised teacher for genuine spiritual process and the necessity of belonging to a genuine tradition of those who know. He spoke of his own master, Gaudapada, who was known simply as 'the Great One':

"Actually, I can hardly speak of my Guru Dev, his greatness is beyond words. When I first saw him I knew that this was what I had been waiting for, even without knowing I was waiting! He was so sublime there was just not one particle of doubt, not even the possibility of one particle of doubt. Total surrender, and a different life started. Yet at the same time, paradoxically, it was all very natural, no fuss. It was like..." he paused for a long moment, "you know when you have been hearing about the glorious taste of a mango, and you go from garden to garden and you get some good peaches or grapes but you don't find the mango, but then one day you do find the mango and you think 'Aha, so *this* is what the mango is like!' And then you think 'Well, perhaps I should build a hut under the mango tree so I can enjoy these delicious mangos all the time' – well, like that I met my Guru Dev, and that was it. This was the luck of a seeker of Truth, all working out naturally enough.

"But even for those who were not fortunate enough to be in his presence, his legacy was assured by his brilliant commentaries on the texts. Before my Guru Dev took *sannyasa* he had studied with the greatest of all grammarians, Maharishi Patanjali, and in his commentary the reasoning was so polished, and the language so succinct, that people joked that he got more pleasure from the omission of an unnecessary syllable than a normal man got from the birth of a son!"

Govinda chuckled, and closing his eyes began to recite:

This state is unborn yet always awake,
 quite free from illusion, beyond name or form.
Pure intelligence, unbroken and whole --
Ah yes, that's how it is, that's just how it is![16]

He went on to speak of Gaudapada's own Master, Shukadeva, who was born already established in the enlightened state. Up to that point the teaching had only been passed down from father to son as no stranger to the family was trusted, but such was Gaudapada's stature that he became the first person to receive it from someone who was not his own father. And then came the other great names in the tradition stretching far back into time: Shukadeva's father Vyasa, 'the Compiler' who set down the texts from divine dictation and wrote matchless commentaries on them, then Parashara and his father Shakti before him and back to Vasishtha, and from Vasishtha back to Lord Narayana[17] and the birth of creation. Together these names comprised the tradition of majestic teachers of the unity of life, the supreme knowledge of Vedanta, in which all the different spiritual paths are united in their own extinction.

Govinda then spoke on the many aspects of renunciation: the rules, the expectations, the etiquette. He described how an itinerant monk should live off alms: he must avoid the houses of known drinkers of alcohol and those who eat flesh, also criminals and those without children, for a childless couple will not have the means to support a mendicant. He spoke of how suitable houses should only be approached after the smoke from the kitchen fire has ceased to rise, for then the inhabitants will have taken their meal and their donation will not be an undue burden, and of how the *sadhu* must first chant the names of God as he stands outside the door, to alert the mistress of the house, and then the *Gayatri* mantra to purify the atmosphere. If no one has answered after eleven recitations he must move on, but, if the woman does come, the *sadhu* must ask for only a little food as that way four or five houses will yield enough leftovers. And before he begins his meal, he must divide it into four equal portions: setting aside one for the animals, birds and insects, the second for unexpected visitors, and only the remaining two for himself.

Finally, as the afternoon light began to fail, his voice filled with affection:

"The state you are about to embark on is very precious, a great blessing. Only a few are ripe for such a step. It depends on various karmic conditions – the subtle physiology, the temperament, the allotted destiny of this birth. In all of these you have been fortunate. You have the possibility of a great destiny, I would almost say a unique destiny..." Here he stopped himself abruptly and concluded in a tone that was almost offhand:

"Anyway, let things happen as they will, everything will sort itself out nicely in the end. You need not strain towards the future, it will come to you of its own accord. But remember one thing: don't be too hard on yourself. Even if you occasionally fail in your vows, be gentle, for there is always the danger that an ardent young *sannyasi* can lose his humanity in the search for divinity. Renunciation is a means to allow us to become more fully human, to realise our real potential and be an example to the rest of the world of what it is to be fully human. Nothing is achieved by over-exertion or straining. After all, enlightenment is the natural human state, so all we need to do is unlearn some unnatural habits that we have picked up in the past, purify them, release and be done with it. What we *sannyasis* call renunciation is just the precious opportunity to focus wholeheartedly on this necessary purification, and get it over and done with as soon as possible. And never forget, in the end it is not really we ourselves who do anything, it is all the grace of the Divine, in whose hands everything, without exception, rests.

"There will be times when you feel unsure, your way will seem bereft of meaning or direction, and the grace of the Divine may seem to have deserted you. This is in the way of things, there are always moments when one feels empty and estranged. Actually, these arid times are really most desirable, for they signify that the soul has really cast off its turgid moorings and is sailing for far distant places. This feeling of having no safe and solid ground under your feet is the first taste of real detachment, when the old is over but the new has not yet been born. This state may well be uncomfortable and you may even be afraid, but there is really nothing to fear. You must learn to welcome what the world calls disillusion, for such a state is just the shedding of illusions, no matter how consoling they may have been. Above all, in any situation, always remember the instruction: 'Whatsoever you come across, let go and move beyond, let go and move beyond'. This is the *dharma* of those who are destined to wander, without whose movement the settled world would lose its balance and topple into chaos. That is why the *sannyasi* roams free as a warrior through this great web of illusion; he walks upright without a backward glance, alone on the edge of madness.

"So" he finally concluded, "your time has come to die to everything you think you are, and whatever is left will be the seed of the work that is to be. But for now, that is quite enough! Go and have a good rest and take only milk until I see you again. Meet me over there" – he indicated a flat mound at the river's edge that served as the local cremation ground – "freshly bathed, at midnight tomorrow." The boy prostrated and left, his head swimming and his heart beating wildly.

It was Mauni Amavasya, the fifteenth day of the dark fortnight of Magh[18] when the sun and moon join together, an event so auspicious that the holy ones refrain from speech and food to show their respect. All the sacred rituals observed during the holy month of Magh come to an end to honour this day. The boy's head was freshly shaven, with only a knotted tuft of hair left at the crown. As he approached the mighty river he could only just make out the sitting figure of the Master silhouetted on the bank, illuminated by many small oil lamps. His mind full of the steady sound of the river's insistent flow, the boy approached, prostrated before his *guru* and took a ritual bath, submerging himself three times in the icy water. Govinda indicated a pile of wheat flour beside him. The boy began to knead little balls to offer with prayers to his departed ancestors, for he was now to participate in his own funeral rite as a preparation for re-birth into the life of the spirit. And when the time finally came for him to leave his earthly body, no more such rites would be needed.

A little back from the riverbank, a square had been marked out by sacred leaves and flowers. Within this square a second *mandala* had been drawn in coloured powders: red – the colour of blood, earth and the Great Goddess who rules all material things – and white, the pure, untainted spirit of Lord Shiva himself. Stepping carefully into its centre, the boy sat down facing his Master. After some minutes of silence, the older man began to offer water from a small clay pot but using his left hand, for the rituals pertaining to *sannyasa* reverse the normal ways of the world. Then he lit a small heap of sandalwood and placed it between himself and the youth. Each movement was calm, conscious, authoritative. Handing the boy two handfuls of sesame seed and keeping the same amount for himself, Govinda began to chant. It was a sonorous refrain, ancient yet strangely comforting, and the boy felt the hairs on the back of his neck stand up:

> I offer this oblation of sacred sesame, its crushed pieces and sweet-smelling juice, may they soothe my mind... and so be it!

May cattle and gold, and good food and drink, be offered to Lakshmi, Mother of Abundance... and so be it!

May these sesame seeds, black and white like my karma itself, liberate me from all my blemishes... and so be it!

May I henceforth be free from all the karmic debts I owe to the gods, to my ancestors, to my parents, to the world at large... and so be it!

May the five life-breaths within me be purified, so I may become the light of pure consciousness, pure, free, unattached... and so be it!

May I become That which is beyond the pairs of opposites: beyond success and failure, happiness and misery, beyond even life and death... and so be it!

'And so be it!', 'And so be it!', time after time, as the sesame seeds, herbs, *ghee* and many other oblations were tossed into the sandalwood fire. With each offering the flames leaped in response, hissing and spitting like a ravenous creature rising to snatch its prey. Finally, leaning over with a knife, Govinda grasped the boy's sacred tuft of hair, severed it deftly and tossed it into the crackling blaze.

Then he rose and, motioning to the boy to follow him, walked the few paces to a second square which was again fenced-off by leaves. "Lie down on that" he said, pointing to a heap of wood in its centre. Then taking some burning coals, he approached the pyre and, murmuring *mantras*, moved his hand over the seven *chakra* points in the small prone body and set light to the wood. After what seemed like a long time, almost choking on the smoke curling up around him, the boy saw the shadowed figure of the older man motion him to get up and then he himself had to chant the *mantras* for the dead over the smoking wood. Thus was he symbolically freed from his born limitations: the obligations of caste and creed and family, the inborn habits of body and mind. From now on he was irrevocably on the open road, set fast on the path to join with the universal cosmic spirit that is beyond all personal limitation, beyond the round of birth and death. Throwing off his white novice's robe, the young man strode into the sacred river for his first bath as a free being.

As he emerged, shivering, he was handed a folded ochre robe which the Master had himself dyed from the traditional *gerrua* clay.

When the boy had donned it, Govinda bowed down before him. "All victory to you, young Shankara. May you prove yourself to be a fitting embodiment of your namesake, Lord Shiva himself! May you become the greatest of teachers, renowned in all three worlds as the purifier of the Ancient Way! I wish you all success in your mission!" He then handed the boy his new skull and a new spine: a gourd shell as an alms bowl and the bamboo staff that symbolises the wandering recluse's upright way of life and his connection with the heavens. And thus was it done.[19]

Govinda signalled the boy to return to the ashram alone. As he was doing so, he was met by a group of three women from the nearby village who had heard on the grapevine that a young man was taking *sannyasa*. Hair freshly oiled and plaited with white jasmine flowers, they stood shyly at a respectful distance, gaze averted, holding plantain leaves heaped with food, eager to have the honour to offer the newly-ordained *sannyasi* his first meal. Diffidently, the young man waited while each woman touched his feet in turn. Then he took a little from each offered leaf, so none would feel left out, and continued his solitary walk back. Behind him, left at the edge of the initiation area, lay a small white stone, his sole companion since he first stood on the bank of the mighty Goddess Narmada.

The self-transcending nature of the young Monk's service to Govinda was so completely satisfying that it had never occurred to him that one day it might end and he would have to leave that blessed hermitage where only the present existed. The place was so deeply steeped in the infinite depth of each moment, where was there to go, and for what? Everything was already here, not in the sense that all material possibilities were manifest in the community around the Master, of course, but that whatever was here, simple though it might be, breathed infinity through and through. Every particle of the place was saturated with that peace, that nourishing plenitude which wanted for nothing. Such fullness of being admitted no lack and no addition, for what could be greater than the infinite? In comparison to a life in the ashram spent serving his *guru*, the outside world seemed nothing but a sea of mud. And so it came as a shattering blow when, one bright May morning, Govinda summoned the young monk and told him the time had come for him to leave. He was to go to Kashi,[20] spiritual capital of the Land of the Veda, and Mother Nature would guide his steps once there.

The young Monk reached Kashi after several months on the road. Leaving Govinda's hermitage had been nothing less than a desolation, for he was greatly attached to his Master and life without his presence seemed to have no meaning or purpose. But his first duty was obedience, and gradually the pain had ebbed enough to be tempered by a new sense of aloneness that turned into a freedom from all influence, an almost invincible self-sufficiency. It was as if all the wisdom and power accumulated and stored during his years of service was beginning to rise to the surface and emerge, coaxed out by his interaction with the life that lay waiting beyond the ashram walls.

And now, he felt an urge of excitement as he finally came to the forest of sacred *kadamba* trees[21] that ringed the city, protecting it from the impurity of the outside world. They seemed to tower towards heaven itself with their offerings of brilliant red and orange flowers, and behind them rose the line of magnificent golden pillars that announced the entrance to the holy citadel. He had reached, at last, the goal of every pilgrim and the spiritual home of every believer. The place was the living temple of the Vedic religion, established by the Noble Bearers of the Ancient Knowledge when they first arrived from the rugged lands beyond the northern mountains at the dawn of time. It was here that those mighty ancestors had had their first sight of the Divine Mother in her earthly form as Ganga Ma, and it was here they had decided to renounce their wanderings and settle down to build the greatest civilisation known to mankind.

Kashi, 'the City of Light', was the first of all cities, standing in a forest carpeted with sacred *kusha* grass. All the gods migrated here to be blessed by Ganga Ma and to receive their due worship from the pious. And here too Shiva himself, Lord of Transformation, came to visit. Pleased by the scented smoke of a thousand fire-offerings, he was refreshed by the sonorous waves of Sanskrit recitation and charmed by the repetition of countless *mantras* buzzing like nectar-intoxicated bees. Finding himself delighted with the natural beauty of the women and the dedicated knowledge of the men, he decided to stay and make Kashi his earthly abode. And ever since then, the entire city, from the magnificence of its most sacred temple to the ash of its cremation pyres, has been his playground. Kashi, the absolver of sins and granter of liberation, Kashi, the city of diamond light where every contour is etched in gold, Kashi where the veil between the human and the Divine is at its thinnest. Kashi, the very navel of the world!

The sun was beginning to set by the time the young Monk had his first glimpse of the river: a vast, limpid expanse glowing gold and pink and soft turquoise in the crepuscular light. It seemed to stretch forever. All along the *ghats*[22] people were making their devotions. Bells and gongs and chanting sounded everywhere, whilst singly or in groups, the devout offered prayers, bowing and bending this way and that, with the natural elegance of grasses caressed by the breeze. Everywhere in the water glowed little leaf cups, each one bearing flowers, incense and a single flame, carrying a prayer, a wish or a vow downriver, towards the open sea. And as these little lights gleamed and sparkled, bobbing and winking their way into the deepening darkness, as if in response, the first stars began to twinkle overhead. There were larger fires too, burning in front of shrines all over the waterfront in readiness for the *pujas* that would soon begin to honour the Goddess and her many courtiers. More and more people were streaming out of the narrow alleyways that led to the riverfront, and the young newcomer was almost swept off his feet by the purposeful press that surged forward as one body, individualities cast aside, down, down the wide steps to the sacred water. Reaching it along with thousands of others, he continued onwards without hesitation, to immerse himself in the sun-warmed softness, floating free in a delirium of happiness and self-abandon.

Those first days in Kashi passed in a breathless ecstasy. Not only was the young Monk himself lost in divine intoxication, but the entire place seemed dedicated to just that state. A spiritual fervour raged here such as he had never encountered: the alleys were full of incense and worship; bells, gongs and conch-shells kept up a constant refrain and everywhere the air was stirred by the virile, sombre sound of the recitation of Vedic texts. *Bhajans* greeted the rising and setting of the sun, classical *ragas* soothed the dark hours. A continuous stream of devotion seemed to flow through the temples and shrines, along the riverside and in and out of the boats going up and down the river. In the open squares of the city, and all along the *ghats*, were held well-attended performances of dance, mythic drama and popular plays enacting episodes from the lives of the gods and heroes, and almost every street corner seemed to host a debate between priests, pundits and philosophers. Groups of spectators looked on, doing their best to follow, and even if they couldn't – which was most of the time – they stood and squatted, enthralled. Everyone was fully engaged in their role, absorbed in an intense interior reality that embraced all humanity. All hours of the day and much of the night, colour, noise and celebration mingled seamlessly with the mundane business of buying and selling, looking and leaving, and all the time-honoured rituals of weddings and births and stages of life. And all the while, like a sombre chorus commenting on the whole drama, was the hiss and crackle of the funeral pyres at *Manikarnika ghat*. For Lord Shiva's favourite habitation, with all its intense vitality, is also the City of Death.

At the heart of the old town, like a great twin-peaked mountain, towered the imposing complex that housed the two temples where the parents of the cosmos dwelt: Shiva Vishvanath 'The Lord of All' and the gentle companion of his pleasures, Annapurna Devi Ma, 'The Goddess Who Gives Nourishment'. The royal couple watched over the city with an unceasing and benign attention, releasing their blessings to all who made the effort to visit them. A huge retinue of attendants maintained a well-regulated and continual pattern of worship throughout both the light and dark hours: feeding, washing, entertaining, hymning and honouring the deities several times a day. Scurrying purposefully here and there throughout this vast sacred anthill, these attentive servants ministered to the invisible sacred presences installed so sumptuously at its heart.

Thronging the arteries of the city that extended out from the temple were the pilgrims, an ever-changing yet always similar tableau of thin limbs, cloth bundles and brass pots jostling together alongside faces bright with expectation. Each separate area of the waterfront was dedicated to a particular part of the country and was supervised and organised by priests who spoke the language of that region. These *pandas* knew well the tastes of those who arrived, their ways of living and eating, their preferred routines and chosen deities. They held records etched on bark and palm leaf that stretched back generations, chronicling the family members who had come to Kashi over the decades, and detailing which gods those long-vanished visitors had worshipped where, and when and why, and how much they had given to the shrines. Worn smooth by the steady stream of pilgrim feet, the wide stone steps of the *ghats* were like a vast loom on which was woven an extraordinarily variegated tapestry of tongue and dress, stitched by face and feature, and embroidered by hopes, and fates and fears.

It did not take long for the newcomer's reputation to spread. It was his age of course, together with his ardour and uncompromising intensity, that created such a shock wave. Before long a small group had gathered around him. Some were *brahmacharis* loosely attached to monasteries or other religious institutions in the city, others young men free of commitment and full of idealism. Among these, there were those who wished to debate or be instructed in meditation; others would later go on to undergo full initiation into *sannyasa* by the newcomer. Astute observers wondered if they were witnessing signs of the sort of revival that the ancient stones of Kashi had seen many times before. They remembered tales of the stir created by teachers such as Mahavir the Conqueror, who refused to sit anywhere until the seat had been gently swept clear of insects, or to drink any water until each minute creature floating in it had painstakingly been lifted out and placed in safety. They recalled the arrival of the aristocratic Gautama Siddhartha, the royal prince from the northern hills who had given up his throne and family to find the Truth, and had delivered his first pellucid discourse in the Deer Park not far outside the city. But there were also those who felt threatened by this young firebrand and his uncompromising advocacy of living spiritual experience. Many of the great scholars for which the city was famous were dry intellectuals, weighed down by tradition and imprisoned within the high walls of their narrow speciality, proud of their superiority and devoid of the human sympathy that is the lifeblood of the spirit. They were right to feel uneasy, for in time the clear light shed by the newcomer would reveal them to be as dust to living soil.

For his part, the young Monk had no inhibitions in expressing his view on the paucity of mere book learning. One morning as he was walking through the crowded alleys leading down to the river, he heard the sound of a scholar reciting grammatical rules by rote in a bored, lacklustre style. Rounding the corner and coming across the man sitting in a doorway with his text in his lap, he spontaneously burst into song:

> Adore the Divine, adore the Divine, oh just adore the Divine, you fool!
> When your time comes to leave this earth, old man,
> Repeating all that grammar won't help you at all, you know.
> So just adore the Divine, adore the Divine, adore the Divine!

So contagious was his fervour that, so it is said, each of the disciples that were with him added his own verse. The resulting composition remains even today one of the most popular devotional songs throughout the Land of the Veda.[23]

In those early days the golden youth carried with him an extraordinary and infectious spiritual energy which had a palpable effect on those around him. Many of those he came into contact with would have visions or fall into states of bliss. His own behaviour was completely unpredictable. Often he would sink into a state of deep introversion to emerge, sometimes hours later, radiating laughter and happiness. At other times, he would shake or shiver or swoon with ecstasy, or roll on the ground seemingly weightless, his body buffeted here and there like a leaf in the wind. Mantras would spring from his lips, or his limbs perform spontaneous yogic *kriyas*[24] while his joy welled up in a stream of poems and songs addressed to various deities, particularly the Divine Mother. Above all, he loved to take part in *kirtan*[25] in which the names of God were chanted and praised. These sessions would sometimes go on for hours and, while others became worn out, his energy seemed inexhaustible. It also became clear that he often knew what people were thinking, and could foretell the future; not infrequently there were reports of his being seen in two different places at the same time. Somehow, it was as if the normal laws of time and space were bent out of shape in his case. Curious, and some said miraculous, events would manifest around him. It seemed as if he was surrounded by a sort of force field that ensured appropriate consequences for those actions performed – and even those thoughts entertained – in his vicinity. These consequences could sometimes seem bizarre, or random, and inexplicable to observers, as they appeared out of nowhere, their cause remaining hidden.

One example will suffice: A rich wool merchant was in town on business from the tundra lands beyond the high mountains to the north. It was winter and cold, and he was dressed in his native garb of a long woollen tunic over high laced boots. A thoroughly secular man, unfamiliar with the subtle customs of the Land of the Veda, he has been doing the rounds of a few shrines but in the manner of a tourist, quite unmotivated by any spiritual interest. On hearing of the young Monk and his growing band of followers, he decided to visit him in the riverside house where the group was then encamped. Arriving at the gate, the merchant was very put out to learn that if he wished to have an audience inside he would have to remove his footwear. 'Why should I degrade myself by taking off my boots to visit this young man? Surely I am his superior in every way.' he thought. Nevertheless, on learning that he would not be granted admission unless he complied with a ruling that was everywhere observed in such situations, he very reluctantly agreed to do so. However, as he started to unlace his boots they would not come off his feet. The more he tried, the more he failed and the more frustrated he became. Still, he struggled on, motivated now more by his anger in trying to overcome his own ineptitude than by any desire for *darshan*. After many minutes spent trying to wrest the boots off, to his acute embarrassment he was eventually reduced to crawling on the ground in his attempts to do so. And so it transpired that he ended up 'degrading' himself far more than if he had observed the simple courtesy of removing his footwear in the first place.

Amongst those who kept the young Monk's company at that time was a pious middle-aged man who had come to Kashi on pilgrimage in his twenties and never left. Sincere and conventionally religious, he became very uneasy about the untameable power of whatever was being manifested through this newcomer from the south. Fearing it would create a bad reputation for him with those who held power in the city, he voiced his concerns about what he called the 'growing atmosphere of madness'.

"Madness?" the young Monk replied, shaking with laughter. "Oh no my friend! Normal worldly life is the real madness, but because everyone slavishly agrees to act in the same way, no one recognises it as such. Everywhere you look people are mad for gold or power or lust, but these infatuations can only shrivel the heart and ruin the body. Only if you become mad for enlightenment will this madness of the world take flight. So, we must become mad for God, and then there will be no ruination and no loss, only fullness and increase and happiness. Pray to the Almighty that he will visit such madness on you; I can assure you, it is the only way to become sane!"

Some early teachings:

The fire will have its way

Amongst the first of the young Monk's patrons was a local nobleman who offered him an old and rather run-down palace to stay in. Located in Avimukta, the sacred heart of the city,[26] it soon became an impromptu ashram. At that time the youthful teacher enjoyed going to the nearby Manikarnika Ghat with a few disciples to spend time amongst the funeral pyres. Although as an ordained *sannyasi* he had renounced fire - both of the householder and the wandering ascetic - he seemed to feel at home with the *sadhus* who congregated there, those who had broken away and lived regally, the lions of renunciation. Devotees of Lord Shiva and his motley army of spirits, the *sadhus'* preference for the cremation ground silently mocked the febrile preoccupations of worldly life. These holy madmen were spectral figures, smeared grey with ash from the pyres and huddled around the flickering half-light of their fires. Passed on from *sadhu* to *sadhu*, teacher to pupil, generation after generation, these flames were considered living beings, kept fed with offerings and never allowed to die. They burnt the folly of worldliness to nothing and opened the portals to the invisible realms where time and space are elastic and the subtle entities dwell, waiting to be commanded. It was believed an advanced *sadhu* could accomplish almost anything through his fire.

One morning that winter the young Monk was sitting at the burning *ghat* with four or five followers when a well-known philosopher from the east of the country, who had recently acquired quite a following in the city for his startling views, approached. He was a clever man, tall and confident with a theatrical manner and skilled in public debate. But there was little love in him and a trace of self-satisfaction in his bearing suggested a latent arrogance. He had with him a small group of disciples. Those who observed them closely would have seen there was something strained and unnatural about their demeanour, as if they were engaging in a hidden effort.

The philosopher raised his palms high in the formal greeting offered to a superior and, after introducing himself, sat down opposite the young Monk and began to speak:

"Tell me, Sir, is it not said in our scriptures that the universal Self is present in all places and at all times?"

"Indeed it is" smiled the young Monk.

"And is it not said that therefore the Self is our own nature?"

"It is".

"And is it not further the case that the Self, as our own nature, our given and inherent birthright, must lie beyond the mind and all individual effort?"

"Yes, that is the case" the other replied patiently, as some present wondered where all this was leading.

"Then what, Sir, is the use of all these spiritual exercises – meditation, yoga, *puja* and all the rest? What is the use of *guru* and tradition? If the Self is our natural state of being, then all we have to do is realise it, and all the rest is just nonsense kept in place by those who wish to profit from the accepted pattern of doing things. The time has come to do away with all this mystification about enlightenment. All we need to do is just wake up to our own nature, awaken from the dream of *not* being enlightened and recognise the Self that has always been there and always will be there. There is nothing more that is needed".

He paused to get his breath. The young Monk, sensing that there was more to come, kept silent.

"You yourself teach that the ego is unreal, do you not?" continued the philosopher.

"That it has no abiding reality, I do" came the careful reply.

"Then if the separate 'I' has no real existence, there is no 'person' to become enlightened! Any effort to become other than what we already are is a waste of time and all the paraphernalia of the spiritual path is also a waste of time, just polishing the bars of the prison. What is more, these so-called authorities tell us it takes time to tread the path and reach the goal, but how can there be a gradual growth to enlightenment through time when enlightenment itself is the timeless state? Therefore when we realise there is nothing to do, as everything is in reality the Self, then whatever happens at any moment is quite complete and appropriate, however it may appear to us, and any attempt to change it or improve it is just a misunderstanding of the real nature of things."

With this he turned with a triumphant final flourish to his people:

"And this means that the spiritual life and what are valued as spiritual experiences are no better than anything else that happens! Just ordinary life right now, *this* is the Reality – just as it is, here and now, everything is alright just as it is. Your ordinary awareness – the one that hears these words – this is the infinite Self perceiving itself; just realise this and there is nothing else to do!"

Somewhat flushed from his speech and hoping he had stoked the fire of a heated debate, the philosopher sat back and fixed the young monk with a quizzical expression.

The latter remained silent for some time, as if to let the atmosphere settle a little. Then he began quietly:

"What you say about the nature of the Self is all very fine, and it certainly accords with the descriptions of the realised ones. And you are right in your implication that one cannot achieve the Self by mere will-power or strenuous effort. On the other hand, those who are unwilling to undergo the fire of purification will always look to find a teaching that reassures them they are fine as they are. However, our Holy Tradition is the record of those who have gone through all those disciplines that burn away the obstructions to the natural state and prevent its shining forth; it is because of this preparation that they were, in the end, able to live the real Self and describe it to inspire others.

"But a partially evolved being cannot live the experience of one who is fully evolved any more than a dog can live the life of a human. There will be no end of mischief if we take descriptions of the enlightened state and somehow try to hold them in the mind over and against the reality of our actual experience. Such an attempt will be quite unnatural and the strain will wear us out in the end".

The philosopher shifted a little uncomfortably, and his tone became more defensive, but he was still in full flow:

"Yes, what you say is fair enough," he replied, "but it does not apply to one such as I. I know very well that in reality, I am not the body but the Self, invincible and immortal, about which the scriptures tell us:

Weapons cannot cut him, fire cannot burn him, water cannot wet him, wind cannot dry him away![27]

"Well, you know the text well enough" came the answer, "but in your particular case I'm afraid it is like a poor man proclaiming that he is rich. He may go on declaring his wealth for so long that he eventually comes to believe it himself. But this is a type of self-hypnosis – the real fact is that he is not wealthy. He remains without money and when the day comes that he has to settle all the bills he has incurred in foolishly trying to live like a rich man, he will find out very swiftly that he is, in truth, still poor."

After a moment's pause he continued:

"What stops a man from experiencing the bliss of the Self naturally in his daily life is the accumulation of unresolved experiences deep in his mind and heart. These give birth to endless unfulfilled desires, which in turn cause him all sorts of attachments and repulsions that prevent him from seeing clearly and living happily. The enlightened one is free of the burden of the past and so he is free of desire. His mind is like a burned-up log: no matter what happens to it, it will not start burning again because there is no fire left in it waiting to come out".

So saying, he leaned forward and picked a smouldering branch from the fire.

"But if an unenlightened person tries to emulate a saint, his mind will be like this half-burned wood here. The fire of suffering and delusion may not be seen, but when the winds of *karma* come along, as sure enough they will, the flames soon flare up again".

So saying he blew on the branch and it crackled into flame.

"Now, you were saying that fire cannot burn you?"

He tossed the flaming branch towards the philosopher, who crying out in fear, scrambled to his feet and left hurriedly, taking his crestfallen followers with him.

Some of those present found the whole incident puzzling. Later someone asked:

"Swami-ji, were you angry with that philosopher fellow?"

"I was not in the least angry" came the reply. "This body just did what had to be done, that is all."

After a pause, he added with a chuckle: "And after all, isn't fire needed sometimes to burn the rubbish?"

Another follower asked:

"Swami-ji, what if by some chance the situation had been reversed and someone had tossed a burning log towards you, would you have moved out of the way?"

The young Monk laughed out loud now. "Of course I would have – and quickly! Why not? This body has no more desire to get burned than any other body does. But mark well, whatever might happen to this body in the outer world, it could not disrupt the inner peace, that's all".

The followers looked at one another; there were no more questions.

Eight virtues conducive to Enlightenment

The following comes from a formal teaching session, typical of those given by the young Monk to religious groups at this time:

Q: "Maharaj-ji, what is humility?"

A: "The absence of self-esteem".

Q: "And what is modesty?"

A: "Not proclaiming one's own virtues".

Q: "And what is innocence?"

A: "Doing no injury to any living being".

Q: "And what is patience?"

A: "Not being affected when others have done you some injury".

Q: "And what is service of the teacher?"

A: "Doing acts of service to the spiritual guide, he who teaches the means of attaining enlightenment which is liberation in life".

Q: "And what is purity?"

A: "Outwardly, cleansing the body of dirt by the use of water and earth. Inwardly, cleansing the mind and heart of attachments and other passions by the practice of discrimination".

Q: "And what is steadfastness?"

A: "Focussing all one's efforts on the path to liberation".

Q: "And what is self-control?"

A: "Directing the restless body and mind exclusively to the spiritual path".[28]

Concepts

One day during a *darshan* session in the Avimukta ashram the young Monk remarked:

"You see, the normal man is imprisoned in a dense forest of concepts and stumbles around as if blind, unable to get even a glimpse of the clear blue sky overhead".

"What is the place of the *guru* in all this?" came the question.

"The *guru*? Oh, he is just some madman who wiles away his time by chopping down the trees with one hand and pointing to the sky with the other".

So saying, he pulled a comical face and exaggeratedly mimed the actions of chopping and pointing.

Everyone in the hall laughed.

Faith and works

A prominent merchant asked:

"Surely faith is enough to reach the goal?"

The young Monk replied:

"Certainly, faith may bring spiritual wisdom but it could take a long time. That is why it is taught that as well as having faith the spiritual seeker should also always focus on a specific means to gain wisdom, such as devoted service to a *guru*. What is more, a person who has faith and devotion may still not have mastery over the senses, therefore it is also taught that meditation should also be practised so as gradually to withdraw the senses from their objects. This gives us the whole picture: one who has faith and devotion and has also mastered the senses will certainly attain spiritual wisdom".

"Yes, young Sir," came the slightly impatient reply, "but these are all inner disciplines, suited to the monkish way of life. I am an active householder, fully engaged in the world. Surely good works play a part?"

The answer came as a surprise:

"Actually, external acts count for little. They may even mask hypocrisy. But a person full of faith and the rest cannot be hypocritical".

The merchant countered:

"And what then are the practical results of this spiritual wisdom?"

"One result is all that is needed" came the reply, "and it is the most practical thing of all, that supreme peace which is liberation, enlightenment"[29]

The role of the guru

A well-known musician came for *darshan*. Used to adulation, he was confident, suave and good-looking and his finely brocaded shawl announced its origin from the most expensive Muslim looms in the city.

He began in a strong melodious voice:

"You are a newcomer to our ancient city young Sir, so you may not be familiar with our local saying:

'*Gurus* are easy to find but worthwhile students are rare'?"

When there was no response, he continued:

"Well, my question is this: how important really is the *guru* in the spiritual search?"

"The role of the real *guru* is crucial" came the reply. "The teacher is absolutely woven into this fabric of enlightenment. That is why the Vedic literature tells us that 'There is nothing greater than the *guru*'[30] because the *guru* is the embodiment of all that is greatest. In our *pujas* we say, do we not, that: '*Guru* is Brahma, *Guru* is Vishnu,

Guru is the great Lord Shiva?' These are not just flowery words, this is the literal description of the reality of the *guru*. The *guru* is on the level of the Absolute, but personified. When the *guru* speaks it is the Absolute that speaks through him".

"And holy scriptures ..."

"Likewise, the words of the *guru* are the words of the Veda, indeed, it is only from the *guru* that the Veda is properly heard. So in effect the *guru* means the Absolute, that from which the Veda emerges. If one holds the *guru* fast in this esteem, then one is in turn held fast by *dharma*, the Natural Law that organises the entire universe. What could be more important than that?"

Five bodies

She had been a beautiful woman in her time, in fact her beauty had been so exceptional that she had made her living from it. Originally from the southern foothills, her family were agricultural labourers who had come to Kashi looking for work at the time of the great famine. She herself had entered service as a courtesan attached to one of the palaces of a local *raja*, rising in time from her humble beginnings to enjoy a life of luxury and refinement, with fine living quarters, her own servants and a retinue of admirers. Life had been a heady round of clothes, music, dance, feasting and of course the bedroom. Her skills had won her many lovers but also enemies: men soured by the knowledge they had not the money or power to win her favours, women poisoned by the slow, steadily dripping venom of envy.

But now it had all come to an end. The *raja* had dissipated his money and died; she herself had not aged well. Most of her friends were already dead and her children had long since moved away to better themselves by erasing the circumstances of their upbringing. All she had left were her memories and even they were fading, chipped and tarnished like the mirrored decoration on her once-glittering saris.

Despite her worldly lifestyle, the woman had always felt a tentative desire to penetrate the veil of luxury and know the real meaning of things. In her younger days she had stifled this inner voice, partly because she considered herself unworthy to become involved in anything religious or spiritual but mainly because, like the other women, she feared any disruption to her comfortable existence. But now all that was over, she was spending her last years seeking out the company of holy men to see what comfort they could offer that might help her make some sense of her life.

Feeling herself immediately drawn to the young man sitting opposite her in the large reception room which was serving as the *darshan* hall, she began with a refreshing honesty:

"Young Maharaj, I have heard you follow the Vedantic teaching that we are not really the physical body but the spiritual Self, and here am I sitting in front of you as one who has lived only for the body and by the body. And now it has all come to an end. Have I just wasted my time in this life? It has all passed so quickly..." her voice tailed off and sadness hung in the room.

"Well" replied the young Monk smiling gently, "I suppose it would be a problem if you only had one body".

"Only one body? Oh, I suppose you are talking of reincarnation. I don't believe in all that, I'm afraid".

"No, no. I mean it would be a problem if you only had one body in this life".

"I'm sorry, Sir? I don't understand..."

"Didn't you know you have more than one body?" He smiled playfully at her surprised expression.

"No? Then listen carefully and you will learn something really worthwhile today, for this is the wisdom the god Varuna gave long ago to the sage Bhrigu. Now, in truth, you have no less than five bodies, one within the other, each made of successively finer matter and each of increasing subtlety. Yet, none of them is the real you. It is as if you are dying of thirst, and you come across a well but the water you crave is covered over with several layers of duck-weed and you can't get to it. Like that, what we are all seeking is our real Self, but it is covered over and obscured by these five bodies, whether we realise it or not".[31]

The woman looked quizzical, but he had caught her interest.

"Let's begin with the physical body anyway, what is called 'the food-body.' By your own admission, you are an expert in this area, so we don't need to spend much time on it. But this gross body is the least of what you are. Viewed dispassionately, this body is a meaty conglomeration of fat, flesh, blood and bones. Even with due care and the right food it is a false friend, changing day by day, constantly subject to all sorts of impurities and decay. This body can give great pleasure, but equally great pain, can it not?"

She nodded, smiling wryly.

"Only those whose mind is dull and confused identify themselves with this physical body; those of clearer mind will realise they are something else. In fact, it is said an unintelligent person identifies with the body, a cultured person identifies with the body and soul, while a great being realises 'I am the spiritual Self '".

"But good Sir", she interrupted, "this may be the way for great scholars, but what about us normal people?"

"The realisation of truth has nothing to do with learning. You can be thoroughly versed in the Upanishads and all the other great texts but unless you consciously unite with your deepest Self, you will never become free. And once you do, you will be no more attached to your body than you are now attached to your shadow".

She nodded slowly; her interest aroused now and all trace of self-pity gone.

"Within this 'food-body' lies a subtler one, a subtler level of self. This is 'the energy-body' which is the vehicle of the life-energy, the *prana*. This *prana* flows through the physical body and gives it vitality and the ability to act. *Prana* is a subtle modification of the air element, as you can see from the fact that all living beings depend on the flow of breath to live".

"Then what form does this energy-body have?"

"The same as that of the food-body, which it fills as air fills bellows. It assumes the same shape as its outer covering, just as when a temple-image is being cast the molten bronze assumes the shape of the mould. Each of the subtle bodies has the same contours as the physical by adopting the shape of its predecessor in the series".

The woman nodded again, wondering how this brilliant youth could be so fluent in such esoteric topics.

"Now" he continued, "within this 'energy-body' lies a third: what we call the 'the mind-body'. This is made up of the perceptions of the senses combined with the thoughts, feelings, concepts, ideas and images that are entertained by the mind. All this varied information is held together with the idea of 'I', 'me' and 'mine'. This mental body is very powerful, very tenacious and it is the cause of the fundamental ignorance that keeps us bound to not only our physical shell but to the cycle of repeated rebirths in the world. What is needed is to go beyond its activity".

"I understand your words Sir, but the whole thing is becoming rather abstract for me ..."

"Well, look at it this way. You know that when you are dreaming, the mind creates a whole world of fantastic experiences and events, none of which is ultimately real, as becomes obvious the minute you wake up. Actually, the situation is no different when you are awake; everything then is also the play of the mind. We can see that this is the case from the simple fact that when you are deeply asleep and the mind is dissolved, nothing exists, whereas the moment the mind comes back when you wake up again, the outside world returns once more.

"Yet whatever we may experience while awake or dreaming does not last; it has no permanence. Imagine the clouds passing over the sun. One cloud comes – it is the experience of suffering. That passes away and another cloud comes along – it is the experience of happiness. Like that, the mind creates the whole world of duality, and in doing so binds the soul down to the body and the senses and keeps it wandering through successive reincarnations, all the time labouring under the burden of 'I' and 'mine'. These mind-made limitations are superimposed on the real Self just as the clouds cover the sun and they are the cause of all our problems. But this imaginative play has no ultimate or abiding status and what we call Enlightenment is just waking up to this fact.

"Now, to be free of all this unreality you must dedicate yourself to do all you can to purify your mind and thereby transcend the condition of embodiment. When you start on the path to liberation, the mind is attached to everything in the world, like an animal bound by a leash, but, as it matures, it starts to expand and become free of those binding objects and experiences. When your mind is fully purified then liberation will be there, easily and naturally, as tangible as a lovely ripe mango sitting right in the palm of your hand!"

"Well, this all sounds marvellous Maharaj, but how is this 'waking up' achieved?"

"That is exactly the question, and to answer it we have to go a little deeper into the thing! Subtler than the mental body is the 'knowledge-body'. This is a deeper level of self, containing all the seeds of our past experiences, our memories, desires and impressions that have been accumulated through countless lifetimes. It is the sprouting of these seeds that make us identify with the limited body and compel us to act, and because we are fixed on obtaining the result of our actions, we remain attached to them. Deep in this 'knowledge body' resides the intellect, which is what gives the light of consciousness to the mind and what gives us our sense of who and what we are, our sense of identity. In the usual person, because the intellect only faces outwards, it identifies with the sense of a limited 'I' and gives rise to feeling of being an isolated individual operating in the world. But the intellect can also be trained to face inwards to its source, which is the real Self and then it can begin to reflect that limitless light. Therefore our task is to purify the knowledge body and free the intellect to reflect our true nature, which is the immortal consciousness of the Self".

At this the woman held up her hands, exclaiming: "Sir, this is all becoming too abstract for me, too theoretical".

"Alright."

A pause. Then:

"Look at it another way: imagine you see a piece of rope in the darkness and mistake it for a snake. What a lot of shouting and crying and running about! But the idea of the snake lasts only so long as there is darkness; as soon as someone brings a light, you see clearly that it is a rope, not a snake. What is needed is to clarify the intellect so it can naturally discriminate between the real Self and the world, and then all ideas of limited individuality and identification with action, including the concept of a personal soul and the need for reincarnation, will vanish".

"I can see that, but how to get this discrimination?"

"It is born of all those spiritual disciplines that destroy egotism and the tyranny of the deluded mind".

Still a little lost, but carried along by the brilliant force of his conviction, she continued:

"This is indeed a wonderful teaching, Maharaj! And you said there is yet another body?"

"Deep within the 'knowledge-body' lies another, even subtler level of the self, that is called 'the bliss body'. This level is characterised by happiness. This body is enlivened in those fortunate souls who enjoy good fortune in this life due to the *karma* of their virtuous deeds in previous ones, especially their devotion to meditation and ritual. But we all have some experience of it. We retire to the 'bliss-body' in dreamless sleep, which is why everyone loves sleeping! Don't we all wake up feeling happy and refreshed, saying 'Ah, I slept so well' even though nothing at all has happened? This inherent happiness can also be felt in dreams and on the point of waking. It is even there in the waking state also. When you attain something you wish for, or enjoy some gratifying experience – such as meeting a loved one after a long separation – it is the bliss-body vibrating within that gives you the feeling of happiness. But when this body is purified, it can function much more powerfully and at that stage, one's ability to experience joy from every side is vastly increased".

A long pause followed, as if to let the weight of so much powerful knowledge sink in.

The young Monk had not finished:

"Yet even the 'bliss-body' is not the real Self, because it is also part of the changing, limited individuality that is subject to the effects of *karma*. The happiness it enjoys is but a pale reflection, a mere particle, of the eternal joy of the real Self. This bliss surpasses everything in all the worlds, gross or subtle, because as our own deepest nature it is quite independent of any external cause. To reach that, one must transcend all these five bodies and reach the place where one can go no further. The real Self is an eternal field of Consciousness, the infinite witness of all that is, was, or ever could be. And when you are anchored in that state, you will no longer identify with the body at any level. In this state, one feels spontaneously and permanently joyful, with no effort or cause whatsoever".

"I cannot conceive of such a state".

The young Monk nodded.

"Well, look at those earrings you are wearing. As long as you have them on, you think 'I am the person with the earrings'. But you can take them off at any moment, and then that limited identification ceases, does it not? Like that, beyond the ever-changing body there is the divine unchanging Self and, in truth Khutumbay,[32] that is who and what you are".

The two sat silently for some minutes before the woman bowed down low in front of the young teacher. She remained a long time in that position, then got up and left the hall, sobbing uncontrollably.

Being is impersonal

A religious devotee said:

"I am very attracted by your teachings Swami-ji, but I cannot accept your claim that the supreme reality, which you often call pure Being, is impersonal".

The young Monk smiled serenely.

"If pure Being were not itself impersonal, then how could it contain the infinite number of impure personal beings and yet remain unsullied?"

Karma or God?

A well-educated visitor was in the throes of a conflict:

"You seem to explain the workings of the world by the theory of *karma* – the mechanical law of cause and effect – whereas I was brought up to see everything that happens as being ordained by God. I cannot reconcile these two positions".

"Each position is correct from its own perspective" came the reply. "There is no inherent contradiction between the two. In its attempts to understand life, the limited human mind forms all sorts of concepts, all types of models. Each explanation will reflect the mind that made it; some will seem compatible, others not. But it should never be forgotten that life is ultimately a mysterious, inexplicable and wholly Divine process. If the mind's models appear to contradict each other, too bad for them! Their incongruence and the resultant confusion demonstrates nothing but the limits of human understanding.

"And, as regards the workings of the world, look to the play of puppets. At first glance they appear to be moving themselves and to be independent actors, but without doubt there is someone holding the strings and moving them. The whole creation is actually very much like a puppet show. It is the Divine will that operates through the chosen actions of apparently autonomous individuals and apparently separate events. And whatever may happen, because it is the will of the Divine, it is always wholly consistent, right and unimpeachable, however it may be judged from a particular perspective".

Kitchen duty

The young Monk would often help out in the ashram kitchen work, and his presence there gave a great boost to the workers. But the other side of the picture was that he demanded wholehearted effort and constantly used the occasion to instruct people in going beyond the limits of what they had thought possible. At the same time, the mundane everyday experience of kitchen work would serve as a vehicle for spiritual teaching.

An example:
"Your hand may be doing the work – peeling, chopping, washing – but your mind can remain silent. This is *karma yoga*, remaining ever aware that you are That which never moves, no matter what else may be happening. If you realise this as your natural state, work will not tire you and anything can be accomplished".

Knowledge and Ignorance

The discussion had turned to the Bhagavad Gita. A visitor from the great central plain read out a Marathi version of some famous verses which were translated back into Sanskrit so that the young Monk could comment. The passage distinguished between 'ignorance' and 'knowledge'; there was confusion over what this meant exactly.

The young Monk explained:
"The ignorance mentioned here is nothing to do with education or intellectual ability. The ignorant man is simply one who does not know who he is. And if a man does not know himself, how can he know the world?"

"What is the cause of this ignorance?" came the question.

"To begin with, there is erroneous identification with the body and the mind. Once this initial collapse of awareness has taken place, there automatically follows the assumption that one is the doer of action, the active agent. This misperception is the root of all suffering".

"But if one is not the doer, how is action accomplished?"

"Whether we say that activity is carried on by God, or Nature, or the three *gunas*[33] the important point is that we are the Self and the Self has nothing to do with any activity. The Self just witnesses everything while remaining eternally silent; it is an uninvolved spectator of the whole show. Now, for all practical purposes we must of course keep on acting and we will be motivated by our action's intended results, but as spiritual practice matures we will become more and more even-minded, whatever the outcome of an action may be. This even-mindedness is what is meant by *yoga*, and it culminates in the experience of the complete separation between the Self and the non-Self, between inner silence and outer activity. This separation is described as the difference between *purusha* and *prakriti* in the teachings of Sankhya and *yoga*[34] and it forms a central part of the Gita's teaching also".

"But young Sir, I need a motive for acting!" came the heartfelt response.

"Fine, then dedicate your action to the Lord".

Another asked:

"I don't understand this, Maharaj. If one is unattached to activity, how can one live in the world which is nothing but constant activity?"

"Extremely well!" laughed the young Monk. "Just look at the marketplace. The merchant who works for himself is always running around here and there, worrying about prices rising or falling and concerned whether he will enjoy profit or suffer loss. But the man who works for another is unconcerned with these inevitable swings of fortune. He just keeps on doing his work and remains unaffected by the outcome. Like that, if one is free from the sense of doing and allows another to bear the burden of responsibility, everything turns out perfectly. Rest assured, almighty Nature is more than competent to bear what to you is this huge weight of agency, so why don't you just give it up and be happy?"[35]

Living in 'the now'

A visitor asked:

"You talk a lot about enlightenment, Swami-ji. Is this what some other teachers call 'living in the now', being in the eternal present?"

"Well, you could describe it as such if you so wished, as long as you were not opposing 'now' to 'then' or contrasting 'the present' with 'the past' or 'the future'. That which IS transcends all time; even to label it 'eternal' is a stain on its purity."

Padmapada joins the order

As time went by, an increasing number of people accumulated around the young Monk. Some were lay people from many different walks of life, some itinerant *sadhus* of various persuasions and some *sannyasis* who were already loosely affiliated to established monastic orders but were drawn by his charisma and teachings. Several of the *sadhus* and *sannyasis* moved into the Avimukta ashram, while many of the lay devotees provided practical help in organising the buildings and establishing channels of patronage. Some of them began to spend much of their time around the young teacher; little by little a powerful spiritual centre was spontaneously growing up.

Amongst his new companions, the young Monk felt especially close to a youth called Sanandana, who, like him, was a Nambudiri *brahmin* from the south-west. Sanandana was known for his devotion to the spiritual path and it is said that one day the sage decided to test his sincerity.

A group was returning to the ashram from a ceremony at a temple located on the far side of the River Asi, one of the tributaries that flows into the Ganga. There was only one small boat and the young Monk had crossed first, leaving Sanandana with some others on the far bank. As soon as he landed, the Monk called out to Sanandana saying he needed him urgently. Without a thought for his own safety, the disciple ran into the flowing water to join his teacher and, as he did so, it is said that lotuses suddenly appeared to form a bridge of flowers to support his feet.

When he reached the other side, he was embraced by his delighted teacher who promptly gave him the name Padmapada 'the lotus-footed one'. He had passed the test, was initiated into *sannyasa* and became the young Monk's first ordained disciple and chief assistant.[36]

The qualifications of a seeker

The question arose among a visiting group of *sadhus* as to what distinguishes a genuine seeker after Truth.

"He must fulfil the four qualifications" was the reply.

"And what are these, Sir?"

"Discrimination, non-attachment, right conduct and right desire".[37]

"And what is discrimination?"

"The ability to differentiate between the Real and the unreal".

"And what is non-attachment?"

"The enjoyment of the unlimited Self in the midst of the restrictions of daily life".

"And what is right conduct?"

"Tranquillity, self-restraint, tolerance, endurance, faith and remaining centred. These six constitute right conduct".[38]

"And what then, Sir, is right desire?"

"Right desire is the longing for Enlightenment above all else".

Recitation of the Veda

Each morning and evening at the ashram there would be *Veda parayana*, recitation from the Vedic scriptures, along with other devotional chants. The young Monk would sit motionless and majestic and his face, notwithstanding its radiant youthfulness, often seemed as if carved in ancient stone. Once when asked about the benefit of such chanting he replied:

"It helps to purify the body and to bring the mind to silence".

Suffering

Question: "Sir, I have heard you teach that the individual self who undergoes suffering is an illusion?"

Answer: "From the standpoint of supreme knowledge, such limited selfhood is illusory, yes".

Question: "Then to whom does the suffering occur?"

Answer: "To the one who is asking the question!"

The best profession

It was dusk at Manikarnika *ghat*. A large number of tantric *sadhus* were there, smeared grey with ashes from the funeral pyres, fearsome *aghori babas*[39] with staring bloodshot eyes, drawn to the cremation ground by their desire to commune with the spirits that inhabited the sombre place. The pyres were flickering gently in the fading light; every so often there came a dull popping sound, as a skull exploded from the intense heat of the flames.

A middle-aged man with a dignified air joined the group and sat down.

"May we know what your job is, Sir?" asked someone politely, showing the respect due to an elder.

The man answered that he was a maker of packing cases.

"Aha! You have chosen the best profession!" intervened the young Monk.

The man looked surprised.

"We should all keep our cases packed. Who knows when Yama Maharaj[40] will send his messengers to call us away? And when he does, there is no denying him, it's the arrest warrant! Make no mistake, this whole world is the burning ground, so we should keep our cases packed at all times".

The body

One day a number of people from the Avimukta ashram were walking by the river along the Hanuman *ghat*, a place traditionally used by wrestlers and body-builders for their daily routine of exercises. Here there were also several hermitages of *hatha yogis*, who practised rigorous regimes of bodily purification and taught students there.

One of these *yogis*, famed for his physical prowess and extraordinary flexibility, recognised the young Monk. He approached him, saluted respectfully and asked:

"Maharajji, you frequently say that the perception 'I am not the body', is one of the hallmarks of the enlightened state, yet surely the body is essential to us. It is the physical seat of awareness and through awareness we know the world. Without this body there would be nothing to provide us with experience, with life, whether that life is one of ignorance or Enlightenment".

"Well," came the answer "the body is valuable and yet it is not; it depends on your perspective. Certainly, you are quite right, the body must be kept in good order, for only if it is kept in good condition – healthy, clean and so on – will it be possible to locate the Self, which is the master of the body. As a *hatha yogi* you know well that the whole body, gross and subtle, must be purified so as to reflect the light of pure Consciousness. It as a valuable and needed servant. But, in paying due attention to all the necessary disciplines, it is important to remember that, in truth, you are not the body. Not only are you not the body, you are not the mind, you are not the intellect, you are not the ego. All these limitations of individuality whether gross, subtle or causal, are mere superimpositions that obscure your true nature. In fact, your true nature is unboundedness, the one unobstructed Consciousness which is like open space, transcendent, ever-luminous, unborn, indestructible, stainless, omnipresent and ever free".[41]

Somewhat taken aback by the ardent fluency of the reply, the *yogi* was silent for some moments, before asking:

"Well, what then is the correct attitude to the body in your view?"

"Look" continued the other, indicating the mighty Ganges that flowed serenely beyond the *ghats*. "let's say you wanted to get across the river here. While you are making the crossing, the boat in which you are travelling is of great importance, is it not? Of course; you must look after it, see it is serviceable, has no leaks and so on. But once you have reached the further shore, you no longer give a moment's thought to the boat that took you there, it is gone from your awareness completely, left behind, finished with. Well, it is just like that with the body. Once one has left behind the sense of limited ego, which is marked by identification with the body, then there is no more concern with the physical. In that state one's body becomes just another object in the field of objects, none of which has anything to do with the Self. Then one lives without any body-consciousness. Even something going wrong with the body – an illness or accident – does not impinge unduly, because one has become the Self, which is ever unstained by the body and its vicissitudes. So use the body as your ferry-boat to the further shore, which is the bodiless bliss of the Self, and do not be overly attached to it, however beautiful or impressive it may appear to be".

"Is such a radical state necessary for Enlightenment?" came the question.

"It *is* Enlightenment. The knower of the Absolute is he who knows himself to be the one Self, the witness of all, everywhere the same. Just as you normally have no feeling of 'I' or 'mine' in relation to other people's bodies, so even while apparently located in this body such a knower has no attachment to his own limited selfhood".[42]

"But how does such a person function in the world then?"

"Extremely well! Everything goes on automatically and quite naturally for him, without effort or engagement. He himself does nothing, because the Lord does everything for him. Bodily movements, sense-perceptions, feelings, thoughts, and memories – all are seen to arise in the intellect, but all the while he stands eternally separate, pure and free of even the slightest trace of fear that inevitably accompanies identification with a body".[43]

The ego as Master

One day a mature woman came to see the young Monk. She explained she had studied with a well-known teacher for many years but recently had found it increasingly difficult to go along with what he said and taught. She had therefore come to the realisation that she had outgrown the need for traditional discipline and from now on needed to follow the promptings of the 'inner *guru*'.

"And to be honest, Sir," she continued in an almost confidential tone, "as a woman, I am sick and tired of other peoples' authority. I have obeyed others all my life, and mostly men: first my father and my elder brothers, and then my husband and behind him, his mother. Now I have come to the point where I can no longer follow the directions of another. From now on, I must act on my own inner authority, even on the spiritual path".

"And how do you know this is the right way and not just a mood?"

"It just feels right; that's all I can say".

The young Monk nodded sympathetically but said nothing. Then, after some small talk, the woman rose and took her leave.

Later, when the matter of authority was being discussed by those who remained, he commented:

"Submitting to a genuine *guru* is never an easy option, but this is how the sacred tradition works. By instilling a discipline that frustrates the ego, the teacher gradually aligns the student with something greater than his own individualistic tendencies, his own *samskaras*.[44]

"Some people go along with the spiritual path only so long as it seems comfortable or consoling or seems to yield them some benefit, but they will abandon it as soon as they find it becomes too difficult or testing. At that point their decision is justified in their own eyes by finding fault with the teacher or with the tradition, but never with the ego itself. In fact, it could be said that this uncomfortable tension is what really marks the beginning of the spiritual path. Rest assured, until the behaviour patterns of the limited ego are transcended, there is no Enlightenment. The ego can never be the spiritual Master, however much it might like to be."

Signs of Enlightenment

An eager young man asked:

"Swamiji, what are the signs of Enlightenment?"

"Objectively? Not always easy to say: one cannot know for sure another's state of consciousness, it is a highly subjective matter, not open to another.[45] Nevertheless, you will have some good feeling when you meet an enlightened being. Because they are tranquil in all circumstances, wise and impartial, they will exude something attractive, something pleasant that makes you enjoy being in their company and want to stay near them as much as possible. Something about them feels nourishing. This magnetism will usually be interpreted as an effect of their personality, but it is not to do with that superficial level; it is a natural effect of the fact that they are living and radiating the Self, which is as much your real nature as it is theirs. The Self is the most attractive thing there is, and it draws everyone, eventually.

"But, mark well that enlightenment is nothing to do with external circumstances. Forsaking the demands of the world may concentrate the mind on spiritual progress, but physical renunciation in itself is not the criterion. The *yogi* in his cave may lust after the things of the flesh, while it is perfectly possible for an enlightened soul to live in the middle of the market place of the world. And while there, he may even not be recognised, like a great mountain too high to be seen by those living in its shadow".

"And subjectively? How does a seeker know when he is progressing on the path?"

"In general, there will be an increase in contentment, a native sense of happiness which has nothing to do with outer circumstances. This equanimity will be particularly noticeable when we are not upset when our expectations are confounded and things 'go wrong'. Self-sufficiency will increase, and there will be a growing sense of freedom: freedom from emotional reactivity and freedom from sense objects and their demands on our energy and attention".

The questioner persisted:

"Then is there one thing above all others that characterises the growth of consciousness?"

"It is the effortless discrimination between the Self and the not-Self, between the Real and the unreal, the permanent and the transient. To whatever extent this discrimination is spontaneously and continuously maintained throughout the states of waking, dreaming and sleeping, to that extent enlightenment can be considered established".

"How does this feel?"

"It is the realisation that one is ever beyond birth, death, old age and all sorrow. It is the experience 'I am immortal' even while in the midst of this unstable life and all its insufficiencies"[46]

The necessity of knowledge

Some villagers, having travelled many miles on pilgrimage to Kashi, had now come to have the *darshan* of the young sage they heard about as soon as they arrived in the town. Rather shyly, they sat down on the floor in front of the young Monk's couch and after a few moments their headman opened the discussion with a question:

"Maharaj-shri, the sacred texts always talk of the necessity of having knowledge, yet many of us are simple people with no schooling. Does this debar us from spiritual progress?"

"Certainly not. The knowledge that is spoken of in the texts has nothing to do with book learning or the specialised education of the *pandit*. These are but the superficial levels of knowledge. The essential knowing is to know the Self, by which is meant enjoying the direct experience of that inner happiness which remains unshaken no matter what may happen in the outside world. This type of knowing is as direct an experience as the luscious taste of a ripe mango!"

There were smiles in the group and relief softened some of the lined faces.

Then, a change of direction:

"Without this knowing there is no end to the cycle of birth and death".

"How is that, Sir?"

"Each one of us must endure the fruits of his past actions. Whatever a human being is involved in during a lifetime leaves its impression stored in his mind and this impression acts as the seed from which future desires and actions will in time sprout. These seeds may take many births to come to fruition; like any crop, they need favourable conditions to appear. You are a farmer Sir, so you know well the principles involved here".

The headman nodded, then asked:

"So is this is the cause of rebirth, Sir?"

"It is. An individual may have to take an indefinite number of births to harvest the effects of all his latent impressions, and then, in each fresh lifetime there is further action, which sows further seeds of *karma*".

The questioner looked rather glum. "It sounds a never-ending process".

The young Monk smiled.

"Well, it will continue until the destruction of its cause".

"And what is that, Sir?"

"The way we identify with our body as the doer of action. And this lifelong habit is only destroyed by knowing oneself to be the bodiless Self. This is why it is said that knowledge is the fire that reduces *karma* to ashes".

After a few moment's silence the older man asked:

"And does a person whose *karma* is burned up by the fire of knowledge continue to act in the world?"

"He does indeed, but his action is free from personal desire and attachment. If he is a householder engaged in the world of work and family, then he continues to act to set an example to the people around, even though he does not feel himself to be acting at all. If on the other hand he is one of those who have taken the formal vow of renunciation, then his actions are merely such as are needed to maintain the body. But in either case," he repeated "he does not feel himself to be acting at all. He has become the great silence that is beyond all activity. Once he knows the truth of action and the truth of silence together, his *karma* is said to be burnt to ashes. This is the status of a real man of knowledge, and such a man is quite untouched by the poison of doubt, which is a source of ruin for many on the path".[47]

Another of the villagers, who had been following the discussion keenly, then spoke up:

"But if a person's *karma* has been destroyed, how does he continue to exist as a body at all?"

"Those actions which brought this present body into existence in this lifetime have already begun to bear fruit, and this must continue until their effects have been fully worked out. The experience of the Self destroys only those seeds of action as have yet not begun to sprout. This applies whether those unsprouted seeds were created in this life prior to the arising of spiritual knowledge, or in any number of previous lives, come to that".

A third visitor, feeling the discussion was becoming too abstract, put his own question:

"Maharaj shri, surely devotion to God is also needed to realise the Self?"

"Yes, but if you do not know what God is, how can you be devoted to Him? Real devotion is not a mood you can practice or a state of wishful thinking. It is the direct *experience* of God. When you see Him as ever present, everywhere and in everything, and you perform service to Him constantly and worship Him continuously, that is real devotion".

"How can we bring this state about?"

"Choose one of His many forms and get to know Him intimately. Become familiar with Him in, and as, and through that form. It does not matter which form you choose, be it Narayana, Vasudeva, Hari,

Vishnu or Krishna, all are good and you should just follow the one you feel most naturally drawn to.[48] If you are sincere in your devotion, supreme knowledge will surely dawn and then you will always remain absorbed in God and devoted to Him. He who has drunk the nectar of knowledge and realised his unity with God has done all that is to be done. His evolution is completed; he has attained the final goal of human life".

Three kinds of mind

One day in early spring the young Monk and some of his followers were sitting in a forest clearing on the outskirts of Kashi. A devotee arrived from one of the nearby houses with an offering of some chapattis and a type of honey which was a speciality of the region. While they were all enjoying the food, someone remarked how delicious the honey was. The devotee told them that it was made by a particular local species of bee that is tiny, no bigger than a gnat, and has no sting.

The young Monk seemed delighted by this and remarked:

"See how life is always teaching us! There are some minds that are like the mud-worm. If you take the worm out of its mud and put it on a beautiful clean leaf in the sunlight, it will protest, twisting and squirming this way and that and will only be happy when it is sunk back in the dark mud. Due to its *tamasic* nature, that is where it functions most naturally.

"Another type of mind is like the fly: highly active but one minute feasting on a heap of sweet sugar and the next alighting on a pile of filth. It moves from one to the other with no discrimination – driven by its inherent *rajasic* nature it keeps on moving restlessly – one minute on sweetness, the next on dirt.

"There is yet another type of mind and this one is like the bee. It feeds only on nectar, moving from one sweet-scented flower to another with pleasure and quiet purpose, without getting distracted. This is the *sattvic* mind. It too is active, but its activity is refined and put to good use: from the accumulated nectar comes delicious honey that spreads sweetness, nourishment and happiness all around. So, let your mind be like these bees: directed, co-operative, productive of all that is good".[49]

After a moment's pause he added:

"And without any sting!"

Everyone laughed.

The debate with Mandana Mishra

As the months went by, a name kept cropping up in discussions and *darshan* sessions. It was that of a *pandit* by the name of Mandana Mishra, renowned as the foremost exponent of Karma Mimansa, the 'Enquiry into Action', which is the knowledge of the Vedic science of ritual. The *pandit* lived in Mahishmati[50] a town set on the northern bank of the Narmada river that was a centre of poetry and the arts. Its inhabitants were famed all over the Land of the Veda for their independent characters and sharp minds. It became clear to the young Monk that if he was to succeed in reviving the true understanding of Vedic teaching as being beyond mere ritual, and bring it to the people at large, it would be necessary for him to meet this man and engage him in debate. And so, arrangements were made for him to travel south to seek out the *pandit*. Padmapada and others of his closest followers would accompany him.

After some weeks they reached Mahishmati. The young Monk was happy to see the holy river again on whose banks, in what felt like another lifetime, he had received initiation from his *guru* and spent those extraordinary years in his company. The group found accommodation in a dilapidated but peaceful Shiva temple and the day following their arrival, after the morning bath and meditation, set off to find where the *pandit* lived. Before long they came across a group of local women, whose leader was evidently charmed by the young Monk's looks. She smiled flirtatiously at him, then, seeing his evident discomfort, laughingly pointed out a magnificent mansion with the following ironic couplet:

That house with the pillars is the one that you seek,
They shine green like the parrots who flock there to hear him speak!

Spurred on by her witty response, the group went up to the imposing gateway, only to find it guarded by a large moustachioed attendant. Casting a withering glance at their ochre robes, the door-guardian imperiously informed them that *pandit-ji* was performing *shraddha*[51] for his father and absolutely no-one was allowed in. His size and demeanour left no room for argument.

It is said that the young Monk sent the others back to the temple where they were lodging but lingered a while himself. Then, unobserved by the doorkeeper, he wandered round the side of the building. A tall palm tree was growing next to the wall. A *mantra* used by the toddy-tappers in his childhood village popped into his mind – he uttered it and the tree bent down obligingly towards him. Jumping up into it, he leapt nimbly onto a balcony and climbed into the house through the open shutters of a window.

The young man found himself in a large, airy room, at the far end of which sat a group of people on a low platform of carved wood. At the head of this gathering sat the *pandit*: an imposing and well-built figure wearing several strings of beads around his neck, a heavily brocaded shawl over his wide shoulders and chunky gold earrings under his freshly oiled hair. He was surrounded by the pots and dishes of the *shraddha* ceremony and the family members and *brahmins* needed for such a performance sat beside him on the platform. When he saw the intruder, the *pandit's* brow clouded over. As a prominent leader of the orthodox householder community and an unequalled expert on the Vedic rituals that guided its life, he was well-known for his dislike of *sannyasis* and his disparagement of the recluse way of life.

"And from where has this shaved one suddenly come?" he sneered in mock surprise.

Without a pause for thought the young Monk replied:

"This one has come shaved from the neck right up to the head!"

The *pandit* felt anger flare up at the self-assurance of such a reply.

"And what are you doing in my house, may I ask? You have no business being here uninvited!" he barked. At this, one of the *brahmin* priests leant over to whisper respectfully that although *sannyasis* were forbidden from attending ceremonies such as they were now performing, the texts also stipulated that any unexpected visitor to the *shraddha* ritual must be fed, whoever he might be.

Overhearing the priest, the young Monk intervened:

"Thank you kind Sir, but I have not come seeking food for the belly, I have come seeking food for mind".

Mandana Mishra now looked at the young man more curiously. "Oho!" he thought "This is quite a bright youth, even though he is a work-shy *sannyasi*".

"Very well", he replied, sighing exaggeratedly, "sit over there, stay quiet and when my rituals are finished you shall get your discussion".

A long time later, when at last everything was duly completed, the *brahmins* fed and paid and the family members finally departed, the *pandit* turned to his young visitor.

"Well now, young master *sannyasi*", he began, in a tone heavy with irony, "you certainly have a high opinion of yourself to barge in here and expect a debate. Nevertheless, I have to admit that you have a certain style about you and what looks like a quick mind, so in honour of my recently deceased father I will accede to your request. What exactly is it you wish to discuss with me?"

"I wish, honoured *pandit-ji*, to demonstrate that the life of knowledge as followed by the *sannyasi* is superior to the life of rituals as practised by the householder".

The older man was surprised at such temerity but there was something in the demeanour of the visitor that warned him not to dismiss him too lightly. "Oh, do you now?" he replied. "Well, you have certainly picked a profound and important subject, young man, I'll grant you that. And may I ask what the prize of such a debate is to be?"

"The loser will adopt the life of the winner" came the unswerving reply.

Now the *pandit* really was shocked. The victor in such ritual encounters was always rewarded by an increase in his reputation and often in material ways – gold, shawls and the like – but a debate whose outcome might entail a complete change of life was something else altogether. He sat in silence for some moments, considering the sudden and unexpected gravity of the situation. He realised that his name as an expert in the knowledge of sacred ritual, on which his ample livelihood depended, was being put on the line. At the same time, this could be a wonderful opportunity. By defeating this arrogant young man, not only would his star rise but many others would be deterred from the parasitic lifestyle of *sannyasa* and actually do something useful with themselves. But if he lost....no, such an outcome was unthinkable! This meeting had obviously come as a blessing from the gods, instant good *karma* earned by his *shraddha* offerings. Of course, that was it! Here was a heaven-sent chance to boost his fame and do some good into the bargain.

"Well now," he responded carefully. "This is a serious affair and if you really wish to go ahead with it, we will need to have a reputable umpire, isn't it? I don't suppose you have anyone in mind?" he asked, his voice tinged with sarcasm.

"No, Sir".

The *pandit* thought for a moment then nonchalantly indicated a woman who was directing the servants clearing up the remains of the ceremony. "Well, as it happens, I have been blessed with an unusually intelligent woman for a wife; indeed local people say my Ubhay-abharati is an incarnation of Saraswati, the Goddess of Knowledge. I suppose she could sit in and judge our debate ..." The disingenuous suggestion was left dangling in the air. The young Monk said nothing.

The *pandit* called his wife over and put the idea to her. The woman immediately felt trapped – how could she remain unbiased in such a situation? She obviously wanted her husband to win, and that of course was why he had suggested her, but there was something about this young *sannyasi* that made her uneasy. She had felt he was a special being the moment she set eyes on him and hadn't he already shown his agility of mind in everything he had said? Not one word wasted and they hadn't even started debating yet. Perhaps he would turn out to be the cleverer of the two. Or, on the other hand, he could be the vehicle of some mischievous spirit come to cause them trouble. Either way, he was potential trouble.

"Honoured Sirs", she replied demurely. "You are both highly knowledgeable in your chosen fields, and to be honest I really do not feel competent to judge between you on such esoteric subjects, especially when you get into all the technical details. However, I have another suggestion. Why do we not let Mother Nature herself decide?"

So saying she picked up two garlands of white jasmine that had been part of the decorations for the ceremony, and weighing them gently in her hands said:

"We shall have fresh garlands like these made for the debate and each of you will wear one. The jasmine will keep your minds cool and your words sweet, but whichever of the garlands begins to fade first, its wearer will be judged the loser".

The two contestants looked at each other and nodded. A brilliant decision indeed, worthy of Saraswati herself. It was agreed that the debate would begin the following day.

The word had gone swiftly around the town that a young *sannyasi* from Kashi was challenging *pandit-ji,* and by mid-morning a large crowd had gathered in the compound where the contest was to be held. In the front row sat many venerable scholars and religious experts, each distinguished by sectarian marks and colourful shawls. A dais had been set up, draped with flowers and shortly after eleven o'clock the two contestants emerged from inside the house and took their places opposite each other on the platform. Incense was lit, each man chanted some *slokas* from the Vedas, and then the *pandit's* wife stepped forward and ceremoniously draped a pristine garland of white jasmine around each neck. To the onlookers this was a ritual courtesy, but the two on the platform knew well that the soft-scented touch could end up being the noose that hanged them.

And so the great debate began. Starting on a personal note, Mishra lost no time in letting the younger man know his low opinion of the recluse way of life. He castigated the unmarried status of the *sannyasi*, saying that to remain unmarried was a dereliction of duty to one's own family and also to society at large, for both benefit from the rites an orthodox married householder must perform. Indeed, everyone benefits, for such rites serve to bring the gods down to earth and elevate human life to heaven.

"Salvation cannot be achieved through spiritual insight alone, because each individual soul is born with a destiny and must exhaust its latent possibilities through action, as a seed fulfils itself through sprouting, growing and flowering. This is the superiority of the householder way: through his work and marriage and all the responsibilities these entail, he is securely embedded not only in society, but in the universal chain of *karmic* action which is existence. Moreover, the householder can have a boy child, who can perform the correct rites to cancel out his own father's debt to the ancestors who gave him his own life. This is how the great tapestry of human culture is woven age after age. It is a perfect system, and that is why it has endured for so long."

"But Sir," countered the young Monk smiling "marriage is surely not confined to the householder. Does not every *sannyasi* also marry?"

The *pandit* could hardly believe his ears at such nonsense. Was the boy an idiot after all?

The Monk went on:

"His spirit is the husband, his body is the wife – these two must marry and sweet words will be the children. And what is more, in this marriage there will never be any quarrelling!"

A ripple of pleasure spread through the crowd; this was going to be interesting.

"Clever words, young man! But please, let us not be flippant. Your answer exactly proves my point – the *sannyasi* is concerned only with himself. What about others, the family and the rest of society?"

"Family relationships are important Sir, no doubt, but they are not absolute. In fact, in the wider scheme of things relatives are no more closely united than travellers who meet at a *dharmashala*[52] sojourn together a while and then part again, losing sight of one another as they continue their different journeys. And actually, a *sannyasi* is far more concerned with family than is a householder. His family is not narrowly confined but hugely extended and stretches right through society – every person who gives him alms is his mother, everyone who gives him spiritual instruction is his father, and every one of his students is his child. In this way the *sannyasi* really lives out the Vedic axiom that 'The world is my family' and, moreover, he is taking care of this hugely extended family continuously. Everyone he meets is part of it".

Realising that such a quick-witted opponent would not be as easy to overcome as he had initially supposed, the *pandit* shifted the tone of his argument.

"Very well, let us not get bogged down in such particulars but consider instead the universal principles involved. After all, every detailed example derives from a more generalised law, does it not? So, to begin with, how can you *sannyasis* deny the value of action?"

Without waiting for an answer he continued:

"Action is the very stuff of human existence. Without it, knowledge is fruitless and happiness impossible. Most importantly, if we do not engage in action our born *dharma*[53] and the duties of *varna*[54] cannot be fulfilled. Make no mistake, we followers of Karma Mimansa are concerned with salvation just as much as you devotees of pure knowledge, but we believe that salvation can only come through right action. The soul is bound to survive this life and be reborn again, therefore the knowledge of correct action and its rewards are absolutely necessary. Mimansa is the guiding light of our ancient culture: all our rituals depend on it, all our moral conduct is guided by it, all our law is founded upon it. Yet, given this obvious fact, not only do you renunciates step off the path of evolution that the gods have laid down for humanity, but you shirk an honest day's work and even expect to be fed by hardworking householders for doing so!"

Seeing that the debate had taken a more serious turn, the young Monk also changed his tone:

"You are quite right, Sir, when you say that action is necessary. As long as one is in the body, one cannot remain without working, as the Lord Krishna himself clearly tells us.[55] So from that point of view, the *sannyasi* works no less than the householder, only his work is not concerned with the accumulation of possessions and worldly comfort. In the material world there are many levels of life, some are gross, some are subtle. Now, is it not the case that the movement of the mind is subtler than the action of the hand?"

"Yes, I suppose that is so" conceded the *pandit*, instinctively beginning to feel a little wary of the young man's direction.

"Just so, we recluses do not abandon action totally but simply chose a subtler form of action than others. Our work is both refined and unceasing – we teach, we advise, we meditate, we discriminate. This is mind-work, but work it certainly is. As it is concerned with the spiritual side of life, such subtle activity is every bit as necessary and as useful as gross material work, in fact I would argue, more so.

"Moreover, each one of us has to engage in work that is appropriate to his temperament, for to do so is to follow his *dharma*, and, as you say, without following his *dharma* no one can succeed on life's journey. All should certainly do their allotted work; I have no interest in confusing the people on that score and unsettling their beliefs.[56]

"However, the texts clearly teach that there are two paths, each valid for a different level of aspirant: the path of action for the less advanced, that of knowledge for the more advanced. The path of action will gradually purify a man so that in due time he is fit for the path of knowledge. But commonly today, men of action forget this, and, thinking that all they ever need to do is perform action, they confine themselves to the transient surface of life. As a result they themselves suffer and they spread suffering. It is to counteract this common misunderstanding that the knowledge and the visible example of the *sannyasi* is so vitally important in society".[57]

"Well, you will admit that every worthwhile action must have a tangible result, will you not? This being indisputably so, just what is the practical result of this spiritual knowledge of yours, my dear young *sannyasi?*" asked the *pandit* with a condescending smile.

"The practical result of the way of knowledge is that one will come to realise that, in fact, nobody really acts at all! To one who sees clearly, the world is going on automatically and we are just witnessing it all. It is only the deluded man who, egotistically identifying with his limited body and mind, thinks 'I am doing this, I am doing that.' The man who knows the truth of life sees that he is not the 'doer', and that all activity is just the play of the three *gunas*. Therefore, he remains quite unattached to action and its fruits, and lives a selfless life of loving happiness even in the midst of this world with all its folly and suffering. As you must know well, oh *Mahamahopadyayaji*, all this is laid out very clearly by Lord Krishna in the third chapter of his glorious song".[58]

An appreciative murmur ran around the crowd. For his part Mandana Mishra was beginning to realise that it was not going to be so easy to defeat this youth. Not only was he quick-witted, he had good knowledge of scripture also and, what was more ominous, he seemed to speak of high states from personal experience. Into the bargain the youth was a good tactician, drawing his references from the most popular of the householder texts, which not only endeared him to the crowd but was forcing his older opponent to look for ever new ways of attack, while he himself only needed to produce counter arguments, thereby expending less mental energy.

The *pandit* began to go even more deeply into the subject, drawing on the recondite texts on Vedic ritual that were his speciality. He spoke of what makes an action correct and in accord with cosmic law; of the structure of *gotra*,[59] the duties of caste and the necessity of fulfilling one's *dharma*; of the use of *mantras* and the meaning of rituals. He spent time extolling the various *yajna* fire sacrifices: those that are a regular duty, others that are performed only at specific times and yet others that are needed for a specific motive and result. He reiterated the fact that it was only the performance of Vedic ritual that kept the world in harmony with the wider cosmos, for without it the gods would be angry, life's natural balance would be destroyed, rain would not come, crops would fail and chaos would erupt in society. Time and again he drew on the importance of the sacred science of sound, backed up by the acknowledged authority of the esoteric *sutras* of the great sage Jaimini and his complex analysis of the magic efficacy of grammar that structures the world and keeps it in harmonious equilibrium.[60]

The young Monk calmly met each of these arguments as they came. He did not deny the value of ritual, but pointed out that it was a limited science because it only covered the changing field of life. Basing his own position on the teaching, found in the most ancient Upanishads, that ultimate Truth lies in the transcendental field beyond all relative limitations, he reminded his opponent that even King

Janaka, greatest of all rulers, who had all anyone could ever wish for in the material world, eventually found the only real satisfaction in life was to renounce his kingdom in order to realise the unbounded Self.[61] Quoting the texts fluently, he reminded all present that there is a lower and higher level of sacred understanding and that those who take rituals to be the limit of knowledge are wandering around like the blind led by the blind. Rituals are unsafe boats to reach the farthest shore of liberation, and surveying those worlds won by ritual, a true *brahmin* arrives at dispassion.[62]

But most of all he quoted the Gita. In particular he focussed on its central message: that life has two halves – the unmanifest and non-dual Absolute and the manifest fields of duality bound by time, space and causation. Taken together these make one wholeness, *brahman*, but the Vedas are concerned with only one half of the picture, the relative worlds of action. As long as a person is only concerned with a better life and greater worldly joys, so long is he confined to the cycle of birth and death in realms that are inevitably hedged in by suffering and limitation. The ultimate freedom we all long for does not lie in the seductive promises of a heaven that can be won by rituals but by passing quite beyond the relative realms and uniting with the Absolute as our own deepest Self. And for one who has realised the Self, the Vedas are of as much use as a small well in a place flooded with water on every side.[63]

And so, day after day, the debate raged. With each point won or lost, the crowd swayed this way and that. Most of them, as householders themselves, had come prepared to support their local *pandit* in what they assumed would be an easy victory. But now many were not so sure. This young stranger from Kashi had a self-assurance and brilliance that was beginning to look invincible.

After debating for many days, some say twenty-one, the contestants were finally beginning to flag. Everything possible had been dealt with; the young *sannyasi* produced his summary:

"So revered *pandit-ji*, we have seen that there are two levels of knowledge. The lower pertains to the relative world and the conventional person, who, identified with his body and limited ego-sense, thinks he is the doer, and seeks to win all sorts of enjoyable experiences for himself, both in this world and the next one. The higher knowledge is concerned with transcending the perception that is the basis of all our suffering, which is the erroneous idea we are an isolated individual in need of salvation. We are not an isolated individual, we are the unbounded, absolute consciousness of the real Self, and therefore we are already saved! It is quite true, there will always be those individuals who need the consolations offered by conventional religion, and those situations will always occur that require the intervention of correctly practised sacred ritual. But if we are talking of ultimate liberation, it does not lie in the self-fulfilment offered by the promise of worldly advancement or imagined spiritual security, it lies in total self-transcendence. From this point of view, any attempt to bolster or continue the separate sense of a bodily self, whether in this life or in some pleasurable realm hereafter, is to remain stuck in the isolated sense of 'I' that is the root cause of all our suffering in the first place.[64] This being so, the real sacrifice is not to offer herbs and *ghee* into the fire-pit but to offer the ego into the purifying flames of transformation. The mind must let go of everything it has known, expected or feared. This is the way of pure knowledge, and only this unstinting surrender can unclench the closed fist of egotism and release the chronically contracted sense of self that is our normal reality".

Suddenly, the older man felt exhausted. The strain of so many days of intense intellectual effort flooded over him. He sat with his head slumped forward on his chest as he vainly sought to dredge up a counter-argument to these fluent words. He could find none. Then, out of the corner of his eye, he noticed that several of the creamy jasmine petals on his garland had begun to curl and turn brown at the edges. Incredulous, he sneaked a sidelong look at his opponent and saw that his garland remained as fresh as the day it was made. The *pandit* cast a despairing glance at his wife, who understood its significance immediately. As her husband was summoning the strength to admit defeat, she subtly motioned him to keep quiet and stepped forward with a smile on her lips.

"Revered Maharaj shri," she began with modestly lowered eyes, choosing her words carefully and hoping to flatter the young man with such an exalted title, "you have indeed proved an extraordinarily knowledgeable and subtle debater, effortlessly able to draw on all the hallowed scriptures of our holy Land of the Veda to make your points. But Maharaj shri, please forgive me if I have missed something," – here she smiled disingenuously – "but I do not remember your referring to the teaching of the renowned sage Vatsayana in your debate?"

"Do you mean the Kamasutra, Madam?"

"Yes, I mean the Kamasutra".

"You are correct, Madam, we did not discuss that text. I am a life-celibate, so how could I know anything of the Kamasutra which deals with the science of sensual pleasure and the relations between man and woman?"

"But Maharaj shri, was not your agreement that each and every Vedic text could be summoned as a witness in this debate?"

A pause.

"It was".

"Well, Maharaj shri" she continued, "you will remember that the Kamasutra is the discourse of Kama, the youthful God of Love, who keeps the world turning by firing flower-tipped arrows from his bow made of sugar-cane and strung with hummingbirds. As such, it is a sacred text on the art of living, is it not?"

"I suppose it could be considered so" replied the young Monk, unsure now for the first time.

"Well then, Sir," and here she arched her fine eyebrows, "could it not be that there is material in the Kamasutra that would support my husband's arguments and undermine your position?"

There was no denying the clever woman's logic.

"I suppose that is possible, Madam" he cautiously replied.

"Then, my dear Maharaj shri", her smile was triumphant now, "if all the witnesses have not yet been summoned, how can the debate be considered resolved in your favour?"

The young Monk sat considering the situation for some moments.

"Give me one month, and I shall return to conclude this debate".

With huge relief, the *pandit* and his wife bowed deeply to signal their agreement, while the audience erupted in prolonged applause.

The *sannyasi* left the *pandit's* house to return to the old temple by the river where he and the others were staying. He had no plan in mind; all he knew was that there must be some way to win this debate, for Truth was on his side. It so happened that just as he was leaving the main path to descend to the water's edge, he heard in the distance behind him the rhythmic *chant* that accompanies a body on its journey to the cremation ground: "Ram nam satya hai! Ram nam satya hai!"[65]

A large procession was approaching, dozens of well-dressed and important-looking men surrounded a sumptuously decorated corpse being carried at shoulder height. Enquiring of a passer-by, the youth learnt that Raja Amaruka, the local king, had recently died by falling from his horse while out hunting. Immediately, a bold idea leapt into the young man's mind. Now he had his plan, and there was no time to lose!

Hurrying down into the temple, he summoned his companions and quickly led them to the rocky incline that rose up behind the ancient walls of the compound. Finding a cave there he went straight in, giving strict instructions that he should on no account be approached unless and until he chose to emerge. One of the followers was always to remain on guard at the cave's entrance to ensure no one disturbed him. With a promise to return within the month, the young man sent them back to the temple, took his seat and closed his eyes.

It is said that there in the darkness, he quickly sank into deep meditation and by use of a yogic *siddhi*, having withdrawn his awareness into the subtle body, directed it to leave its gross outer casing and travel straight to the royal cremation ground. Once there, unseen by anyone he approached the body of the *raja* as it lay on the unlit pyre and entered into it through the fontanel opening in the skull, thus taking possession of the corpse, infusing his awareness into the body from crown right down to toes.[66] As the king's eldest son approached the pyre, flaming torch in hand, he was astonished to see his father's body move. He blinked; it moved again! Excitedly summoning the onlookers, together they quickly began to unwrap the corpse, who then calmly sat up to survey the scene. It was a miracle – the great ruler had come back to life!

The celebrations at the palace were jubilant and prolonged. Special rituals were performed, including the royal lustration with milk, just as Lord Rama had received when he returned to Ayodhya with Sita after defeating the demon king Ravana of Lanka. No one was happier to see Amaruka alive again than his chief queen – who welcomed him into her perfumed bedchamber with added ardour, eager to celebrate the joys of being alive with someone so miraculously snatched from Lord Yama's noose. Over the next few days, the king enthusiastically enjoyed the sexual favours of his minor queens as well – each with her own preferences and particular techniques of the art of love. All of them were delighted and astonished by their lord's renewed vigour and his innocent enjoyment; it was almost as if the whole business were new to him!

Everything went well for some time. But gradually Amaruka's ministers became suspicious; they had begun to notice an increasing number of curious discrepancies between the brilliant character of this 'returned' king and their former ruler. One of them who was schooled in yogic knowledge came to the conclusion that the dead body of their monarch had been possessed by a wandering spirit. At a hurriedly convened council the ministers agreed to issue an edict in the unsuspecting king's name that all lifeless bodies found throughout the kingdom must be cremated immediately. If they located an apparently dead body that had been deliberately left unburned by its close relatives, they would automatically know the identity of the possessing spirit. Into the bargain, the burning of such a body would avoid any further incidents of possession.

For their part, the Monk's companions were also worried. They had heard of Amaruka's miraculous return from the dead and guessed what had taken place. But now the promised month had almost elapsed and their leader had not returned to the body in the cave. Had the unthinkable happened? Had their beloved *guruji* succumbed to the temptations of householder life and sacrificed his life-long asceticism for the pleasures of wealth, power and sensual delight?

A plan was hatched. Several of the followers disguised themselves as musicians and went to the palace, gaining admittance to sing before the king. They began a recital of their young master's favourite songs: some were lines from the wandering *sadhu*-poets on the insufficiencies of material life and the poverty of worldly joys; others were verses from the Veda extolling the incomparable delights of the spirit.

In the middle of their recital, the *raja* dropped dead.

The young Monk swiftly returned to his own body, just as one of the royal search parties had forced its way into the cave and were planning to cremate the apparently lifeless ascetic sitting there in lotus posture. To their astonishment, the ochre-robed figure suddenly opened its eyes and surveying the scene, cheerfully remarked on the benefits of deep meditation.

And thus, so it is said, the young *sannyasi* was able to keep his appointment with Mandana Mishra. His ability to describe each and every nuance of the sensual life and still show that renunciation was the superior path, proved invincible. The astonished *pandit* soon admitted defeat and, with the blessings of his equally bemused wife, was initiated into *sannyasa* without delay. He was given the name Sureshvara and became one of the young Monk's four closest disciples. In time he was to prove to be the most intellectually celebrated among all the followers.[67]

The Meeting with the Untouchable

Not long after his return to Kashi from Mahishamati, an event occurred that was to mark a radical turning point in the young Monk's life and mission.

It had long been the daily routine for him and some of his followers to go down to the *ghats* just before dawn for their early morning bath in the Ganga and to imbibe the blessings of the first rays of the sun. As the blazing ball edged above the eastern horizon, turning the sky first pink and then golden and colouring the wide water aquamarine and turquoise, they would chant the *Gayatri* mantra to invoke the blessings of the Supreme Intelligence, offer prayers to the gods and the ancestors and call for the blessings of the Almighty on all creation. Trickling water in front of their eyes, they stared straight into the growing light, allowing its warm rays subtly to infuse their minds and hearts. Then as a group they would join the swelling crowd moving back up from the riverbank into the heart of the old city, for the first *puja* of the day at the mighty Vishvanath temple.

Although the Monk and some of his followers were ordained *sannyasis*, and therefore technically absolved from the duty to worship the gods, he encouraged them to attend temple rituals to set an example of piety to the people. The *galis*[68] were always crowded at this time. *Sadhus*, pilgrims, the young and the old all jostled with the early morning *jalwallahs* carrying pitchers of fresh Ganga water along the narrow lanes lined with flower vendors, while the smells of boiling milk and freshly baked sweets mingled with the heady scent of incense. There was always an intense atmosphere of excitement and expectation, for what could be better than to begin the day with a sighting of the Lord of the Universe at home in his splendid dwelling place?

It was Shivaratri, the spring festival that celebrates the marriage of Shiva and Parvati, so this particular morning the crowd was exceptionally large. Pilgrims from all over the country had converged on the holy city and the place was thronged by bobbing and drifting tides of people. The time for the beginning of the *puja* was nigh and so crowded were the lanes that there seemed to be no hope of reaching the temple on time. Hurriedly taking a shortcut through a narrow side alley, the young Monk and his group found their way blocked by a ragged beggar accompanied by his four mangy dogs.

To the orthodox *brahmin* meeting such a collection of impure beings on the way to the temple was highly inauspicious, a pollution that augured very badly for the day. Pressing himself against the wall to avoid physical contact, the young Monk gestured impatiently to the beggar to move aside. But as he did so, the ragged creature in front of him spoke up in a clear and pure voice:

"Aha, noble *brahmin*! I do not know if you are addressing your scorn to this body that stands in your way or to the spirit within it. If the body is the object of your displeasure, then you know as well as I that the body is but a superficial form of no great consequence. Both your body and mine were born, both grew and both will change and die, so where is there any difference between us? If, on the other hand, you are speaking to the spirit within, then you and I both know that there is but one universal spirit manifesting as all the differences in the world, so once again, there is no difference between you and I. And so I ask you noble young *brahmin*, just who are you commanding to stand aside and move out of your way?"

For a long moment the Monk stood as if transfixed. Then, uttering a cry, he fell to his knees and prostrated before the dishevelled figure, remaining stretched on the ground for many minutes. When he staggered back to his feet, he was clearly disorientated, hardly able to walk. All ideas of *puja* were abandoned; his companions took him back to the ashram. Once there, he went straight to his room. He spent the next few weeks in silence, seeing almost no one and not moving out from the place. Clearly, something momentous had happened, after which things would never be the same. His followers could only watch and wait.

It was only many years later, reminiscing with his closest disciple Totakacharya, that he spoke of this event.

"That day marked the great turning point. It brought the final realisation of the true nature of Reality. With that man's words, a number of things were impressed on my mind in rapid succession. In fact, there was no succession, only talking about it now, at a distance, can it be said there were stages to it. When it happened there was no time and so no succession; everything happened all at once, as if in an instant. But that instant had many layers to it somehow, which now, in retrospect, can be differentiated and described.

"To begin with, the beggar took the form of Lord Shiva, the great ascetic with matted locks and body smeared with ash, wearing a tiger skin, holding trident and alms bowl. The four dogs became the four Vedas. It became perfectly obvious that the entire universe is his play and that that play is one of infinite possibilities. How then can anything be rejected? Even what is deemed impure and unacceptable is part of his play. Such impurities serve the greater good and actually deserve our gratitude, because in playing their allotted part they exhaust certain possibilities and save others from having to manifest them. In this play of the Divine, the impure are in their essence just as much part of the divine process as is the purest law-abiding *brahmin*. What mankind judges to be good and evil is all part of Shiva's grace, each and every difference is intrinsically part of the total unity. Divisions and differences, purity and impurity, effort and discernment all have their necessary and legitimate place on the surface of life, because without these distinctions the whole process would just disintegrate into disorder and chaos, and yet at the same time, everything without exception and however contradictory, is essentially the manifestation of the Divine.

"And then even Shiva was left behind. It became clear that any vision, no matter how lofty, is limited, because it is predicated on a separation between what is seen and the mind that sees it. Any vision is locked in duality and as such it comes and goes. But in truth there is always and only the ultimate One, displayed in different forms. Every apparent separate object is but a mirror of That non-dual essence, reflecting back the divine nature of its source. In truth there is only that source, the infinite consciousness we call *brahman*. It is all that is; it is both subject and object, it is Shiva, it is the dog and it is the Self. It is everything that exists, and simultaneously it is that which surpasses existence. So there is no need for visions because we are never, not even for an instant, without That, because only That exists.

"This was the Great Awakening communicated in an instant. And with it, everything is changed forever. There is nothing left to learn or gain; all seeking comes to an end. A doll made of salt has returned into the sea and this journey is final, it is impossible to return. Once there is that Unity, there is no coming back to limitation; only the Divine remains."

After a long pause he smiled:

"It takes time to function comfortably in this supreme knowledge. All that has been before is annihilated, the body is flat on its back and it may remain like that for some time. A new way of functioning has to be learned, like a new-born child. But then, after some days the body begins to do little things, move around a little, becomes gradually adjusted to moving in and through and as the blissful Oneness. With time it does a little bit more and then a little bit more. After some weeks or months, it can function, fully conscious in and as the non-dual *brahman*, in and as the transcendental Divine. This is full Enlightenment and it is the greatest gift of all. And bear in mind, we have done nothing of ourselves to merit such a state, all glory goes only to the Holy Tradition of our Masters. All glory goes only to them."[69]

PART THREE:

THE MASTER

The courtyard of the ancient monastery, Kashi's pre-eminent centre of spiritual learning, has been cleaned and swept. At one end stands a great *peepul* tree whose lovely wide-spreading branches give such welcome shade. Crows squawk as they hop from one branch to another and little squirrels dart here and there across the dusty ground beneath them. The simple regularity of the arches and doors of the cloisters around the courtyard give a neat and ordered feeling to the place and the scene has a pleasingly settled atmosphere.

About four hundred monks are sitting on the ground in a wide semi-circle facing the tree and the clusters of ochre, red and yellow robes show the various different schools that have assembled for the event. They are arranged according to rank with the senior monks of each school up at the front while young novices, many in white robes, sit at the back of the gathering. At one end of the arc is a large group of *sadhus* who are not wearing the robe of an official order, but many sport the bright distinguishing colours of their particular lineage. Under the tree a raised dais has been built of wood; it is covered in saffron cloth and strewn with red and orange flowers. On this dais sits the Master with his staff and water pot beside him as he serenely surveys the crowd in front of him.

The proceedings begin with recitation by a group of twenty-one pundits, shaven headed and wearing yellow silk shawls. The verses of Rig and Sama Veda swell and dip in deep sonorous cadences of elemental power: the sounds of Mother Nature herself, like the rolls of distant thunder advancing from beyond the horizon of time. After perhaps half an hour of chanting, the Abbot, a small, dignified man in late middle age with the humble air of a true scholar, rises to his feet formally to welcome the Master.

"Respected Maharaj-ji, it is indeed an honour for us to have your august presence here with us today. Notwithstanding your lack of years, your reputation has already spread rapidly through our ancient holy city and further afield. It is said by some that you are the legitimate spiritual heir of the Masters of the Holy Tradition, those *rishis,* saints and enlightened beings who have taught the eternal truth of life since time immemorial.[70] Indeed some are even saying that you are the Lord Shiva in human form, come to restore the purity of the Vedic teaching in our troubled times. So to open our debate here today, good Sir, pray present us with your essential teaching".

After a pause, the Master begins by chanting a few stanzas in praise of the line of *gurus.* Then he starts to speak in a soft and melodious voice:

"Venerable Abbot, there can be no greater use of our precious human birth than to dedicate oneself to the pursuit of Truth. All of you gathered together here have had the rare intelligence to realise this and to make good use of your limited time in this unpredictable life. You have decided to do more with your existence than just breed, struggle and die, and you have wisely turned your back on the thin yield of worldly pleasures in favour of the rich harvest of the spirit. Your orange robes fly the noble flag of renunciation, proclaiming far and wide that you have chosen to store and circulate the sacred energy within your own bodies and not dissipate it in the market place of the world. And in your nomadic lifestyle you uphold the *dharma* of 'those who are destined to move' without whom the sedentary *dharma* of the householder would lose its balance and be overrun by its own aberrations.[71] I salute you all as the noble warriors who move deftly through this great web of illusion we call the world, and it is a very great joy for me to be here today in such an illustrious company of spiritual luminaries and genuine seekers.

"My teaching, oh forest of ascetics" – here the young man uses the traditional form of address to a company of monks – "is the culmination of all Vedic knowledge. The entire range of sacred wisdom, the knowledge of the subtle powers that govern life on earth, the knowledge of how to contact and invoke their help and support through fire offerings, the knowledge of herbs and healing, the skills of archery and governmental organisation, the understanding of celestial sound and its effects, the insight into the movement of the planets and their effects on earth – all this is both contained and transcended in the Way that I teach.

"For I teach Unity Consciousness, the state of ultimate freedom, liberation and indescribable joy, that those who follow *sanatana dharma* call *moksha* and those who follow Gautama the Enlightened one call *nirvana.* In this state of non-duality, everything from Lord Brahma down to a clump of grass is clearly seen to be a form of the one formless Divine, and that Divine, the immaculate and omnipresent substratum of the universe, is one's very own Self.[72] This formless unity is to be realised here in life, whilst we are still in the body and in the world. It is not, as some erroneously teach, a state that can be reached only after physical death and it far surpasses any of the heavens or celestial realms that are won by the correct performance of rituals. Moreover, this liberation is available, O forest of ascetics, to anyone who truly wishes it and is suitably ripe for attainment".

"And what, respected Maharaj", responds the Abbot, "is the basis for a teaching that transcends the wealth of Vedic knowledge?"

"The basis, Venerable Abbot, is the very nature of life. Beyond the changing world of the senses, beyond the mind, beyond all our normal boundaries of individuality, there exists an ultimate Reality. This field of ultimate Reality is transcendental and silent; it is divine, absolute and all-pervading. As such, it gives rise to the manifold worlds of name and form but is itself ever unstained by its own creations. Our tradition calls it *brahman,* 'the unbounded expanse', but names do not matter, as Truth is one, though the sages may describe it by different terms".[73]

"Respected Maharaj, as we well know, there are many theories and beliefs about the nature of reality and they are not all consistent. How can we be sure that this *brahman* is not just another such theory or belief?"

"You are quite correct, Venerable Abbot, in saying that there are many theories and beliefs about the nature of reality! Because of this there are also many seekers who spend their time accumulating and propagating such theories and beliefs. But to do so is to be like a starving man who seeks to satisfy his hunger by repeating to himself the words 'rice and vegetables, rice and vegetables'. Such words will never cure his hunger; he has to eat rice and vegetables and taste and enjoy and digest and be nourished by them. Like that, a person who merely collects metaphysical theories and beliefs will never be satisfied. Such a one will have to experience the Truth directly, taste it and enjoy it and digest it fully so that it becomes a natural part of him. This is the practical benefit of the knowledge I teach".

"What then is the most important thing for a seeker of truth, respected Sir?"

"Direct spiritual experience is the most important thing for a seeker of truth; true knowledge depends on our direct experience. Of all the means of gaining knowledge that are accepted as valid by our sacred tradition, direct experience is said to be supreme.[74] Indeed, if even a thousand scriptures were to tell me that fire was cold, I would still not ignore my own direct experience of putting my hand into the flames and finding that fire was not, in fact, cold".

At this a ripple runs around the assembly, and a mixture of surprise and consternation appears on some faces, particularly among the older monks. There is some shaking of heads.

"Are we to understand from this, young Sir, that you impugn the authority of the holy scriptures?" asks the Abbot.

"Indeed, I certainly do not impugn the authority of the holy scriptures, Venerable Abbot", comes the measured reply. "Our sacred texts are eternal and true, for they are not just the products of the human mind, but life's record of its own intrinsic wisdom, passed down age after age, time after time. And no-one can claim to be a truly proficient teacher unless he is thoroughly versed in the Veda.[75] But the ultimate role of these scriptures is to inspire, verify and corroborate that direct personal experience of the absolute Self, without which the teaching of *brahman* would indeed be just one of those many theories about the ultimate nature of reality. Truly, the absolute *brahman* lies beyond the individual mind and its concepts or opinions. But the inmost Self, which is one with the absolute *brahman*, can be directly experienced when the mind goes beyond the limits of individuality".

"If it is beyond the mind, then can anything really be said about this ultimate *brahman*?"

"You will all know well that our sacred Upanishads ascribe to this eternal level of life three attributes: Truth, Consciousness and Bliss: *sat – chit – ananda*. Truth is that which does not change, for *brahman* is a level of pure Being that knows no change, no diminishment, no death. This pure Being is a unified field of unbounded Consciousness, it is the divine intelligence from which all creation springs, by which it is maintained and into which it eventually returns. And coming into contact with that unbounded Consciousness is a state of constant loving bliss, compared to which the joys of the senses pale into insignificance. And this pure Being, O forest of ascetics, is your very own Self".

Many in the assembly are visibly moved by the calm authority of the young man's words.

"Well said, respected Maharaj!" responds the Abbot. Initially concerned that he might find himself having to defend Vedic orthodoxy against this young teacher who has defeated and converted the great

Mandana Mishra, he is beginning to suspect that what he sees before him is the Upanishadic wisdom in living form.

"And how, then, is the life of one who knows this Self?"

"The life of one who knows this Self, Venerable Abbot, is one of peace, bliss, wisdom and unity. In this awareness there is no burden whatsoever, all is immaculate, pure and full of grace. Such are the blessings of this level of life. Truly, the enlightened state is the goal of all yoga, all worship and all spiritual disciplines".

The Abbot pauses and looks around at the audience. He can see they are captivated by what they are hearing. It is not just the words that hold them, for many present are accustomed to impressive oratory, it is the fact that the young man on the dais is transparent to the reality of which he speaks. Even the novices are held by his lucent countenance, aware that they are in the presence of something very unusual.

"Respected Maharaj" he continues, warming to the debate and conscious of his role as mediator. "You have spoken very eloquently about the state of enlightenment and we thank you for that. But what about the world? It is well-known that you and your tradition teach that the world is *maya*, an illusion. This is not a doctrine that is easy for the masses to understand and even many of us in the robe who belong to orders renowned for their scholarship and discipline, find such an extreme viewpoint difficult to comprehend. This hesitation is all the more so when, with all due respect, such a radical doctrine is heard issuing from the lips of one as young in worldly experience as yourself. Pray enlighten us further on this cosmic force of illusion that you call *maya*".

"Venerable Abbot, your question is a beautiful one", responds the Master smiling slightly, "for it has gone to the very heart of the whole matter. You have asked what should be asked and your question deserves a fit answer. So, then, listen carefully, O forest of ascetics, to what I have to say".

He pauses a moment before continuing:

"Strictly speaking, *maya* is not a force as such, it is a *concept* that the wise use to describe the true nature of the world and an understanding of the true status of our daily experience. Advaita does not teach that the world is an illusion, though such is often claimed by its detractors. The world is not an illusion, in the sense that it does not exist. Certainly, it exists, it has a phenomenal existence, of course" - here he raps the dais firmly with his knuckles - "the world of matter revealed by the senses exists, and no one in their right mind would deny that. But just because it exists does not necessarily mean it is real in any ultimate sense. And how is it that we can we say so? Well, one thing that is undeniable about the world is that it is forever changing. The world of normal experience is ceaselessly in movement, moment to moment, age to age. Some changes may be as quick as the blinking of an eye, others may be lengthy, like the change in the contours of a mountain, but everything without exception is in movement, changing, evolving. And what is ever-changing is also ever-dying: it is transitory, unstable and it is therefore undependable. No reliable foothold anywhere, no permanence.

"On the other hand, however, the criterion of ultimate Reality given to us by our scriptures is very clear: Reality is that which does not change. Our texts never tire of telling us that Reality is that which does not change. So the truth is that the world has an existence, but it has no ultimate reality. That lordly status belongs only to the transcendental phase of life, that which is never-changing and absolute Consciousness, utterly free of the bonds of time space and causation. And this is why we describe the world of empirical experience as *maya*, which means 'that which is not'. In itself, it has no abiding reality, being a wholly contingent superimposition on the transcendental realm of Reality. And without that underlying Absolute, no relative manifestation would be possible.

"And so" he continues, "to see the whole picture, we must realise that there are two banks to the river of life: one changing, dying, full of limitation and suffering, the other eternal, unlimited and forever blissful. Yet, in some mysterious way, these two together make one life, and the wholeness of this one life, with its two phases, one changing and the other unchanging, is called *brahman*, 'the Totality'. Those that follow the Way that I teach come to enjoy *brahma vidya* – the living knowledge of *brahman*".

"How can these two opposed phases exist together as one life?"

"It is like the waves and the sea. Both are the same water, yet in one phase that water takes a limited and transitory form, which we call 'a wave' while in the other phase it rests deep, stable and silent, and we call it 'the sea'. And though opposed in their nature, both of these phases go on happily together with no conflict! Like that, the Absolute remains hidden and unattached, unsullied even in the midst of its own creation. Such a state is mysterious indeed and this happy coincidence of two apparently opposed values, limited and limitless, is alluded to by another meaning of the word *maya*, which is: 'a magical show, a sleight of hand'".

Pausing to let his words sink in, the Master takes a drink of water from the pot beside him. Sensing that the foundations have been laid for a lively debate, the Abbot bows to the speaker, and, as he resumes his seat, head lowered in thought, he motions to the monks that questions can now come from the floor.

A middle-aged monk, no doubt a senior teacher in his order, stands up immediately:

"Respected young sir, you have just said that the world is a creation of the Absolute, which implies that this pure Being is the cause of the material world, does it not?"

"It does".

"This surely cannot be right. Wherever there is material creation, there is always an assembly of materials and instruments. Here in the world, we see that there is creation only when the appropriate tools and materials have been assembled. Potters, for example, only create once they have brought together their clay, water, wheel and turning stick; weavers only produce when their threads and shuttles and looms are ready. How then can the Absolute create when it is said to be an unbroken mass of pure Consciousness, without parts and auxiliaries?"

"There is no problem here, good monk, for creation is due to the peculiar nature of the causal substance. Take the example of milk. We find milk transforms itself quite naturally into curds. Or look at water, which changes quite spontaneously into ice. There is no additional means or instruments involved here, the causal factor is inherent. And so it is with the Absolute".

The monk counters:

"But Sir, how can you say this? Both these transformations you mention as examples *do* in fact depend on external means: the temperature. Milk depends on the external agent of heat to turn it into curds, and water depends on the external agent of cold to become ice".

"This is no objection either," continues the Master, pleased with questioner's acuity "because it is the intrinsic nature of milk itself that determines its reaction to the temperature and thence its transformation into curds. Heat, or any other external agency, can only hasten the transformation that is already latent therein. And if this potential were not there, then no amount of heat, or anything else for that matter, could turn the milk into curds. If you heat up the air, for example, it will not turn into curds! So the auxiliary factor of heat merely enhances the already latent potential of milk to become curds and, in the same way, the auxiliary factor of cold merely enhances the latent potential of water to become ice. Like that, the Absolute, which by its very nature is a field of infinite possibilities, can undergo myriad transformations without the need of any external agency".

Feeling himself being backed into a corner by such clear logic, the monk attempts to shift the argument sideways:

"Well then, let us approach the matter from another angle. The difference is that milk and water are not conscious entities, so it may well be the case that they can be transformed as part of the natural order of things without any external agent being involved. But the potter and weaver I mentioned *are* conscious beings and as such they need external means to help them create. Now, if the Absolute is itself conscious – which as the causal cosmic intelligence it surely must be – how can it then create without recourse to some external means?"

"As you know well" comes the answer, "our *puranas* and *itihasas* describe the antics of the gods and the great *rishis*, *siddhas* and the rest.[76] All these beings are certainly conscious, yet they can create and dematerialise at will: they manifest different bodies, glorious palaces, even whole kingdoms. And they do this just through the power of their thought-force, spontaneously, without any recourse to external means. If they can do this, how much more can the Absolute, which is Consciousness itself? Take note here, oh forest of ascetics, no general rule can be established that causality is always bound to operate in the same way that we have observed it operating in any particular case in the past".[77]

The next contribution comes from a teacher of the yoga philosophy who is well-known in the city.

"Revered sir, we are discussing how the world of becoming arises from the absolute level you call pure Being. As regards this question of causality, in the teaching that has come down from our Master, Maharishi Patanjali, the apparent causes of a change do not actually bring that change about, but merely remove the obstacles to an inherent potential's being expressed. He likens it to a farmer who removes the stones in order to allow his crop to emerge and sprout.[78] Is this the same as what you are saying about the process of causality?"

"It is the same mechanism at work, described from the point of view of the perceiver" replies the Master. "Your Master has spoken well on this".

Another, younger, monk stands up and asks:

"Maharaj shri, forgive what may seem like a repetition, but I still do not understand how can there be modification of the one eternal Being when the scriptures clearly and repeatedly say it is 'without parts, always at rest, ever pure and indivisible'?"[79]

"There is nothing amiss here" comes the reply "because parts and modifications *do* indeed arise. But the point is that the nature of these will be misperceived and misunderstood by an ignorant mind that does not see the truth, just as a rope lying on the path can easily be mistaken for a snake when there is not enough light available to see clearly. An uncultured mind will generally perceive these parts and modifications to be independent, self-sufficient and even unrelated entities. This is because the typical man lives ensnared in a world of concepts and his dull mind takes these concepts to be real, whereas in fact they are largely the result of habit and convention. It is like a man who thinks his dream is real because he is not awake.

"All such partial perspectives notwithstanding, from the established platform of ultimate truth there is only the Self, one without a second, ever at rest even in the midst of this turbulent world of effects.[80] The one Being maintains its integrity and persists under all its apparently different configurations. It is a question of one substance assuming various different forms, like a snake that assumes various different coils or the self-same clay that can be perceived as powder, or as a lump, or a pot or some broken shards".

At this, another monk, known to be skilled in dialectics, jumps up:

"Respected Maharaj-ji, you use the analogy of a lump of clay and a pot made of clay, but these two are surely separate realities, as distinct from each other as they are from the original unshaped clay. In the same way the relative universe, being an effect, is a distinctly separate reality from its cause which is the Absolute. Surely they are quite different, as different as, say, a cow and a horse?"

A ripple of amusement runs through the assembly, relieving the intellectual tension that is beginning to accumulate.

"Ha! Not so!" responds the Master, smiling as the laughter subsides. "For while the lump and the pot exclude each other, in that they appear to be quite different things, yet even in their difference both unequivocally remain clay. When there is a pot there is no lump and when there is a lump there is no pot, but neither the pot nor the lump exclude the clay, as both are, essentially, nothing but that self-same substance. Now, a cow can very well exist without a horse, and *vice-versa*, but neither the lump nor the pot can exist without the original clay, for it is their essential cause and they are merely the temporary forms of it".

"Very well, revered Sir, so are you then saying that what we call the relative world of time and space is in fact the temporary form of the infinite Absolute?"

"Exactly so".

"Well, if that is the case, then what, exactly is it that *produces* this temporary form? It must have some germinal cause that is more specific than the Absolute ground that is its source. Even if there is no external agency, as you have shown in your answer to a previous question, still there must surely be some internal agency, some little thing somewhere, to cause the limited to emerge from the unlimited. I just do not see how what is limited and partial can emerge from that which is taught by all the holy texts to be undivided and seamless".[81]

"Well said, O. monk!" The Master is really enjoying the debate now, as each new question brings out fresh aspects of the teaching.

"You are very right, this *maya* is indeed a mysterious business! Somehow, the limited and partial world can emerge from that unlimited and seamless absolute intelligence by virtue of the very nature of that intelligence. We have already seen that that pure intelligence can be characterised in a threefold manner as Being, Consciousness and loving Bliss. Now to say it is Consciousness implies that it is conscious of something, does it not? There must be some object-subject relationship – howsoever subtle it may be – present within that Consciousness, for to be conscious implies that there is a subject that is aware of an object. So this singularity of pure consciousness is conscious of something, yet it is by nature transcendental, quite beyond the material world of empirical experience, beyond all objects. So what can the absolute Consciousness be conscious of, if there is nothing but itself existing?"

The Master lets the question hang rhetorically in the air a moment; no one answers.

"It is conscious of itself! It is conscious of itself. So the absolute intelligence, as Consciousness, is conscious of itself, it is aware of just itself, nothing else. It is the subject aware of itself as its own object. And it is in this miniscule junction point of subject and object, as the absolute intelligence contemplates itself, that the possibility of something other than its own pure unboundedness is born. In this way, embedded in the very structure of pure intelligence, lies the seedbed of all the possible expressions of its own nature – its own *prakriti*.[82]

"This *prakriti*, we can call it Nature, is an archetypal organising energy, a fecund field of all possibilities from which all manifestation arises. The seeds of manifestation are lying there, ready to swell and sprout. These are the causal powers that create and maintain the universe and they take form as the laws of nature conducting the countless gross and subtle worlds. Just as all has emerged in this way from the absolute Self, so every object and every event in manifestation can be reduced to the conditions from which it proceeds, and every condition can itself be traced back to its cause, and every cause can in turn be traced back to the Self, which is the uncaused cause of all causes".

There is a pause while all present attempt to digest this abstract knowledge. Eventually, the direction of the debate changes as the next question comes from a devotee of a theistic school:

"Sir, these may well be fine metaphysics suited to rarified intellects, but we are taught that the universe is the creation of a personal God".

The Master nods.

"And so it can be seen. As the scripture says: 'Know then that *prakriti* is *maya* and the one who orchestrates *maya* is the Great Lord. This whole world is pervaded by His many parts'".[83]

Another monk, bent with the weight of years, returns to the previous subject:

"Young Sir, if I understand you correctly, you are saying that everything is a manifestation of the primal energy which, in its essence, is nothing but the Self?"

"That is correct".

"And you say that the nature of the Self is consciousness and love-bliss?"

"I do".

"Then, Sir, why is it that so much of the world is sunk in suffering and displays very little consciousness and very little love or bliss?"

The Master nods sympathetically as if to acknowledge the practical value of the question, then stretches over and delicately selects a red rose from the flowers that lie around him. Such a down-to-earth question merits a clearly illustrated answer.

"See, it is like this beautiful rose, which they say is Lord Vishnu's favourite flower. The colourless sap flows everywhere to form all the various aspects: leaf, stalk, flower, petal, thorn. At various points the silent, self-sufficient sap thinks to itself: 'I shall become the green leaf; I shall become the straight stalk; I shall become the soft petal; I shall become the sharp thorn'. Just like that, the creative, organising power inherent in absolute intelligence unfolds all the inherent expressions of that intelligence. And because that intelligence is infinite, it is a field of all possibilities. And because it is a field of all possibilities, it has the potential to give rise to expressions that, without for one moment ceasing to be that intelligence, can even appear to be its opposite. See here how the innocent sap becomes both the fragrant, pleasing petal, so soft and luscious and delightful, and then see there how it becomes the sharp, dangerous thorn! And so it is that the undying, absolute and blissful Divine can take expression as the mortal, relative and suffering world. Mark well, O. monks: the unchanging and the changing, the general and the specific, the abstract and the concrete, what is spirit and what is matter, the Self and the apparent non-Self – all are complementary aspects of the one undivided Reality; they do not exist apart from one another".[84]

The next to pose a question is an impressive-looking *hatha yogi*. Tall, handsome and youthful, with black matted hair falling to the ground, he is well-known in Kashi as a teacher of the rapid path to enlightenment through rigorous purification of the body. His whole air is straightforward and his approach is equally direct.

"This is indeed a valuable theoretical teaching, Sir, but what is your opinion of *yoga*?"

"You mean *hatha yoga*? Its value lies in kindling the fire of knowledge".[85]

"Is there no real value in doing *asanas* then?"

"Yes there is, but not just for themselves. *Asana* postures help to purify the body and steady the mind. When the mind is steady and the awareness is settled in that which stands pervading all existence, the posture is perfected. So the best *asana* is actually *nididhyasana!*"[86]

"I do not know that *asana*, Sir".

"It is the most important of all, the foundation of real yoga. True yoga consists in making everything that one has learnt in theory about the spiritual path become a living experience. This is Supreme Knowledge: when awareness of the ultimate becomes a direct and immediate perception.[87]

"How then does this knowledge develop? What are the means to it?"

"Listen carefully, *yogi raj*. This knowledge proceeds in three stages. First there must be 'hearing', the seeker must hear about the truth from the scriptures or a realised teacher. This is the first point of contact, indispensable. But not everyone is capable of such 'hearing', they might misinterpret what is said or have intellectual or emotional resistances to accepting it or they may even reject it outright. This is all a matter of their *karmas,* what they bring to the situation. A man may listen to his guru for twenty years and still not *hear* him. Nevertheless, however long it may take, once a person has really heard the teaching, then they have to reflect on it, think it through deeply, contemplate the meaning of what they have heard. Many people stop here and think that by persisting in such intellectual contemplation, they will eventually come to the Truth. But this is incorrect. The seeker has to become really absorbed in the import of what he has heard and contemplated and through this absorption enter so deeply into it that the mind transcends meaning and goes beyond thought. So eventually the yogi's awareness must embrace the transcendent experience of Reality and not merely be left directed to the tip of his nose!"[88]

Laughter lightens the atmosphere again, but the Master continues:

"Mark well, these three stages are all necessary and must be practised together on the path. They are all necessary because they involve different faculties: hearing involves both sound and meaning, whereas reflection involves just meaning and absorption just sound. Taken together they nourish the mind holistically and eventually lead it to transcend all its habitual limitations".

The next question:

"Young Sir, you speak of this apperception of Reality as Supreme Knowledge. How does this differ from what we normally experience and understand by that word? And how does this intellectual analysis fit with the actual experience of the enlightened ones?"

"We were discussing just now the two values of intelligence – subjective and objective. If these two values of intelligence can exist, both dedicated to themselves and separate from one another, then surely there must be a third value of intelligence which can entertain both these together? They do not exist in a vacuum, after all. So, this third value is the ultimate structure of knowledge, it is the Reality containing and reconciling within itself the two contrasting modes of subject and object. The Sankhya school identifies these two modes as on the one hand *purusha,* which is unmanifest and totally self-sufficient spirit, and on the other *prakriti,* the energy-matter which is ever ready to manifest its limitless possibilities. These two taken together can be called the ultimate structure of knowledge, which is known as *brahman,* 'the Totality'. This is lived directly in the state of enlightenment. The liberated one knows directly that 'I am that

Totality, that Totality is infinite consciousness and you are That, all this is That and That alone is'".

The power of these *mahavakyas*,[89] runs around the assembly like an electrical charge.

After some moments of silence, a venerable monk stands up with the words:

"Maharaj-ji, we have heard very beautifully from you of the relationship of the Absolute and the relative and the creative show of *maya*, and in your descriptions you have managed to reconcile the old adversaries of Sankhya and Vedanta. For this we are all grateful. What I would like to ask is by comparison a simple question: if what you have so eloquently explained is actually the case, if it is the reality of our daily lives, then why do we not realise it? Why is this perception so rare?"

"The cause of our ignorance of the reality of life is the deluded nature of the mind and its false imaginings".

"So what then is the cause of these false imaginings?" continues the questioner.

"These false imaginings come from the activation of latent impressions laid down by past experience deep in the mind. You are familiar with the process of dying cloth – of how, for example, a cloth dyed in turmeric becomes orange? In just the same way the mind becomes 'dyed' with an impression when it comes into contact with objects that present themselves to the senses. When these objects are pleasurable, such as the experience of a beautiful woman, the impressions they leave stain the mind with attachment; equally, when they are unpleasant, the mind becomes coloured by aversion. Now these impressions are of differing intensity: they can be light, influencing the mind like a cloth dyed pale grey, or they can be vivid, like a cloth dyed brilliant red with cochineal.[90]

"The emotional reactivity inherent in these impressions can be born from both from the qualities of the object itself and from the nature of the person's mind. Either way, the person is trapped in a cycle of action and reaction. And by the same mechanism, just as a white lotus is a pure object, so do some peoples' minds assume impressions of purity and these are conducive to freedom.

"Now, these dormant impressions of past experience can flare up into life in the present, just as a smouldering ember can suddenly burst into flame, and when this happens the mind loses its present clarity and is governed by the force of the past impression. It is by dwelling on the details of these sense impressions that attachment arises; from attachment comes desire; from frustrated desire comes anger; from anger rises delusion; from delusion one forgets all that one has been taught; from forgetfulness of all that one has been taught comes lack of discrimination between what is right and wrong, and from lack of discrimination between what is right and wrong, a man is ruined. In short it is the dulling effect of *karma* that veils the light of intelligence and impels us to act in ways that are all too often un-conducive to mundane happiness, let alone supreme liberation".[91]

"Can you be more specific about these mental impressions? Are there different types and categories?"

"There must be, why not? But they are essentially unknowable – no one can determine their beginning, middle or end, their number or the place or time or immediate occasion of their rising up. They are innumerable and their causes are innumerable also. This is the reason our Upanishadic texts take a practical line on this matter and do not waste time trying to enumerate the specific types of impressions that exist. Instead they discuss their typical characteristics and the general forms they assume.[92]

"It is to purify the mind and heart of these latent impressions that we undertake spiritual disciplines. These in turn lead to non-attachment and the mind begins to transcend the bias, partiality and suffering that is the legacy of the weight of its past experiences. Then we can see the truth of any situation impartially as it really is. Ultimately, this clarity reveals that the changing finite world is permeated by the eternal Reality that cannot be fathomed intellectually. When the mind's contact with that level of life is unshaken, we live in the unchanging infinite, and the very world of multiplicity is experienced as the non-dual Divine which is always pure, ever untouched by experience".

Many more points come up; the Master deals painstakingly with each one, whether abstract or practical, with the same easy and serene fluency. Finally, as the sun begins to dip and the sky above the sacred Ganges turns pink and orange to salute its departure, the Abbot steps forward once more.

"Maharaj, you were asked to explain your teaching and you have graciously and faultlessly instructed us in the glory of the Self, the mechanics of creation, the nature of *maya*, the cause of ignorance and suffering and the beatitude of one who sees clearly. For this we shall always be grateful. Can you, by way of a final summary, describe for us the essence of this Vedanta for one who knows it directly?"

The Master nods slowly.

"The essence of this Vedanta teaching is that everything without exception is *brahman*, the one Divine Consciousness. The visible, manifested realms of time, space and causation and the hidden un-manifested Absolute are the two complementary aspects of the one *brahman*. As everything is essentially that Divine Consciousness, humankind is naturally that also. We are born to live that, to radiate that, to enjoy that. We should live divine unity in the midst of diversity. This is the import of all the Vedic teachings and the ecstatic confession of our holy tradition of Vedic Masters. All glory to them".[93]

So saying, he bows his head.

Following this highly prestigious *sammelan*[94] a fresh wave of the master Vedantin's reputation spreads through the narrow lanes and crowded salons of the ancient city. Huge crowds now begin to assemble wherever he is teaching. Even those who had no previous interest in spiritual or philosophical matters, long since made cynical by the fact that so few teachers really live their message, begin to attend his discourses. 'The young sage from the South' as he is known, begins to galvanise the whole city. 'Here, at last, is one who really embodies the ancient Vedic teachings!' goes around the bazaars and *galis* and numbers attending the daily *pujas* in the temples rise, and donations to religious causes increase. Teaching with an effortless grace and ready humour, he is always gentle and patient with his opponents, simple in his expressions, but devastatingly to the point. His mind is as calm as silver, while his words are golden. Coming from the immense silence that is the fully enlightened mind, they are imbued with its power. The Master speaks the Truth because he lives it.

A binding separation

One evening not long after the debate at the monastery, a logician renowned for his debating skill comes for *darshan* at the ashram. A vain man, he is secretly hoping to outwit the Master and has chosen for his topic the question of identity. While he can accept that an embodied individual soul exists, the idea of a universal Self eludes him. The Master's position is that they are one and the same but that in our usual state we are unaware of this identity and fall prey instead to a limited sense of 'I-ness'. This mistake is known in Advaitin teaching as 'ignorance', which means not lack of learning but ignorance of our real nature.

The visitor begins his argument confidently:

"Sir you claim that there is only one non-dual Self and yet the sacred texts talk at great length about the embodied soul. They describe it as being smaller than a grain of barley or a grain of paddy or the tip of a goading stick and so on, and they counsel that if we want to realise this soul we should meditate on it at the heart."

"Yes, these recommendations are all just practical guides for meditation. It is indeed taught that the Supreme should be meditated on in the lotus of the heart, just as we are taught to worship Lord Vishnu in the symbol of a stone. Once the awareness is refined enough, it can certainly catch a glimpse of the omnipresence there, localised deep within. But actually, the Self is just like space: in itself it is universal and unbounded but it can still be located in the tiny eye of a needle. So for practical purposes, as long as the cosmic Self is overlaid by various conditioning factors – the individual body and mind, with its weight of personal and cultural images – we can certainly speak of it in an approximate way as the individual soul".

Scenting victory, the logician replies:

"Then Sir, if the two are one as you say, it follows that the universal Self must also suffer the effects of pleasure and pain that afflict the limited individual self. And furthermore, this being so, it then follows that there is in fact no supreme Self distinct from the reincarnating individual self!"

"Not so! Just because the Self is intimately connected with the hearts of all living beings does not mean it is the same as the embodied self, because they have quite different natures. This limited, embodied 'self' acts and enjoys, acquires merit and demerit and is affected by pleasure, pain and all the rest. The Self, on the other hand, is infinite consciousness, which enjoys freedom from all relativity, all action, all suffering. The *karma* of one does not touch the other. To conflate the two just because of their proximity would be like seeing an object in flames and concluding that the surrounding space in which the object is situated is also on fire."

"So the Supreme exists in the body then?"

"Indeed he does, but not in the body alone! The individual self is defined by the body, which is the seat of all its experiences and it does not exist anywhere else other than the body. Now while we cannot attribute all-pervasiveness to something that is spatially limited in this way, it does not mean that what is unlimited cannot also be found within limitations. After all, one who is the king of all the world cannot be denied to be the king of a particular city as well! Indeed, being simultaneously both here and there, inside and outside at the same time, is exactly what omnipresence means".

The visitor still looks unconvinced; patiently the Master continues:

"As I say, the Supreme is eternal and omnipresent, like space. Now, is the space within a pot or a jar essentially different from that space which is all around? No, these vessels are just limiting conditions temporarily imposed on what is, in itself, all-pervading. So before the individual is ripe to be instructed in the Upanishadic revelation that he is in fact cosmic, it is not incongruous to talk from the point of view of duality, which includes the apparent separation between the embodied soul and the universal Self. When the truth dawns, however, all those false imaginings just evaporate. At that point, even the duality of ignorance and enlightenment no longer has any ultimate meaning".[95]

Absolute, ego and Self

One afternoon the Master is sitting by himself on the ashram terrace that overlooks the garden, beyond which the great river lies quiet, glinting in the soft light. A visitor arrives. He is a tall, imposing figure in his middle years, very straight in his stance. His light skin betrays a northern origin. He seems a pious man, and soon shows himself to have a clear, thoughtful mind and great sensitivity to the folly and suffering of the world. He explains that he has spent most of his adult life on a search for truth, studying with various spiritual and philosophical groups in whatever spare time he has managed to find from the demands of his job and family. For many years he regularly attended the public *satsangs* at a local community of Buddhist monks, but has recently left, disillusioned with the hierarchical nature of the monastic organisation. Now, aware that time is passing ever more rapidly, he is wondering if any of the offered paths really lead to the truth he is seeking or whether the whole business of looking more deeply into life is in fact the waste of time that most people think it is.

"One invaluable thing I have learned from my lengthy study with the Buddhists is that the world is a process of interlinked causality. Each event is relative to everything else and none of these events is permanent. This universal impermanence seems to me the only undeniable truth, yet I hear you teach that there is a permanent Absolute underlying this ever-changing world. Much as I would like to, I just cannot accept the idea of permanence. So perhaps this subject can be the starting point of our discussion today?"

"Indeed" the Master nods. "So, you have learned that the relative world of our experience is ever-changing?"

"Yes, that much I am sure of".

"The world is always unstable, always changing and transient?"

"Yes".

"And you really believe that everything is always changing?"

"It is not a question of belief", replies the other sharply, beginning to feel irritated at the Master's repetition. Is this young man really the genius he has heard about or is this just another case of reputation exceeding reality? "It seems perfectly obvious to me, from my own observation".

"Now," continues the Master evenly, "let us look for a moment at this 'always'. This element of 'always' – the 'ever' in 'ever-changing' – what is it? Surely, 'always' is something that continues, persists. So this abstract context of continuity within which the process of change is always operating, in which phenomena are always coming and going – that persists, does it not? And because it always persists, it is unending, and what is unending, unchanging, that we can call absolute. So when you talk about the changing, you are describing a partial aspect of life, the changing, relative side, but there is another aspect behind the scenes, which is the unchanging absolute side."

"Well, I can see your logic, Sir, but I do not get the picture exactly".

"It is just like the waves and sea. Waves come and go one after the other, one after the other, but after one wave falls and before the next wave rises – what is left? It is not nothingness, not the vacuum of non-existence or non-being, it is just the flat, calm ocean, silently witnessing the rise and fall of each wave. Like that, change exists on the basis of non-change, the relative world rises and falls on the basis of the Absolute. Indeed, the very words 'relative' and 'absolute' are inseparably connected; as soon as we use the word 'relative' the sense of an 'absolute' is involved, because absolute means non-relative, and *vice-versa*. So in terms of both experience and logic the existence of the relative necessarily implies the existence of the Absolute."

"Yes...I think I take your point". He is hesitant.

"Now, the fact that life is ever-changing is not the end of life as such – change continues eternally. In fact, we could even define life as the continuity of change. So change, which is brought about by time, takes place on the basis of eternity; the relative is upheld, and validated, by the Absolute. The finite and the infinite are embedded in one another and together they make one life."

The visitor is not convinced.

"I cannot deny your lucid reasoning, Sir, but my quest has not just been a philosophical one. I am searching for enlightenment. The other fundamental point I have grasped from my Buddhist teachers is that the barrier to enlightenment is the ego. Destruction of the individual ego is the way to liberation. You must agree with this, at least?"

The Master nodded but said nothing.

"How do you define the ego, Sir?" the visitor continues.

"We can describe the ego as the sense of being a 'self' that is contracted around a limited or fixed centre that calls itself 'I'. This contraction is a moment-to-moment process of recoil from our natural state of openness. In fact, it is a mistake, an hallucination, but it has become habitual, so nobody questions it".

"And how does the ego operate?"

"By associating itself with the body and appropriating what the body experiences. From this appropriation follows a sense of agency and a sense of ownership; we say 'I do this', 'I feel that', 'I like this', 'This is mine' and so on. The ego is called *ahamkara*, the 'I-maker'".

"And it is the inflated ego that gives rise to the egocentric, selfish behaviour that is the cause of the world's suffering, is it not?"

"Well, such behaviour certainly contributes to the suffering of the world, but it is not the result of a large ego. Actually, it is the consequence of having a limited sense of self. Those who have to dominate, exploit, control and always be the centre of attention, such people do not have strong egos, they have weak ones. A restricted sense of self is always fearful of its own demise, it is always insecure and it is this chronic insecurity which leads a person to act in ways we call selfish or egocentric, disregarding the needs and rights of others and all the rest. A strong ego is confident, secure and generous; it has no need to behave egocentrically. So from this point of view, it can be said that the task of spiritual life is to build a strong ego".

The visitor is clearly shocked to hear something that so blatantly contradicts much of what he has learned hitherto.

"A strong ego...? " his voice tails off.

"Yes" continues the Master "an ego that is strong enough to die to its limited individuality and embrace its universality".

"So you are saying that the sense of 'I' still exists in enlightenment?"

"Why not? Expanded to all infinity. Have you not heard the Vedic text: 'Aham brahmasmi – I am the Totality?'[96] This is the essence of Vedanta, and there are many such proclamations throughout the scriptures that celebrate the triumphant state of enlightenment".[97]

Astonished now, the man sits silently for some moments. A silent presence seems to engulf the terrace where they are sitting.

He continues hesitantly:

"So enlightenment is only possible with the destruction of the normal ego-sense. Do you agree with that, at least?"

"I do, but let us look at that word 'destruction'. Who is it that will destroy the normal ego-sense?"

"You mean who is prepared to undertake such a difficult task?"

"No, I mean which part of the individual personality will split itself off from the rest to 'destroy the ego'? Surely it will just be the ego again, under another guise or another name? The ego is not a solid object, a separate thing that the mind can somehow grab hold of, conquer or kill. It is a mental process itself, a mode of perceiving, and no mind can bring an end to itself by an act of will. Indeed, the ego has no intention of bringing itself to an end, that is the very last thing it wants. Will a thief betray himself? Not if he can help it! The ego cannot bring an end to itself; it must be transcended without effort or self-centred struggle, then what is the essence of the little ego, its real nature, will have the space to shine forth spontaneously".

"And what is the essence of the little ego?"

"The absolute and infinite Consciousness, which is self-luminous, eternal, without qualities, non-dual, the witness of all. Unbounded, it is reflected in the limited human nervous system as what we call the individual ego. Ego-consciousness does not come from the ego-mind itself, it is a reflection of the pure consciousness of Self. The situation is similar to the brilliance and heat of the sun being perceived as reflected in water, when in fact those qualities do not belong to the water but to the sun".

"So are you now saying that the mind is not the source of consciousness? I don't follow, Sir".

"Well, we cannot say that the mind is self-luminous, because to say so infers that it is not a perceivable object. To be self-luminous means the mind is not illumined, and therefore not perceived, by another. But this is palpably not the case. On the contrary, we know that the whole activity of human beings arises from their awareness of the operations of their own mind. They are aware: 'I am angry', 'I am afraid', 'My desire is for that one', 'My anger is against that one' and so on.[98]

"So, just as the light of consciousness does not derive from the mind, in the same way the ego-sense stands in proximity to the Self as its limited reflection, which then becomes superimposed on its source. In normal experience the two become, as it were, mixed up together and this gives rise to idea of '*my* mind', '*my* body', '*my* senses', '*my* wife', '*my* possessions' and all the rest of it. In this way the unlimited Self gets overshadowed by the limited realm of the non-Self and this superimposition is what the Vedic texts call 'ignorance'. It is a universal condition and in this regard humans are really no better than animals".

Again, the visitor looks shocked; this young man is devastating in his clarity. Seeing his discomfort, the Master smiles sympathetically:

"Well, just look at your cow. If you make nice noises she will come towards you, if you shout at her she will back off. And if you advance towards her with a raised stick she will run away thinking 'Oh! he wants to hurt me!'. But if you hold out some sweet green grass she will happily come towards you. In the same way, if a gang of evil ugly people come at you with raised clubs you will turn and run, whereas you'll be naturally drawn to a person who is gentle and friendly. So, where is the difference? In both cases there is perception and behaviour based on a lack of discrimination between the body and the Self".

"Yes Maharaj, but those are rather particular examples..."

"Particular examples of a general fact" replies the Master. "As I say, this superimposition is universal. If you think 'I am healthy' or 'I am ill' you are superimposing the characteristics of the whole body on the Self, just as you are when you think 'I am thin', 'I am fat' or 'I'm staying', 'I'm going'. It also happens in the case of the senses, as when you say 'I'm deaf' 'I'm blind' or 'I'm dumb' and in the case of the organs if you say 'I have lost an eye' or 'I am a eunuch'".[99]

Both men smile at the last example.

"Similarly, mental attributes such as desire, will, doubt and so on are superimposed on the Self. All of this comes from the limited ego and its thinking 'I', 'me' and 'mine'".

There is a long pause. Sensing the approach of evening, flocks of kites begin to wheel overhead. Thin trails of smoke begin to rise from fires on the distant river bank.

"How, then, is the Self, Sir?"

"It is beyond hunger and thirst, without any distinctions or differences, beyond birth and death".

"Can you describe it further?"

"The Self cannot readily be described because words refer to objects or actions and the Self is neither. Words can be used approximately to indicate the Self but we should never forget that they cannot designate the Self in its real nature. It is like the saying: 'a torch burns' when what we actually mean is that the fire inside the torch burns, not the torch itself, which is only the inert vehicle for the burning flame".

"Yes, I can see the limits of description. Can we go back to the ego, then? Could you explain more about how the Self is reflected in the individual ego?"

"Well, let us imagine a face reflected in a mirror. Now, the reflection is not the face, because the reflection conforms to the qualities of the mirror. So if the mirror is dirty or cracked the reflection will suffer accordingly but the face itself remains quite unaffected. And likewise, the face is not the same as its reflection because it remains untouched by whatever qualities or distortions the mirror may possess. Like that, the Self is reflected in the ego as the face is reflected in the mirror, but the two are not the same thing at all. Nevertheless, they get muddled up together in common empirical experience".[100]

"Yes, I can see that".

The Master calls for water for his guest. Clearly enjoying how the discussion has dived deeply into the nature of reality, he continues, eyes sparkling with vitality:

"Now, let us take this a little further! What exactly is the nature of this reflection? What is its status? If we look closely, we see that the reflection belongs to neither the face nor to the mirror. If it did, it would continue to exist in one or other of them when they were separated, which is not the case. Now, it might be thought that because we refer to the reflection as 'the face in the mirror', the reflection belongs in some way to the face. But this also is incorrect. Why? Because on the one hand, as we have just agreed, the reflection is effected by the characteristics of the mirror, which would not be the case if it really belonged to the face. And, on the other hand, if the mirror and the face are somehow separated, say by a cloth put in between them, the reflection disappears altogether, even while the face still exists!

"So" continued the Master, "if it is agreed that the reflection cannot be said to belong to the face, it might further be argued that it in some way belongs to the face and the mirror jointly. But again, that is also incorrect. Why? Because if the two are both in the same room but they are not aligned, then again the reflection no longer exists".

The visitor nods his agreement; this young man's logic is as inescapable as it is relentless.

"Thus our reasoning brings us into accord with the teaching of the Veda: there is the Self, the ego and the individual nervous system, just as, in our analogy, there is the face, the reflection and the mirror. And mark well, the upshot of all this is that the reflection has no ultimate reality, in that it is temporary and wholly contingent".[101]

Smiling broadly, the Master signals the end of the discussion:

"But to reach final understanding about the Self, we do not only have to use our own reason. We also have recourse to the sublime teachings of the Upanishads which continuously point us beyond all misperceptions of duality. This is something those Buddhists you have studied with do not understand when they reject Vedic scripture. Either way, the end to the ego's false perceptions of 'I', 'me' and 'mine' can come only from the dawning of the Self, for this awakening will remove the very fuel that feeds the fire of ignorance. Such is the time-honoured teaching and we offer all glory to the holy tradition of Masters who have realised the Self, extracted this nectar of immortality from the ocean of wisdom and proclaimed it all mankind!"[102]

Absorption

The woman looks solid and healthy, full of vitality. She exudes an air of self-confidence as she walks into the *darshan* hall and takes her seat on the mat spread out on the ground in front of the Master's couch. She is accompanied by half a dozen others who, to judge by their demeanour towards her, are followers of some sort.

The woman begins by explaining that since the premature and unexpected death of her husband she has had the time and money to focus seriously on her spiritual growth. Having practised meditation for several years, she is now seeking out those teachers she feels could help her progress. One has emphasised the need of fire sacrifices to gain the support of the gods, so she has spent a great deal of money sponsoring *havans* and *yagyas*.[103] This teacher happens to know someone who is an accomplished Vaidya, so under his guidance she has embarked on a lengthy and complex series of Ayurvedic purification treatments and medicinal regimes, special diets and so on. Then the same teacher introduced her to another friend of his who, it just so happens, is an astrologer who has exclusive access to gemstones that are of such a purity that if they are worn on the body they will transform the wearer's life by deflecting malign planetary influences and encouraging benign ones. Gems were duly purchased and worn. Then it was strongly advised that building a new house according to the Vedic architectural principles known as *Vastuvidya* would be the last link to ensure her speedy evolution into enlightenment. All the arrangements were made and now the new house is almost ready.

All these remedies have cost a considerable amount of money, but the woman feels they have truly advanced her spiritually. As evidence of this she has begun to have powerful astral experiences – seeing visions and having powerful intuitions about her past lives – and she begins to relay some of these in detail to the assembled company. All the while she keeps one eye on the Master, clearly hoping for some acknowledgement from him. But he says nothing, just nods abstractedly every so often. To those who know the young sage well, it is clear that his attention is no longer fully on what the woman is saying.

And nowadays, she continues, she feels she is being permanently guided by higher beings who are ensuring that her life goes well. Indeed, it has come to seem that the outside world in some strange way exists precisely in order to fulfil her needs and desires, so easy is her way through life. The truth of the Bhagavad Gita's teaching that the world is really one's very own Self is becoming clear. Of course, there are occasional setbacks, mainly in the form of people who disagree with her or whose actions or desires run contrary to her own, but she sees these as being less evolved souls who do not have the level of consciousness needed to see the whole picture, as she herself does. In short, she has begun to realise that, due to all her intense efforts over the past few years, she has pretty well reached the goal of enlightenment. And so she has come to the Master to seek his confirmation.

Finally, the monologue is over. Somewhat breathless from so much talking, the woman sits back, waiting expectantly.

The Master sits serenely for several minutes without speaking, quietly radiating the plenitude he seems to carry wherever he is, no matter what the circumstance. Then, when he focusses on some ashram business that a couple of *brahmacharis* bring to his attention, it becomes evident he is not about to respond to the visitor immediately. Visibly annoyed, she suddenly rises and leaves the hall, followed by her bemused companions.

Later, the Master comments out of the blue and to no one in particular:

"Mark well, there is a world of difference between being self-absorbed and being absorbed in the Self".

Activity

The monsoon has been full and heavy this year and now it is over there is an abundance of bright flowers and foliage everywhere. Everything feels optimistic: the sky is clear and cloudless, the earth is refreshed and the air full of joyous bird song. At sunset the frogs take over, filling the still scented night with their croaking. Work is being done on some of the ashram buildings to repair damage done by the rains and this sparks a discussion among some of the older devotees about how as time passes they are wearying of the relentless demands of always having to be active just to maintain life.

"Indeed, but it is not only a question of age" responds the Master. "The whole world is ceaselessly driven to activity, even though life's essential constituent is by its very nature inactive. This goes beyond the bodily fatigue. It is because we have lost our own restful nature to the activity of the outside world that we are basically unhappy beings".

"How is that Master?"

He gestures to one of the workers in the compound.

"Well, it's like this carpenter fellow. I have been watching him and it is clear that as long as he is busy, axe in hand, working away for someone else, he is not effortlessly at ease and naturally happy. But each evening, when he returns home and hangs up his tools, able to relax at nobody else's beck and call and enjoy his own company, then no doubt he has some contentment. Like that, when the soul is overshadowed by the waking and dreaming states and the world of duality, it becomes as if a hired worker, fatigued by always having to be active for the body and the mind. And as a consequence it is not really happy. But once the individual soul has returned to its own home in the universal Self, which is always free from the demands of cause and effect, then it is as if a lamp has dispelled the darkness and it remains ever fresh, happy and luminous.

"So take note: just as in his true nature the carpenter is not an agent for someone else but only functions in that mode when he takes up his tools and goes out to work, so in its true nature the soul is not an agent for another, but only when it labours under the superimposition of the mind and body. And those two can be hard task masters, no doubt of that!"[104]

Being resides beyond the three states

The master Vedantin is discussing with his companions the different states of awareness and how they relate to the Self. Draped in a white shawl, he is in a radiant mood, vibrant and clear.

> "Now, let us consider your dreams. They do not stay with you after you wake up, do they? Nor do they persist when you pass into dreamless sleep. Like that, all the variations of the three states – waking, dreaming and sleeping – come and go continuously. But behind them the blissful Self never ceases to be and it remains ever untouched by their changes. So to think that the Self is a state of awareness, or that it is in some way characterised by variations, as are these three transient modes of the mind, is as much of a delusion as seeing a piece of rope lying on the path and imagining it to be a snake!"

With evident affection, he quotes 'a very great teacher in our tradition who realised the truth of the Upanishads', as if the man were sitting there next to him as a friend:

127

When the individual soul finally throws off the hypnotic delusion that has held it enthralled for endless time, it awakens to the One without a second, the unborn Reality that resides forever beyond both sleep and dream.[105]

Bliss

Devotee:

"What is the difference between normal worldly happiness and the bliss of the Self that the texts describe?"

Master:

"What we call worldly happiness arises as a result of the contact of a subject and an object and thus certain external conditions have to be there for it to blossom. When these conditions change, the happiness that depends on them withers and dies. The bliss of the Self is of a far different order. It does not depend on anything objective but is inherent and unchanging. It is an absolute, subjective principle found deep within one's own being. The earth is very beautiful, no doubt, but it should not be allowed to block out the light of the sun".

"How can those of us who have not had such an experience understand this?"

"Well, although worldly joys are as nothing by comparison, they can give us an indication of what the beatitude of this pure subject might be like. We can consider worldly joys as splintered fragments of the joy of the Absolute. When the Absolute creates the world, the supreme joy that is its own nature is manifested through creation in decreasing degrees, starting with Brahma the Creator, down through the hierarchy of all beings. Our scriptures describe the details of this hierarchy, each with its own degree of happiness".[106]

"And what accounts for the difference between these various degrees?"

"Their opacity; the different density of ignorance that each manifests".

"And what then is the cause of these different densities?"

"The degree of merit of past actions and present behaviour" comes the reply. Then with a chuckle, "After all, the words density and destiny are very close, aren't they?"

Another questioner continues:

"Can the bliss of the Absolute be directly experienced?"

"Most certainly, it can be experienced directly by one who is schooled in Vedic wisdom and free from desire, selfish activity and ignorance".

"And how is this accomplished, Sir?"

"The individual is made up of different levels, successive layers nested one within the other. By taking the awareness from the grossest level, the body, and moving inwards – through the layers of *prana*, mind and intellect – one eventually reaches the subtlest level of individuality, which is intense joy.[107] This joy is but a pointer to what lies beyond it: the bliss of the non-dual Self, dwelling deep in the cave of the heart. The Self is the root of that joy and it is the culmination of the increasing happiness experienced by the mind as it travels the path inwards from gross to subtle. It is the unchanging foundation of the entire world of change, the seen and unseen realms, all of which evolve from it. It is the Absolute. And those enlightened beings who know it do not know it as an object separate from themselves, but know it so intimately that they *become* it. Such ones do not derive their joy from external causes or through external organs; they do not make any effort to procure joy, indeed, they do not even desire it! And yet, they are spontaneously blissful, as if they were obtaining joy from all external means all the time. And why is this? Because they continuously enjoy the bliss of the Absolute through all outer circumstances. They have no want, no lack. When spiritual insight has abolished the false separation of subject and object, then the uncaused bliss of the Absolute, infinite and natural, is what remains, and everything without exception is bathed in its light".[108]

Boundaries and boundless

Two friends have come to the evening *darshan*. One is small and wiry with a bright, intelligent face that carries a rather mischievous expression, while his companion is large, plumpy and has an amiable demeanour. The smaller man begins:

"Sir, you teach that everything is a manifestation of the one universal Self and that the world is not different from this Self. But if this really were the case, there would be no distinction between things, no difference between subject and object. For example, my fine friend Devadatta here" – he indicates his companion – "is a great enjoyer of food. But if there is no difference between him and what he eats because they are both the one Self, then he would just merge into the dish and its contents. Now this might well be a very enjoyable experience for Devadatta but it belies all common sense!"

When the laughter has died down, the Master, still chuckling, begins his reply:

"It is all a question of surface and depth, substance and essence. Now, you have given us the excellent example of your gourmet friend Devadatta here, so let us take another example from your everyday experience. Imagine the sea. If we look at it we can distinguish the waves, the foam, the bubbles, the spray, and yet we see that these are all just different modifications of the same seawater. These various forms of the seawater cannot be said to be different from it and yet each one has its separate identity, its own boundaries. Now, just because they are all forms of the same seawater, does it follow that they are obliged to merge into one another? Not at all; they remain quite separate from each other even though they are all forms of the same essential material, all are still water. So it is with your example. Neither those who experience, nor the objects of their experience, are different from the one transcendental Self, yet this does not mean that they all have to merge into one another, does it?"

The questioner nods his agreement.

"So, once the Self has entered into its manifold effects it appears as the state of diversity, because these effects act as limiting superimpositions on its essential unity, the transcendental field of life. Again, look to the example of space. Space is omnipresent and invisible, as we know well, yet it appears to be divided when it comes into contact with the various solid objects of the world even while, in itself, remaining all the time unbroken and undivided. Like that, we see that it is perfectly possible for those who are enjoying experience to appear quite separate from the objects of their enjoyment, while both in fact remain one with the transcendental Self, which is forever their mutual cause and essence".[109]

Cause of all suffering

An intelligent and practical woman who works as an assistant to a local official asks:

"Maharaj-ji, why is that there is so much suffering in this world?"

The answer is startling.

"Suffering, however variegated it may be, has only one cause, and that is superimposition" comes the answer.

"And what is 'superimposition' Sir? I have no idea."

"'Superimposition' is the way we describe what takes place when our real nature, which is boundless and absolute consciousness, free and always happy, is overshadowed by anything that is less than what is boundless, absolute, free and always happy. When the Self is overshadowed by things which lie outside it, we forget our real nature and in that forgetting, suffering is born".

"Can you be more specific, Sir?"

"Well, for example, if a person thinks of herself as being fat or thin or fair, or as standing or walking or jumping around, then what are only attributes of the body are being superimposed on the Self. And if she thinks 'I am dumb or deaf or one-eyed or blind' then attributes belonging to the sense-organs are being superimposed on the Self. And if she thinks herself subject to desires, intentions, doubts and so on, then various attributes of the mind are being superimposed on the Self.

"In this way, assorted fluctuations of the individual self are superimposed on the unlimited consciousness that is the real Self. As a result, the Self, which is actually the unattached the witness of everything, appears to become mixed up with the individual mind, the senses, the body and so on. This is what is called 'superimposition' and it is endless. It is the primal ignorance and from it stem not only day-to-day misperceptions but metaphysical errors also. Thus what is called the individual soul falsely appears to be located in the body and as such seems to be the doer of action and the one who suffers its results. In truth, however, our soul is not limited and individual but unlimited and cosmic, because it is in essence one with the universal Self. In short, ignorance of who we really are is the cause of all suffering and it is maintained by what we call 'superimposition'".

The woman considers for a few moments. Then:

"This is certainly a radical analysis, Maharaj-ji. What is the way out?"

"The only way to free oneself from suffering is by attaining direct knowledge of the absolute Self".

"And how can this be done?"

"By applying oneself sincerely to the teachings of Vedanta".[110]

Change

A middle-aged widow comes to the ashram one afternoon as part of a group. Acting as something of a spokesperson for her friends, she begins rather diffidently:

"I have always wanted to practice yoga, but when my children were young I felt I had no time. Now they are grown up and have their own families, the desire has become even stronger. But I have also come to realise that the children were just an excuse. If I had really been motivated I could have found the time. What was really holding me back was the fear that yoga is said to lead to non-attachment, which sounds terribly cold to me, so unemotional and devoid of feeling".

"You are not alone" smiles the Master "either in your avoidance of spiritual practice or your misunderstanding of its effects. You mentioned your children, why not let them be your teachers in this? Do you remember when they were small how they were attached to their toys and how upset they would get if one got broken or damaged?"

The woman smiles and nods.

"Then they progressed to their studies and learning about the wider world and the toys of yesterday were forgotten. And then later still, their school studies were left far behind and they became adults, working in the world, soon to have children of their own. At each stage, did they suffer from leaving behind what was of no more use to them? No. On the contrary, as they grew their horizons expanded, and they naturally progressed to greater responsibilities, greater understanding, greater fulfilment.

"Like that, as one grows spiritually, one naturally loses attachment to what is no longer useful or relevant to the new state. Imagine you have lived all your life in a hut and you have the chance to move into a palace. To begin with your new home may seem rather strange and unfamiliar and initially you might even miss the old place, but would you continue to cling to your hut and bemoan the loss of it? No. Such a change is not a loss but a gain, bringing more life, more understanding, more joy. So there is nothing to be afraid of in all this, it is the natural process of change that comes with growth".

Character of the Master

It was always hard to pin a description onto the Master, for he did not present a fixed persona of a predictable consistency or partiality; what was constant in him lay beyond the limits of personality. Certainly, he was relaxed and confident in all circumstances, but on every occasion he seemed to speak and act according to the needs of the moment. It was as if the individual that people perceived was in some curious way a reflection of the general need or desire at that time. Not infrequently, people would find that his discourses answered their unspoken questions, sometimes even using images or phrases that they had silently formulated in their minds. In this way, his words formed a compassionate manifestation of appropriate possibility rather than the opinion of a solidly defined character in the normal social sense. Given this, he could be highly unpredictable and, for those closest to such a mercurial intelligence, this vitality was both a constant delight and a continuing challenge. His presence was like a transforming fire: while those too far away could feel left out in the cold, those too close could get burned.

Concepts and models

An expert in legal matters asks:

"You seem to explain the workings of the world by the mechanical law of cause and effect. I come from a religious family and was brought up to see everything that happens as being ordained by God. I cannot reconcile these two positions".

"Each is correct from its own perspective; there is no inherent contradiction between them. In its attempts to understand life, the human mind will exercise itself this way and that to form all sorts of concepts and they will in turn reflect the mind that made them. Some of these concepts will seem compatible, others may not. But it should be remembered that life is a mysterious and wholly Divine process, ultimately inexplicable. If the mind's models appear to contradict each other, then their incongruence and the resultant confusion, demonstrate nothing but the limits of human thinking. People who have not even seen the lotus feet of God exhaust themselves by getting involved in interminable arguments about His face! But rest assured, the will of the Divine operates ever benignly through the actions of apparently separate individuals and events and is always wholly consistent, right and unimpeachable, however it may be judged by a limited human consciousness".

"If I understand you correctly, you are in effect saying that what drives the world is God's grace. If that is so, what must we do to gain it?"

"We do not need to do anything to gain God's grace; it is already with us. The grace of God is already permeating every fibre of our being and the being of the entire universe, at this very moment. We only have to open ourselves to it. Divine grace is omnipresent as the transcendental Self of everything. And, being beyond time and space, it is eternally present everywhere. There has never been an instant when it is not, nor will there ever be".

"So you are saying then that we have no need to practice spiritual disciplines like morality and meditation to unfold the Self?"

"Not at all. Practice there must be, without doubt, but in the context of the understanding that nothing you can do from your side will actually have an effect on the Self. Spiritual practice destroys the ignorance and darkness that obscure the Self, but it cannot throw any light on it. Practice is like the wind that does nothing to the sun but acts to clear away the overshadowing clouds. Then the sun, which is always there independent of both clouds and wind, stands simply revealed. The Self is light itself, ever radiant in its own self-effulgence. Our task is to remove the obscuration".

Company of saints

Everyone who comes into contact with the Master becomes aware of the extraordinary transforming effect the proximity of a realised being can have. Almost all who meet him feel their *karma* has been quickened in some way and that their life will never be quite the same again.

One day someone asks him to comment on the phenomenon of a saint's *darshan.*

"Look to the mongoose and the snake" comes the reply. "They are eternal enemies, though they often live side by side. Whenever they meet they will fight to the death but each is strong and clever and so their enmity is a lengthy affair. Sooner or later, however, the mongoose will get bitten and then he leaves the fight and hurries to the nearest hillside where a particular herb grows that contains an antidote to the snake's poison. Once the herb has had its effect, he feels strong again to return to the contest, until he gets bitten once more. Again he leaves the fight to seek out the herb, again returns and so it goes on. But little by little the snake loses its power; its poison runs out and eventually it succumbs to the mongoose's tenacious attacks.

"Like that, a person living enmeshed in the world will sooner or later begin to feel miserable. Then, like the mongoose and the herb, he goes to seek out the restorative balm of a saint's company. Some time spent there in the peaceful and pure atmosphere heals and strengthens him and, feeling better, he returns to his normal life. But again, after some time, the poison of attachment to the world enervates him once more and back he goes to his teacher. Purified again he returns to his usual activities and so the pattern continues. But little by little, just as with the snake, the world's poisonous grip begins to loosen and the seeker comes less and less under its thrall. Eventually it loses all power to trap him and he remains free and blissful even in the midst of the world and its demands".

There is a rich, extended silence; only the crows can be heard.

Then, the Master adds firmly:

"Make no mistake, some time spent in the company of one who is liberated is indispensable on the spiritual path".

135

Creation

A master logician from one of the academies in the city arrives to debate with the young sage. He has with him with a number of his best pupils. He addresses the Master in a rather pompous tone:

"Honoured Sir, you teach that the transcendental Self, in its capacity as the supreme Lord, is the intelligent cause of the world. But surely any act of creation presupposes a motive? We know from ordinary experience that man, who is an intelligent being, begins to act only after due thought. He does not engage even in an unimportant undertaking unless it serves some purpose for him and this is particularly so if the activity is an important one. Now, the creation of this world, with all its huge variety, is certainly an important affair! So because all action serves some purpose, then the Lord must have had a purpose when he created the universe. And if he did have a purpose that served to activate him, this presupposes an inherent want and this want necessarily undermines his self-sufficiency, which is an attribute the scriptures are always emphasising. If, on the other hand, the Lord really has no motive or purpose, as you seem to claim, then it follows that he cannot act at all. Therefore, he cannot have created the universe. Either way, the accepted religious traditions are shown to be in error".

Warming to his task, he continues without waiting for reply:

"On the other hand, even if we allow that the Lord really did create this world without any motive then his action must be similar to an otherwise intelligent person who falls into a mindless frenzy and acts without a motive, irrationally as it were. But if this were so, then the Lord cannot be called omniscient as the scriptures claim; he is just like any other being, fallible and imperfect. No, I'm sorry, I have to say that altogether there are just too many contradictions here to take these authorities seriously".

He finishes with a flourish:

"Thus I submit that the only logical conclusion is that the doctrine of the creation proceeding from an intelligent supreme Self is untenable".

The Master smiles; he has been enjoying the intricacy of the man's arguments and is amused by the display he is putting on for his students.

"Well said, Sir, well said! But actually, it is not so. As to action presupposing a lack or need, let us consider, as a counter example, those princes in their pleasure palaces down in the old city – as we all know, they do nothing but enjoy themselves! The same is true even for their ministers or other men of high position who have achieved everything and have no unfulfilled desires left. They too act without any extraneous purpose or want but just for the fun of it. Life is an unending sport for them, and why not?"

Then, sensing the other's objection that grandees or royalty could be considered to constitute special cases with little relevance to normal people, he continues:

"Or, let us look nearer to home. Consider how your own body breathes. The process of inhalation and exhalation goes on continuously without reference to any extraneous purpose, the body is merely following the law of its own nature. Like that, the activity of the Lord is without desire, it is the effortless and spontaneous expression of His nature, without any purpose beyond itself.[111] So our reasoning does not find fault with scripture as we can find no purpose discernible in the activity of the Lord. Similarly, it cannot be said that He does not act, for scripture clearly affirms the fact of the creation. Nor can it be said that He acts like a senseless person as you say, because scripture also teaches that the Lord is all-knowing".

"So then, you base your argument on the infallibility of scripture?"

"Well, unless and until reasoning shows scripture to be false, what better basis could there be?"

After a silence, the Master adds carefully:

"And anyway, we should not forget that the many teachings about creation and its nature to be found in the Vedas and the Upanishads do not deal with the highest Reality itself. They only refer to the impermanent world of appearances, which is characterised by names and forms and all the trappings of ignorance. Nevertheless, the ultimate aim of these scriptures is always and only to point towards the Lord, which is the silent Self that wholly transcends the material world and its limitations".[112]

Curious incident

News is coming in daily from the far reaches of the Land of the Veda concerning fierce invading tribes from beyond the Western mountains. They are the followers of some new Prophet and, set to convert the world, are destroying temples, laying the countryside to waste and converting by the sword. Meat-eaters and unshaven, they have mastery of the horse and seem well-nigh invincible. Many take them to be the manifestation of Kalki, the last incarnation of Lord Vishnu, who rides a white horse, wields a flaming sword and heralds the end of the world.

A middle-aged woman pushes herself forward in the *darshan* meeting, prostrates herself and begs the Master to intercede for her son, who is in the army and has been reported missing in the latest bout of fighting. The Master continues talking to those around him and ignores her. The woman begins to shout and sob in near-hysterics. Saying nothing, the Master brushes her aside with a single gesture and, still crying, she is led from the hall.

Death and dying

It is the evening of the first day of Pitri Paksha, the autumnal festival marking those days when the spirits of the departed ancestors come nearest to earth and should be honoured by offerings of food in the rite known as *shraddha*. All along the *ghats* lanterns are being lit and hoisted up on long bamboo poles, to guide the spirits down to earth to receive their due. As the sun dips low, these little lights start to glow in the darkening water, while along the river bank *brahmins* and cows, symbolic representatives of the departed, are being fed. Objects becomes touched with gold in the fading light and high above the lanterns the first stars begin to twinkle overhead.

On the balcony of one of the grand riverside houses overlooking the *ghats*, the Master is sitting with some disciples and followers. It has been a day replete with questions and answers, a *satsang* punctuated by Vedic recitation, devotional chanting and prolonged, vibrant silences. Now, without speaking, the group watches the peaceful yet purposeful scene below, the enactment of time-honoured rituals designed to nourish and strengthen that ever-precarious continuity between the visible and invisible worlds.

At some point the elderly aristocratic woman who is acting as hostess to the group asks softly:

"Master, what actually happens at the time of death?"

"Death?"

The young sage seems to be returning from a long way away to answer her question. After a pause he continues:

"You want to know about death? What we call death is just the departure of the subtle body from its gross material shell".

"And what then is this subtle body?"

"The conglomerate we designate as an individual. The five senses, the five faculties of action, the mind, the ego, the intellect, the life-breath *prana* – all these components taken together constitute what is called the subtle body. It is a structure composed of a subtler energy than the grossly physical body, very, very fine matter, imperceptible to the normal vision. We can call it a second nervous system, an aerial nervous system if you like, that exists within and around the physical body. When negotiating the material world, this subtle body functions through its gross companion; the faculty of sight works through the eyes, the faculty of hearing operates through the ears and so on. So the combination of these two structures working together form the machinery of normal material experience. Then at the time of death the subtle body just withdraws from the physical shell, that's all. Now, here is your question: how does it go?"

A look of great compassion comes over the Master's face, made all the more remarkable by his youthfulness.

"Look to the example of the beehive. You have all seen that when the bees leave the hive, it is the queen that flies out first. She takes the lead and then all the other bees follow her and the hive is left behind, a dry and empty shell. Like that, the queen bee is the *prana*, the life energy in the individual body and when the *prana* comes out it is followed by the subtle body. And where does this bundle of awareness go? It goes to a field that corresponds to the last desire at the time of death, where it will be most easily fulfilled. That is why it is taught that the last desire in life is so important and one should think only of God at that time. Whatever that desire may be, good or bad, doesn't change the process, it is this last desire that promotes the *prana* to come out, but it is the quality of this impulse that gives a direction, a momentum, to the departing subtle body".[113]

Someone asks:

"Master, you are talking of the subtle body but we have heard that it is the soul that survives death".

"You can call it soul if you like, individual soul, no harm in that" comes the serene reply, "but strictly speaking it is the mind in the form of the subtle body. See, just as the tiny seed of the *banyan* contains the totality of the mighty tree, so does the mind contain the totality of the life it has lived, all life's experiences are concentrated there. And wherever the last desire points, that is the direction the individual takes and he goes to wherever that desire can be most easily fulfilled. This is the passage of rebirth: another womb, another body, another family, another life – it goes like that, time after time. In whatever circumstances one is born, one is born there because that environment is most conducive to the realisation of the last desire".

"And what is so important about the last desire Master? Why just the last?" asks the woman again.

"The mind has been created bit by bit throughout the course of the life that is just ending. What it has thought, what desires it has entertained, how it has reacted – all these create a certain quality of mind. The actual circumstance of birth in the next life is due to the last desire in this, and then whether we are born blind or deaf, rich or poor, lucky or unfortunate, whatever it may be – all those details are the result of the total influence of our *karmas*".

Smiling, the Master added:

"Now, do not imagine that by just thinking a good thought at the time of death, all will be fine!"

Everyone laughs and the serious atmosphere is relieved a little. Then:

"To die well is not a child's play" he continues. "At that time the mind will unravel very quickly, quite beyond our control and whatever is stored there will just come out, just as a flower's scent spontaneously emerges as its petals unfurl. When the body ceases to function, it happens gradually, step by step from the gross to the finer layers, but at the very end, when awareness is quitting the gross physical vehicle, the whole process is quite beyond our control. Therefore, the last impulse or desire is not a conscious decision made under our volition, no, it is the spontaneous expression of the overall quality of that particular mind.

"And as the *prana* is leaving the body, it takes some time for the heart to fail and the brain to die, and as this collapse is happening it is the faintest memory traces that go first. So when the brain begins to fail, one starts losing memory and as the physical machinery continues to fail the shallowest lines of memory laid down in the mind are the first to unravel and dissipate, fade away. And the last memory to fade will be that line which is laid down deepest in the mind-stuff, the essential impression that gives the mind its overall quality."[114]

"Now, this whole process could be very rapid when viewed from the normal crude understanding of time, perhaps in one second the whole range of memories from shallow to deep could be erased, the process could be almost instantaneous. You have heard how it is said that at the time of death the whole life passes before one's eyes?"

There is a general nodding.

"So it is; in one instant maybe a thousand layers of memory could unravel. But however long it may take, or may appear to take, the deepest groove of memory laid down in the mind will be that desire of which we have had maximum experience and indulgence in our life. That will be the impression most deeply etched in the mind-stuff, the deepest *samskara* and last to unravel, and it is this that will form the last desire at the time of death. So you see, the process that occurs at our death is just the appropriate and inevitable fruition of how we have lived".

Smiling gently like a father with his children at bedtime, the young man continues:

"You remember the story of when King Karna the World-Conqueror died in the Mahabharata war? His soul went to heaven, and when he arrived he was offered gold and jewels as food. However, he needed real food to eat of course, and so he asked Indra, the lord of heaven, why he was being served all this inedible stuff instead. Indra replied that as he had generously donated gold throughout his life, but had never donated food to his ancestors at the time of *shraddha*, now he was being given gold himself. Karna pleaded with the lord that he had never donated anything to his ancestors because he had been unaware of them, and had not been properly educated in such matters, and so he was permitted to return to earth for fifteen days so that he could perform the *shraddha* rite correctly and donate food and water in their memory. This is the origin of the Pitru Paksha festival we are observing during these autumn days, but the inner meaning of the story refers to just those habits of the mind I was explaining".

A long pause follows, as if to allow the import of the teaching to settle and sink in.

The Master continues:

"This is why it is so important to engage in spiritual practice while still alive in this body and not postpone doing so to some indefinite future. The more one practises, the more the bliss of the Self flows into the mind and that bliss is so refined, so glorious that it naturally creates a deep impression of calmness and peace that has greater force than the impressions of happiness gained from outer things in worldly life.[115] The charm of this experience just surpasses all others gained when the attention is extraverted. So that memory of spiritual bliss, that devotional mood will naturally become the last desire at the time of death and as such it will inevitably take the soul to a field where he will find increasing happiness".

The next question follows naturally:

"Master, are there heavens and hells as the scriptures tell us?"

"There are" is the reply.

"And where are they?"

"All around you!" laughs the Master, before continuing, "See, whatever you experience is the creation of your mind and this is true both before and after the death of the body. Indeed, whatever deeply entrenched illusions which may possess us up to the moment of physical death will persist as our experience after death too, such is their power. Now, we know from the scriptures about the many divine realms in which it is possible for our attention to operate, and we know also that there are other realms, degraded, less than human, demonic even. Some of these realms are states in the subtle planes of this world, some are forms of worlds other than this present one, So there are many, many locations with which the mind can become associated. But whether in this body or in some discarnate state after the physical vehicle has failed, whatever we may experience is always the appropriate result of how we have thought and how we have lived".

"Are there also intermediate realms that the subtle body can go to?"

"As I have just said, there are. After all, each realm could be called intermediate in relation to those in its proximity. Some of these planes are very chaotic and they will be appropriate to those who could not take a direction while departing. Accidental deaths, sudden or violent deaths, suicide – all these may lead to such a confused experience.

"You see, it is as if you are in a house that catches fire and the roof is falling in, everything collapsing all around you. Naturally, you run out and if you see a friend, fine, you naturally go in that direction for some help, some support. But if you leave very quickly and in confusion, without having made any arrangements, you will be bewildered which way to go and may run this way and that, disoriented. Like that, it is their lack of clear direction that makes souls hover around in the atmosphere, unsure of what has happened, where they are or what their present status is.

"Now, there is no need to be alarmed! It is because of all this business that our scriptures have described the correct way to handle one's own passing[116] and the right way to deal with a dying or a recently dead person. It is all clearly set down in the Vedas – what to do at what time, what rituals to perform, and so on. And this is why we read the scriptures to the dying person, to help the subtle body depart in a benign direction. You remember at the end of the Gita when Krishna counsels Arjuna to abandon all duties, all rituals, and surrender totally to Him? This is the most benign direction to take at the time of death – surrender to the Lord alone, total surrender to that one undying radiance.[117]

"Is there any other specific help available at that time?" asks another.

"Yes, there are also words only the dying man should hear, something from outside that creates a certain feeling, a suggestion, which could help and elevate a departing soul. History records some dying souls receiving liberation by hearing just one word at this time and we know that here in Kashi, Shiva himself can come to whisper this ultimate truth to the one who is leaving. This is a very delicate point: where can one find help when everything is falling off and nothing can stop it? You remember the proverb: 'Even a straw floating on the surface is a big help for a drowning man'? In the same way, when the memory is failing, when everything is dropping off, one faint word may be picked up by the attention, even in the midst of its distraction and that one word can help. But such words are only for those who are going, who are in that truly helpless state, they will not be suitable for one who is still attached to the body. Indeed, they may only confuse such a one. But when all attachment is falling off and when that body which has been held so dear for so long comes to the point at which it must be cast off, then, in that desperate state, there are some words that can help. But this must not be talked about in the ordinary state of embodied life and this is why these words are not common knowledge. It is better that way".

A long silence follows. The distant sound of music drifts up from the riverbank below. A servant comes onto the balcony with some message for the hostess. She excuses herself and leaves the gathering.

Then another question:

"Maharaj-ji, we have heard that some already departed souls of friends and family members come to help the dying as they cross over".

"As the mind unwinds at the point of death, many experiences can occur, all of which are mental forms, the expressions of the tendencies which have structured that particular form of consciousness, held it in place as it were. But, fundamentally, no one can help anyone in this. No one can help, it is a matter of our own *karma* – that is what one is left with. So this is one inviolable law of life: an unfulfilled soul reincarnates time after time until it finds fulfilment; whereas for those that have found lasting fulfilment, their journey has come to an end. And that lasting fulfilment is what we call enlightenment".

"Master, if all this business is indeed the case for each and every one of us, why do we not remember our past lives? You would imagine such memories to be common, but they are not".

"Well, to do so would require a clear continuity of awareness, and most people do not even enjoy such continuity as they pass from waking to sleeping or back again to waking! Think about it. Each night you lose that thread of continuity as you fall asleep, and then you regain your sense of being an individual self on waking up. Isn't it so?"

Rueful smiles lighten the atmosphere once more. As the Master expounds these deep truths, a powerful charge seemed to pulse through the assembled company, like the ebb and flow of some mighty, silent tide.

"Certainly," he goes on, "if the mind is strong and clear, it may well be possible for there to be some sense of continuity that yields memories of past lives. But even in such a rare case, is that really so important? Isn't there more than enough going on in your mind already to do with this life, without all the additional clutter of remembering your former ones? But the main point here is that the sum total of everything manageable that happened to you in your previous lives is operating right here in this one – this is the *karma* of your present circumstance. So if you really wish to know about your previous lives, look very closely at the one you have now. The important thing is to get on with this life as best you can, not to spend precious time wondering about all those former existences. And anyway, each of them was less evolved than the present birth; that is all you really need to know. Rest assured, everything is being taken care of, just as it should be".

"Master, why is it that people are so afraid of death?"

"Just this attachment to the body is the cause. All beings suffer this attachment and so are prey to fear, both in life and death. Even the lowest species, even the newly born worm suffers it! And among humans, it is not only the ignorant who fear death. For them, such a fear is logical enough because they identify with the body and so think they are wholly destructible, but we also see that even the wise can fear death. How could this be so? In their case, it is because they have all faced death so many times in the past and they retain that instinctual memory. And from this memory comes also the instinctive lust for life, for continuance, that is everywhere observable. This is why it is said that birth and death are without beginning.[118]

"So we see that loss of the body means loss of the separate sense of individuality and this could cause the typical person great fear. Identification with the earthbound body will trap the soul, fasten it to its material covering, and this deep sense of attachment, the feeling of possessiveness towards it, is such an intense influence that it makes it harder for the subtle body to leave when the time comes. It has no wish to be driven out of familiar and cherished surroundings through which it has enjoyed so much during life, but it has no choice, because the physical perch simply cannot survive any longer, it is worn out. It is as when you are building a house, you can make one to last for twenty years or fifty years or a hundred years. Whatever it may be, the builder uses materials according to the desired life of the house and that's it, finish".

Another long pause ensues before the Master continues.

"But what is death anyway? It is a process of change, radical to be sure, but actually not so unfamiliar. The body is continuously changing throughout life, so, if at death it changes completely, what new is happening? Nothing new is happening, because what we call death is just another change – albeit an extreme one – and change is a process that has been going on moment to moment, all through our life anyway".

Just then the hostess quietly reappears and the Master takes this as the signal to bring the discussion to an end.

"So, do not forget that all of this talk of reincarnation and states of after-death experience and so on is provisional, for it is only spiritual dullness that allows you to limit yourself by thinking you are identical to the body. In truth, you are neither the gross body nor the subtle body, nor are you any of the conventional attributes and obligations that bind these limited vehicles.[119] You are the Self, that pure spirit which dwells within all bodies, eternal and invulnerable. It has never been born and has never died, because it is quite separate from the impermanent material world. If this is too abstract to grasp, for the sake of understanding we could say that the Self casts off worn out bodies and assumes new ones just as easily as you change your worn-out clothes and put on fresh ones.[120] So, let us all take this evening as an opportunity to renew our commitment to real spiritual practice without any further delay!"

The hostess signals the servants to bring food and drink for her guests, while the moon rises silently over the still, black water below.

Desire, action and liberation

While the Master vigorously promotes the life of his monastic order, he is also greatly in demand as a teacher of householders. As such he tirelessly points out that the *shastras* do not explicitly debar householders from enlightenment but only advocate a different path for them in accordance with their karmic tendencies. While the recluse advances through following the rapid path of renunciation and detachment commonly known as the 'Way of Knowledge', the householder pursues the slower path of worldly engagement, the 'Way of Action' which includes scrupulous observance of Vedic rites and working through whatever attachments he or she may have in order finally to transcend them. In this manner they will eventually qualify for Knowledge.[121]

For those active in the world the Master generally advocates practices that enliven devotion to the personal god in whatever form is suitable, together with a life of right action and service to others. This, over the course of time, will purify the mind and heart and thin out the stock of *karmas* that the individual has brought into this incarnation, resulting eventually in fitness for the realisation of the universal Self. Accordingly, he teaches householders that the problem is not desire itself but the direction in which it is employed. What follows is a typical discussion on this frequently misunderstood subject.

"Sir, we have been taught that the great ones are forever inactive and therefore renunciation of action is the only path to freedom".

"Then you have been taught incorrectly! We cannot muddle up the way of the householder and the way of the monk or the recluse, they are different paths suited to different types of people. To begin with, we cannot completely renounce action even if we wanted to, for the body is always active and needs activity to maintain itself, even if we are sitting doing nothing. So merely refraining from action gets us nowhere, it leads only to dullness and hypocrisy. In fact, performing right actions is itself a means to freedom from action, because it purifies the actor. This is what is called Karma Yoga and it is taught as such in all our great texts – the Vedas, the Upanishads and the Gita.

Moreover, the inactivity of the saint is a subjective, inner state, not an outer condition. Even the Self-realised ones, who have nothing to gain personally from action because they have transcended egotistic desire and are free of the sense of individual agency, even such great beings may very well be active, because their activity benefits humanity and helps prevent others from going astray".[122]

"So are we not to relinquish all desire then?"

"Human life proceeds through the dynamism of desire and the average person cannot give up desire just like that, even if they are aware that desire inevitably brings suffering. To do so would be a strain and unnatural for him and go against his karmic tendencies that have been accrued in many lifetimes. There is also the question of his *dharma* – the social role he has been born to play in this present life. So both the individual and society would suffer if everyone just struggled to give up desire in the vain hope that by doing so they would somehow enter the desireless state. No, desire itself is not the problem; what we have to look to is the direction of desire and the attachment associated with it.

"The typical desires of a householder are directed to various aspects of his daily life: his wife and children, friends and relatives, the accumulation of money, reputation, fame and so on. These are the points of attachment for a normal man and they work to bind him to the world of the senses, with all its joys, its limitations and shortcomings. So, in order to set such a man on the spiritual path we must add yet another type of attachment – the attachment to the personal form of God. Through steady devotion to his chosen deity through meditation and worship, the man will eventually be led to the experience of the impersonal and formless Absolute of which that deity is but a personal form.

"So the householder should not treat desire as an enemy but continue in his life of action, steadily practicing devotion to his deity. Little by little his attachment to the deity will increase until its importance will naturally begin to outshine his attachment to the other things that previously claimed his attention. As he continues to practice, this divine attachment will go on increasing until the man comes to that point when he feels his god is always with him no matter what outer activity he is engaged in. In this way we can use desire to transcend desire, just as when a thorn is stuck in the flesh we can use another thorn to remove it. This is how a normal man can gradually be led to God without having to engage in a lifestyle that is not in accord with his level of evolution. For one who is unsuited to it, the attempt to pursue the renounced life can only bring strain and will not further his spiritual advancement. Indeed, to do so is a great danger because it risks wasting a precious human birth".

Devotion

Many of the common people who come before the Master are pious believers, devoted to one of the various forms of God. They come seeking guidance on how to further this devotion, which they generally understand to be an emotional affair, a cultivating of feeling. But the Master teaches otherwise, positing devotion as an appropriate means for the average seeker to attain right knowledge and thence ultimate spiritual insight.

An elderly widow, her face an eloquent testimony to a life of hardship, asks in a self-effacing way:

"Master, what is the role of devotion in the spiritual life?"

"Devotion? Devotion gives us the strength of mind to bear suffering. This fortitude is nurtured by other qualities such as earnestness and steadfastness which are conducive to purity of mind".

"This sounds a difficult path for normal people, Sir".

"Oh no, Mother, not at all! After all God is present in each one of us as our own Being, so devotion is something quite natural to us".

"Then how do we develop it?"

"Visit the temple, worship your chosen deity, keep good company and listen to the stories of the divine beings. Devotion will naturally flower and this will enable you to see the world more clearly and eventually to distinguish between what is real and what is not".

"And how do we know if devotion is maturing in us?"

"It is a very practical thing, Mother. The test of your devotion is how light each tribulation appears".

After a few moments of silence, someone else adds:

"I am confused by this, Sir. To my mind devotion is the direct relationship between the deity and ourselves, but you seem to be saying something else. How exactly would you define it?"

"Devotion is the tendency of the mind which goes one-pointedly towards the lotus feet of God. And from that journey one gets naturally merged in God. And why not? As we have just seen, we are already God; the task before us is just to realise this identity as a living experience. This is the glory of *sanatana dharma*. It shows us how to become what we really are. And what we really are now, we always have been and always will be".

Differences

A young woman is concerned with the problem of inequality and suffering everywhere observable in the world. She has a very direct manner and asks:

"How can you say that the world is created by some benign intelligence? Whoever the creator may be, if you study his creation with your eyes open, you surely have to come to the conclusion that he is guilty of being arbitrary, unfair and even sometimes malicious!"

Some of those present are uncomfortable at such a strong tone being used to address their spiritual teacher, but the Master himself is quite unfazed.

"How so?" he asks, with genuine interest.

'Well, look at the disparities in creation. Some beings, such as the gods, have a blissfully happy life; others, like most of the animals, have a pretty miserable existence, and we humans are stuck somewhere in between these two extremes. Any creator responsible for such discrepancies stands accused of bias, malice even, just as would any common person who promoted such an unequal state of affairs. Yet the scriptures constantly refer to the goodness of the Lord, his kindly nature and so on. What is more, the Creator is also responsible for horrendous destruction, so he must also be charged with being guilty of great cruelty and indulging in a quality that is abhorred by even the lowest among us. So all in all, I just cannot accept that some supreme Lord is the benign and well-disposed intelligence that brings the world into being and conducts its operation".

"Well," begins the Master, pleased by the woman's heartfelt concern, "if the Lord acted on his own account, without any extraneous means to produce this varied creation, he would indeed expose himself to the sort of criticisms you have voiced. But as the scriptures tell us, in creating the world even He is bound by certain laws. He has to work with the law of *karma*, taking into account the mechanics of action and reaction whereby any behaviour entails its necessary and appropriate consequence. So the unequal circumstances of life are in fact due to the accumulated merit and demerit of the living beings involved and they cannot be blamed on the Lord or attributed to some arbitrary whim on His part".

The woman looks unconvinced, but the Master continues in the same vein:

"So in this, the Lord's position is like that of the rain. Rain is the direct cause of the growth of rice, barley and all the other different plants, but in itself it is quite impartial and nourishes all equally. Now, there are enormous differences between the various species of plant but these are due to the various potentialities lying hidden in their respective seeds, and have nothing to do with the rain or the one who sends it. Like that, the Lord is the common cause of the creation of gods, men, animals and so on, as you have rightly said, but the differences between the quality of life enjoyed by these various classes of being are entirely due to the different levels of merit or demerit belonging to the individual souls in each class. All the scriptures are clear on this point. So, considering all this more closely, we are lead to the conclusion that the Lord cannot rightly be accused of bias, malice and all the rest as you claim".[123]

No answer.

Difficulties on the path

Many of the people who approach the Master are not learned philosophers, priests or *pandits* but ordinary householders, people who are simply trying to find some means of incorporating a spiritual dimension into their demanding and often difficult daily lives. A frequent observation of such people is that despite their best intentions, they seem to be making very little discernible progress on the spiritual path. This is a situation that often leads to disillusion or even, in some cases, to despair.

In response, the Master will frequently point out that even though everything without exception that we experience is the due result of some action we have performed in the past, we should never see ourselves just as hapless or passive victims of an unjustly difficult situation or circumstance. Moreover, the power of *karma* notwithstanding, we also always have the ability and the responsibility to make positive choices in the present. Such choices may not always be easy, but they are there for us to make if we really desire our circumstances to change. This fact applies as much in our spiritual as our material lives.

A woman is lamenting the fact that despite going regularly to the temple, praying at home and visiting *mahatmas* whenever she can, she still seems no nearer to having her desired vision of God. The years are going by, and all her spiritual efforts seem to have been in vain.

"You know", begins the Master gently, "there were once two ants, one of whom lived on a heap of salt and the other on a heap of sugar. They would meet from time to time in the fields, chat about how their lives were going on, and little by little they became friends. One day the ant that lived on the salt, who was a little lonely, invited the other to come over and visit her the next day. The other happily accepted and the following day arrived at her friend's, who straightway took her to the freshest part of the salt heap and offered her a meal. Being used to sugar, the visiting ant could hardly stomach the taste of salt, but to avoid giving offence she gamely ate a few small mouthfuls before making her excuses and leaving. As she was going she begged her new friend to come over to her sugar heap the next day. 'I can promise you, you will love it, and once you have tasted the lovely sweetness of sugar you will never want anything else. Come and stay a few days, see how you like things at my place, and if you want, we can then arrange for you to move over permanently'.

"Despite her timid nature, the salt-eating ant agreed. But that night she lay awake worrying. She was used to her surroundings, she was happy with her salt and what was her friend's place going to be like? She might not like this stuff called sugar at all and, if so, what was she to eat all the time she was over there? The next morning, she decided what to do. If she carried a good lot of salt in her mouth, then even if the sugar was not to her taste, at least she wouldn't have to go hungry; she would have her familiar food with her and could last out the visit without giving her friend offence.

"And so she duly arrived at the sugar heap. Delighted to see her, the hostess immediately took her new friend to the freshest part of the heap. 'Here,' she exclaimed 'just tuck into this and see what you have been missing!' The visiting ant began to eat, but of course all she could taste was the salt she had brought with her in her mouth. But, trusting her friend, she persevered and eventually worked through the salt and began to taste the sweetness of the sugar. Of course, she never went back to her salt heap!

"So" smiles the sage, "it is like that. All seekers bring with them the legacy of their past *karmas* when they set out on the spiritual path. They may be lucky enough to meet one who has experienced the fruits of that path, who can tell them of the joy that awaits them but, even so, depending on the strength of its *vasanas*[124] the mind will cling onto its old habits out of fear of losing the familiar. In that case, what is needed is great patience, great perseverance and a determination to continue no matter what obstacles may come up. All is being worked out just as it should be; we only have to continue and not concern ourselves unduly with the eventual outcome. Do your duty to the best of your ability, remain even-minded no matter what the results seem to be, and all will come out well in the end, there is no doubt of that".[125]

Discrimination

Question:
"How does one develop discrimination?"
Answer:
"Good actions, good company and an ever-alert mind".

Dreams

The master Vedantin is in a sublimely abstracted mood today; it is clear that his every glance penetrates deep beyond the surface of whatever is around him, rendering his world transparent to its source. A *sadhu* from the eastern hills who practises shamanism arrives at the ashram for an audience. He sets great store by the interpretation of dreams and is interested to know the Master's opinion on the importance of dreams and dreaming.

"None!" is the straightforward answer. "Dreams are a result of the waking state and actually come to much the same thing in the end".

"How so, Swamiji?"

"Everything seen in a dream is unreal and purely internal, seen within the limited body, so to speak. This is so even with things that appear to be vast, isn't it? We may cover huge spans of distance and time in dreams in a way that is quite impossible in reality. Or, you may have a long conversation with a friend or some other people in a dream, but you will be hard pushed to get them to confirm the discussion once you are back in the waking state! And then the moment we wake up, the dream personality with all its attributes vanishes. So dreams are insubstantial and highly subjective and in this regard they are of the same nature as most people's waking experience".

Many of those present are surprised to hear dreams dismissed so lightly, as it is well known that some people are visited by the gods in dreams, while dreaming gives others psychic communication or reveals glimpses of the future. And anyway, how can the waking state be so denied?

As if to answer this unspoken question, the Master concludes pensively:

"Actually, the whole world of change is much like a dream. All beings and all their doings, whether we consider them higher or lower or equal in the scale of things, they are like a dream projected by the magical play of the Self. Seen in the light of Truth, they are no more real than is a dream".[126]

Duty

There are many orthodox *pandits* in the city who are becoming disturbed by reports they have heard of the young teacher from the South who is teaching that Self-realisation is the most important goal of life. As the hereditary custodians of society's spiritual welfare, they feel that this teaching poses a threat to the performance of Vedic ritual and the observance of duty, upon which rest both the evolutionary journey of the individual and the stability of the community at large. In addition, they are also concerned that this charismatic new teacher, who had already managed to convert none other than Mandana Mishra, the foremost exponent of the Mimansa ritualistic system, might jeopardise their own positions of privilege in the city.

A number of these senior *pandits* have assembled together to form a committee dedicated to the preservation of cultural integrity. They request a formal meeting with the Master as they are determined to test the young teacher for themselves. Their spokesman – a large imposing figure – is revered both for his formidable knowledge and the political power he wields amongst the city's elite.

Despite the somewhat confrontational situation, it does not take long for the atmosphere of tension that the group has brought into the ashram to subside. Once they have seen the Master, noted his unfeigned attitude of respect towards them and sat in his presence for a few minutes they begin to realise that, whatever he might be, he is not merely an irresponsible iconoclast trying to make a name for himself. Nonetheless, their questions are forceful and direct.

The spokesman begins simply enough:

"Young sir, do you accept that the Vedas are the ultimate spiritual authority for mankind?"

"I do."

"Yet we gather you are teaching that the goal of life is to realise the Self and that therefore there is no real need to follow the age-old duties laid down by the Veda. How can this be?"

"The two are not incompatible, honoured Sir. Certainly the duties laid down by tradition and the texts are to be followed; all I am saying is that the ultimate aim of such duties is to prepare a man to realise the Absolute. Performing his duty refines and purifies a man and one whose heart and mind are thus cultured is well prepared to overcome the obstacles to realisation of the Self."

"Is this your own idea?"

"Not at all! Our sacred texts, such as the Upanishads, are very clear that duties act to prepare a man for Supreme Knowledge by dispelling the negative effect of his past actions. They also go on to say that it is only when he has achieved that state of freedom that ritual actions cease to have any further role to play".

At this the spokesman's eyes narrow:

"Are you saying then that there is no need for a teacher of Upanishadic knowledge to inculcate the necessity of performing duty?"

"I am not saying that, Sir. The teacher should have his pupil learn the relevant ritual texts by heart, because in such matters memory always precedes understanding. Then he should impart the appropriate spiritual instructions to the lad. And after that, it is expressly stated in the texts that the pupil should not return home without first being instructed in the practical householder duties enjoined upon him according to his particular stage in life".

"I see. What then are these duties a teacher should impart to his pupil?"

"All the necessary duties that will further his own evolution and the evolution of those around him. These include his private recitation of the Veda and the teaching of the Veda to others. Both these are daily duties and they serve to keep the wisdom lively in his mind and heart and serve to purify the environment. He should offer choice gifts to the teacher in return for the knowledge he receives and also seek permission in the taking of a wife to ensure that his family line continues. Above all, he should not be careless, either about truth or duty, for one who is careless about truth becomes involved in untruth, and duty must at all costs be done. At the same time, the teacher must instruct his pupil to take whatever action is necessary to safeguard his worldly interests and to secure his property and reputation. Duties to the gods and to the ancestors must not be overlooked; in addition, the mother, the father, the teacher and guests who visit the household – all these are to be looked upon as if they were deities".

Surprised by such a fluent answer, the spokesman pauses for some moments before continuing:

"What you say is unimpeachable, young man, but what about the actions of the spiritual teacher himself?"

"Well, as regards the behaviour of the teacher, where it is in conformity with the teachings of the Veda, the pupil should always seek to imitate him. But if the teacher acts in a way that is not in accordance with the Veda, he should never copy such behaviour. And those teachers who are *brahmins* or who exhibit the refined qualities associated with the *brahmin* caste and who are superior to ourselves in rank must be given seats and treated with great hospitality, have their wants attended to and be given gifts with reverence. Such people deserve to be treated with good grace and modesty and never in a perfunctory or insolent manner".[127]

In spite of themselves, the pundits are impressed by the young man's sophistication and the assured tone of his replies. After a few moments' silent thought, their spokesman continues on another line of questioning, and with a softer tone this time:

"You mention the *brahmins*, Swami, What have you to say on the other *varnas*, indeed, our ancient *chaturvarna* system as a whole?"[128]

"*Varna* is Nature's way to manage the variety, strengths and limitations inherent in human life. There is no being on earth, or even among the gods in heaven, come to that, who is not a mixture of different qualities.[129] From the point of view of the Absolute, such distinctions have no abiding reality, for in our deepest dimension we are all equally the one Self, but to uphold the process of evolution and to prevent the world of change succumbing to disorder, the acknowledgement of differences on the surface of life, and the consequent observance of ritual boundaries, is always necessary. Those without the guiding hand of *varna* are confined to living out a random, individualised destiny without centre or circumference. Such a life is alienated from the laws that regulate all existence and becomes dependent on its own casual whims and aberrations. A man's *varna* is an appropriate destiny because it is determined by the mixture of qualities he is born with and these in turn are determined by his deeds in past lives. As these karmic tendencies manifest they naturally dispose him towards his specific duties in this life".

The questioner likes what he is hearing.

"And what are these duties, young Sir?"

"Do you mean specifically?"

"Yes".

With the same effortless fluency, the Master continues:

"The natural duties of the *brahmins*, who are the men of intellect and knowledge, are inner and outer restraint, modesty, purity, forbearance and moral rectitude. In addition they should avoid violence, be good-hearted, speak pleasingly, recite the scriptures and have faith in the revealed spiritual teachings of our tradition".

"And the *kshatriyas?*"

"The natural duties of the *kshatriyas*, who are the men of government, are heroism, energy, strength, skill and the ability to deal with unforeseen emergencies. In addition, they should never turn their back on the enemy and they should be lordly yet open-handed towards their inferiors. Such generous behaviour befits their kingly nature".

"And what about those *vaishyas?*"

"They too conform to their nature, which is to take as real the materiality of things. Thus if he is born as a peasant, the *vaishya* should look after the land and take care of the cows, whereas if he comes from an artisan or merchant family, he should dedicate himself to riches, security and prosperity. He should also cultivate the various skills involved in making, buying and selling. And in the same vein of conforming to one's nature, the natural duty of the *shudra* is to render service".

"And what, in your view, is the reward for following these natural duties?"

"Those who conform to their *varna* will go to the appropriate heaven after death and enjoy the fruits of their merit. When those fruits are exhausted, they will be reborn in an appropriate family on earth to continue their spiritual evolution towards enlightenment. But those who perform all their necessary *varna* duties faithfully while holding to an awareness that doing so is a means of purifying themselves for this ultimate goal, they will thereby become fit for the path of devotion to spiritual knowledge. Performing their duties will be their way of worshipping the omnipresent Lord who ordained those duties, and by doing so they will become ripe for the final freedom".

The spokesman nods his approval; the young teacher's answers have been impeccable. Slowly and deliberately he frames his next question:

"And what then of the *sannyasi*, young man, how does he relate to duty and the other orders of society?"

"The *sannyasi* is one who has taken the responsible decision to step aside from the ordained hierarchy of human society and the duties incumbent on its members. Instead, he has joined an egalitarian group of wandering monks, whose sole aim is to realise the Self. As such he embodies an ideal that can inspire all classes and manifests a possibility that will be open to everyone when they are ripe for it. His constant journeying silently instructs the people in the inconstancy of the world and subtly works to detach them from it. Being solitary, he neither deserts, nor is deserted.[130]

"The *sannyasi* lives a life of purity and restraint, but until the sublime experience of the unity of all things in the Self has been realised, no one can avoid feelings of superiority towards some and inferiority towards others and this is another reason that all should obey the distinctions of *varna*. If a man who does not enjoy the unified vision feigns that perfection, and as a result tramples on *varna*, he lives without proper limits and becomes like an unripe fruit that has been forced to ripen artificially and contains no nourishment".

There is a long pause as the import of the Master's words sinks in. Then comes the final question:

"So, Swami-ji, what would you say are the practical implications of all this for the people at large?"

"As we have seen, *varna* is the natural law governing a man according to his born disposition. Therefore, everyone should perform their own born duty, even if it seems to be humble in comparison with others. To conform to your own nature, whatever it may be, is the surest way to evolve. This way one avoids harm, even as an insect that is naturally born in filth is not harmed by its surroundings. No one should imitate the duty of another, even if it appears more attractive than their own, for the simple fact is that whatever our duty may be, it will have some objectionable aspects to it, because imperfection is the nature of relative life. Until one has realised the Self, which is forever separate from the world of activity, there is no escaping the objectionable aspects inherent in all action. So the best thing is to perform one's own natural duty, faithfully and with perseverance, bearing in mind that our eventual destiny is to transcend such boundaries and differences altogether".[131]

Following this the *pandits* sit for some time respectfully while there is recitation of the Vedas. Refreshments are then served by some of the ashramites. After a suitable time, the visitors rise, make their obeisance to the young teacher and leave, their questions answered and their fears allayed.

Effort precedes grace

A continuing theme of discussion is whether effort or grace takes the seeker to God. One day the Master relates the following story to a group of visiting devotees:

"There was once a pot of fresh curds standing in a kitchen. It was the rainy season and there were many frogs around. A couple of them were hopping around and accidentally fell into the pot. The larger of the two just lost all hope, gave up immediately and sank to the bottom where he soon died. But the smaller frog was made of sterner stuff. He struggled and struggled for hours to get out. Despite his efforts, he could not lift himself high enough and, completely exhausted, he finally floated quietly on the surface, feeling half dead. But his actions had not been in vain. All his thrashing about had churned the curds, so that some butter formed on the surface. This gradually solidified into a lump near the rim, from which the frog was eventually able to hoist himself free.

"Just so, we cannot adopt a lazy attitude and expect that we will be saved – that is a fatal mistake. The struggle involved in undergoing *sadhana* is unavoidable. Nevertheless, it is not that you secure salvation by your own efforts alone, as if it were a mere worldly gain like any other. You should strive hard to find God and when you have done all you can and are completely exhausted and perhaps even hopeless, lying fully surrendered at His feet, only then will He be disposed to come and save you with His grace".

Enlightenment and rebirth

The Master is an inexhaustible fountain overflowing with wisdom and love for those practitioners of varying degrees of maturity that surround him. Frequently one of these followers will find his own need inexplicably fulfilled, whether he has voiced a question or not. And the questions that arise come not only from intellectual curiosity; some are the spontaneous and unexpected manifestation of a process of inner growth that may have been going on for a long time.

Question:

"As I understand it, ordinary people reincarnate, whereas there is no reincarnation for those who have realised the Self of all. Could you explain the mechanics of this?"

Answer:

"It is all a question of perspective. The concept of enlightenment, the opposite concept of bondage and the resultant necessity of numerous rebirths to purify and attenuate the conditions that give rise to this bondage – all these derive from, and depend on, the core concept of 'me', do they not? 'I' am the one who is enlightened, or bound, or destined to reincarnate or whatever. Look into your own life and you will see that this is always the case, isn't it? So, let us examine together this 'me' a little more closely. 'I' or 'me' consists of the idea of being an isolated individual self, a mind and a body that is separated from other people, other things and everything else in the universe which exists 'out there' somewhere. Does this accord with your experience?"

The questioner nods: "Yes, that is exactly my experience".

"Now, this idea of the individual self over and against the outside world disappears entirely when we go to sleep, only to reappear as soon as we re-awaken. This being the case, we can see that the individual self-idea is impermanent and being impermanent, it is ultimately no more real than are dreams, which also come and go. If it were absolutely real, it would persist through all the states of awareness, including deep sleep, would it not?[132]

"Yes, I suppose it would".

"Nevertheless, for all practical purposes, as long there is a subjective identification with the limited self-idea, it certainly remains real to the one who experiences it. And as long as it remains real, everything else pertaining to it – its ignorance, consequent suffering, purification through *sadhana*, rebirths, gradual progress on the spiritual path, eventual enlightenment and so on – all of these must necessarily follow. This is what people understand, this is their reality and so this is what they experience.

"But in truth, the identification with a limited self that is the root of this sequence is actually mere imagination. The thought: 'I am the doer' and 'I am the enjoyer' runs very deep and is very powerful, after all such an opinion has lasted for many births, is the cause of our continued rebirth and is continuously supported by our education and social structures. But in fact it is a type of hallucination that has no ultimate existence. It will seem to be real for however long it continues, just as a dream is real for as long as one is dreaming. But we know that a dream vanishes as soon as one wakes up and in the same way, when this habitual and automatic 'I' thought is sufficiently weakened by a prolonged and spontaneous dwelling in the Self, he who has erroneously identified with a limited, mortal self finally wakes up. He realises he is in fact one with a level of life that witnesses everything, while being itself beyond action and its effects, beyond the succession of events we label time and beyond the 'I' sense of limited individuality.[133]

"So for one who has realised his profound identity with the substratum of everything, how can there be rebirth? Who is there left to transmigrate? Once one has become the omnipresent Self of all, what is there to be reborn, and when and where would it go? As the Veda unambiguously states: he who has transcended desire and loosed the knots of the heart, such a one is not born again.[134] He has the continuous experience 'I am the infinite Absolute' and just as no fruit can grow where there is no seed, and no effect can be manifested when there is no cause, so there can be no more rebirth when there is no more delusion.[135]

"Standing unshakeable as the Self, it is as if the clouds have been removed from covering the sun. With the transcendence of the individual mind, all its concepts are also left behind: there is no bondage, no rebirth, no enlightenment even, because the limited and isolated self who was identified with the body and underwent all these changing conditions no longer exists. There is only the Real, the Absolute, and the realisation: That I am, and always have been and always will be."[136]

"If this is indeed the case, Sir, then what is the purpose of the whole rigmarole of the spiritual path?" comes the question.

"Now, we must be very careful here!" The Master assumes an almost conspiratorial air, as if inviting all those present to share in a great secret.

"What I have just described is the highest teaching, the confession of the enlightened. But for those who are still identified with the limited mortal and evolving structure we call the individual 'I', this sublime truth is just a concept, an abstract idea and, no matter how elevating it may be, it is in no way the reality of their day-to-day lives. So for such people there is indeed rebirth, and if they are seekers after enlightenment, they must indeed follow the prescribed strategies of purification. As we know well, these comprise offering sacrifice to the gods, refining the mind and senses, developing serenity and non-attachment, devotion to the teachings of the scriptures and all the rest of it.

"Mark well, if a normal man tries to appropriate the lived experience of the enlightened by merely adopting the idea that *sadhana* is unnecessary and rebirth does not really exist, such an attitude will never dispense with the necessity of *sadhana* nor end rebirth in his own case. How could it? He will then be on the level of the worst materialist, lazily adopting a concept he finds pleasing in order to avoid the trouble of doing any work on himself! This is certainly not the same as living the enlightened state. Spontaneously living the Self and ignorantly trying somehow to appropriate the experience of the enlightened are diametrically opposed. All sorts of confusion and nonsense will come from conflating them".

Follow the instructions

A young man who has recently been initiated into *mantra* meditation asks:

"Is it possible to reach unity consciousness through meditating on a *mantra* as one of the names of God?"

"It is".

"But surely there are other more direct paths that will get you to the goal quicker?"

"Were you instructed to practice *mantra* meditation or to debate its place in the scheme of things?"

No reply.

Free will or determinism?

An elderly man speaks up in the *darshan* hall. He explains he has reached the stage where he is able to review his life and looking back over the years, he can see that some of his decisions were foolish ones, with regrettable consequences.

"Some people say that everything is determined by destiny, while others claim we have free will. Which is the case Maharaj shri?"

The Master laughingly replies:

"Free will and destiny? Actually, there is no difference, both are the same thing!"

The man looks puzzled but politely remains silent.

"Both are the same thing", the Master goes on, "but viewed from different angles. What we call our destiny of today is the outcome of choices we made yesterday. This is how the law of *karma* works. And from the mountain of our past *karmas*, each person brings a sackful into this life. Technically, the mountain is called *sanchita karma* and the sackful *prarabdha karma*. Now, this *prarabdha* is fixed, it contains certain possibilities, the sum total of which cannot be changed. But what we do with those possibilities depends on our choices, on our free will, if you like. So it is not a fatalistic picture. See, there was once a man who had three sons and when he died he left them each an equal share of the inheritance. One son squandered his portion on a life of excess; the second lived a parsimonious life with little joy and the third used his share to amass a large fortune. Like that, each of us brings a sackful of possibilities into this life, but what we make of them depends on us, on our free will, our choices. Never should we passively feel that our life is an unchangeable destiny. We always have choice; we always have choice".

Freedom and responsibility

A local official announces himself to be a follower of a controversial *guru*. This teacher had formerly gained quite a reputation for his power and charisma; later it transpired that he had been sleeping with some of his female disciples and had also been involved in various underhand financial dealings. Challenged on this glaring discrepancy by someone in the hall, the disciple begins to defend his teacher:

"My guruji teaches that morality as normally understood is simply something imposed by others on you; it is not really religious. It is a form of domination, a form of slavery, because you yourself have not come to the understanding of what is right and wrong; you have been simply told by others and gone along with their opinion. And anyway, one way of behaving is considered to be moral in one society and the same thing is immoral in another society. Given this, how could a true *guru* be bound by any such variable standards? What is more, the scriptures clearly say that the realised ones are beyond the workings of *karma* and attachment to any particular form of action, good or bad and therefore you cannot judge their actions no matter what they may do".[137]

The man who has challenged him replies that, as he understands it, the scriptures give guidelines for action and even the enlightened should not flout them.

"Well, it depends which scriptures you are talking about", counters the official.

"Consider the *Ashtavakra Gita*. It says there:

> For the Yogi, who has attained his fulfilment and who is an embodiment of guileless sincerity, where is licentiousness, where is restraint?[138]

At this point the Master breaks in sharply:

"Texts like these are the confessions of the enlightened and they refer to their subjective experience of the limitless freedom that lies beyond all dualities. They are not prescriptions for the behaviour of the unenlightened. And whatever his inner experience may be, the enlightened man does not exist somehow apart from the outer world, for he continues to live and act among others. Indeed, thanks to his universally expanded sense of being, he is consciously at one with everything and so his thoughts and actions have even more influence on the environment than do those of other people. Therefore, his responsibility to behave well is all the greater. And such altruism is in fact his natural state, because all negative behaviour springs from the falsely imagined attachment to a limited sense of self and an isolated body. If a man has really transcended this attachment he simply will not entertain those selfish, fearful and egotistic preferences that would steer him towards actions confusing or hurtful to others. This being so, why would he not act in a way that is conducive to the general good? This is why the scriptures describe the liberated as being by nature beyond *karma* and free of personal desire. But the scriptures are also very clear that such a one should not confuse the unenlightened. On the contrary, his life should be an example, worthy of imitation by the people at large, who generally like to follow the example of the great. He should act with integrity in the world and not unsettle the minds of the ignorant by attempting to lessen their attachment to action or seduce them away from the norms that necessarily guide society. His lack of attachment is his own inner affair and it can never be copied by those who are not themselves free. Nor can it be used as a justification for behaviour that oversteps the necessary boundaries of civilised human society. To do so would only result in chaos, as scripture reminds us and as we can clearly see in this case".[139]

So saying, he waves away the official who initiated the discussion.

God needs humanity

A group is studying the passage in the Gita which says that the performers of Vedic fire rituals sustain the gods and are in turn sustained by them.[140]

"So it is a mutually beneficial arrangement?" asks one of the *brahmacharis.*

"Yes" replies the Master. "And not only the gods, even God himself needs us as much as we need Him!"

"How can that be?" comes the question.

"Our limited human consciousness is the localised reflection of the infinite intelligence we call God. The physical medium of reflection is the human nervous system, which acts like a pot of water that reflects the sun. Now, the sun's reflection will last only so long as the water is there in the pot. If the pot breaks, the water runs out and what remains is the sun with nothing left there to reflect its light. The reflection is lost due to the absence of the reflecting medium, the individual reflector. Like that, to be located and appreciated, the absolute Consciousness needs a reflector limited in time and space. For the unbounded to be enjoyed, there must be a medium, even though that medium is itself bound. This is the glory of human life and that is why it is such a uniquely precious gift. Take note: even the angelic beings envy humankind".

Greatness

It is Saraswati puja, the annual Spring festival dedicated to the Goddess of Creativity and Learning. Many great musicians are in town and each evening concerts, recitals and competitions take place at various places along the *ghats* and in the city as master vocalists and players paint the canvas of silence with their *ragas*. These events begin around eight in the evening and go on until well after sunrise. The stamina of both the players and audience is astonishing. There are also numerous dramatic performances, with scenes from the Mahabharata, the Ramayana and various Puranas holding the people spellbound with tales of antiquity that are as fresh as if they had been composed only yesterday.

One morning a group of performers comes up from the *ghats* to see the Master who is spending the festival in a Mother Goddess temple on the outskirts of town. They have been performing all night but are still energised, buoyed up by their recent exertions and the crowd's appreciation. Amongst them is a well-known local actor; he is the first to stand up in the hall. Good-looking, rich and successful, the man is the talk of the bazaars, where stories of his dramatic *tours de force*, romantic affairs and ambitious business deals keep the simple people amazed and fascinated. To them, he is a god come down to earth, indistinguishable from the roles he so majestically adopts. Recently though, after a serious illness, he has been spending more of his time visiting holy men and asking their opinions on a variety of topics. Like most actors he needs attention and is fond of the sound of his own voice. In sonorous tones he addresses the Master with a question about the importance of achieving greatness in life; as he does so it becomes clear that he considers himself to have done so. Many present are surprised by the personal nature of what follows.

"Don't think that acting on the stage is your only thing!" begins the Master animatedly.

"You have had a glittering career amusing hundreds of people, so you are considered great. But don't place your claim to greatness on these superficial values of public evaluation. To be really great, you don't have to put on a show, all you have to do is just be, but be substantially. BE what you really are; be your own reality.

"Anything else is just too superficial – you are giving too superficial a value to your life. Life is something much greater; it is that unbounded intelligence that upholds all the universes. And among all the beings to be found in those universes, mankind is unique. He alone is the master of his own destiny, he can arise above the changing winds of situation and circumstance, he doesn't need to be blown here and there like a child's kite. So transcend the glamour of the world and enter the glorious realm of the Self. Anything else, anything worldly, is just too superficial to base a life on. It's a waste of time, a waste of time".

"Are you saying that celebrity and fame have no value then?"

"They have a value and that value is to waste life!"

Stung by the Master's blunt words, the actor counters sharply:

"But my dear young Sir, you yourself have recently become very famous!"

"Perhaps, but that fame has nothing to do with me. Those who feel good from my teachings may well say: 'Oh yes, he is good, he is great' and so on. But I don't become good by their saying I am good, nor would I become bad by their saying I am so. Fame depends on public opinion and all this is just too superficial. Life is so grand, so enormously powerful and unbounded, that all these variable little breezes of fame blowing this way and that are just ridiculous in comparison. Ridiculous! Fame doesn't mean a thing. Life itself is what has substance, for life is divine intelligence, unbounded and invincible. Fame is just a little breeze here or there, it is really nothing".

After a pause he continues:

"The fact is, whatever we gain in the relative world, we won't be satisfied, because that gain will have its boundaries. Those boundaries must go, even the greatest gain in the relative must be exceeded to gain the Divine. And once we have that, there will be nowhere further to go. Only then will our individual life be fulfilled, in that boundlessness. Until that state is reached, there will always be a desire for more and more. Life will not be fulfilled so long as there is still some possibility of further achievement. Only when there is that continuous pristine awareness that is the Self, will we find real fulfilment. Then we will live it in every breath we breathe, and the purpose of all our desiring will be fulfilled. When individuality breathes cosmic existence, cosmic intelligence, cosmic life, then life is really being lived in its innate and glorious fullness. This is the true greatness; nothing less than this".

To his credit, the actor appears to take the words to heart. He is clearly affected by what has passed between himself and the young *sannyasi* and his face wears a sober expression as he leaves the ashram.

167

Happiness is our real nature

"Acharyaji, you say that happiness is our real nature. How can this be, given that there is so much unhappiness in the world?"

"Everybody has the desire to be happy, especially if they are not currently so. This constant desire for happiness is itself a proof of the eternally existing happiness of the Self. Otherwise, how could the desire for happiness arise?"

"I do not understand, Sir".

"Well, take the example of a headache. If a headache was natural to human beings, no one would make any effort to remove it. As it is, when you have a headache, you lie in a darkened room, put cooling sandal paste on the forehead, drink water fortified with special herbs and so on. Why do you do all these things? Because you remember your natural state of having no headache. Like that, you desire happiness because it is natural to you and, being natural, it is not something to be acquired anew".

"But we do all sorts of things to acquire happiness!"

"Actually, if you look closely you will see that these actions are only attempts to get rid of unhappiness. And unhappiness is the realm of the non-Self, the limited ego and its actions, obscuring the ever-present bliss that is your Self. This being so, the loss of unhappiness amounts to the gaining of happiness".

"Can you explain further?"

"Well, we eat in order to remove the discomfort of hunger. We enjoy the food and remain satisfied for a few hours but sooner or later hunger returns and the cycle starts up again. Trying to acquire happiness is like that, whether the happiness be thought to be located in food or drink or sex or power, whatever. Happiness mixed with unhappiness is in the end only unhappiness, just as pleasure which is followed by pain is really only pain. Those who are dull-minded only recognise normal life as painful when they are actually experiencing pain, but the clear-minded see that all the usual endeavours to achieve lasting happiness in the outside world are doomed to fail sooner or later, and therefore they can be classed as pain.

"This is the virtue of non-attachment. One who is truly unattached abides beyond desire, he has no thirst for things seen or heard about, even the realms of heaven or the discarnate pleasures enjoyed by the gods.[141] And why not? Because happiness is his native state. His mind is like a crystal that may register an object presented before it but remains wholly unstained by the object's colour. This is self-mastery, no longer under the thrall of the senses".[142]

This sober analysis is followed by a rich silence. Then someone speaks up:

"What is the way out?"

"The way out is to follow the guidance of all the great ones who have passed this way before. Go within and find the bliss that is your own nature. It is ever fresh, effortless and undecaying because it is your natural state".

How does the Self create the world?

During a particularly joyful discussion on the Self, the Master poses a rhetorical question to those gathered around him:

"Now, why is it that the Self creates? What on earth would make the Self, which is full, blissful and perfect want to create this miserable, insufficient world that is so limited and full of suffering? Well, it is not from any sense of need or to satisfy any purpose, you can rest assured of that! Truly, you know how a child laughs? That wonderful sound like water? It is a natural exuberance that just cannot be contained, it bubbles up spontaneously and overflows. Or imagine a happy man who gets up after a good night's sleep and hops and skips around his room just for the fun of it. Like that, the Lord creates the world as his blissful play, it is all his spontaneous sport, devoid of any need and untrammelled by any tedious purpose".[143]

"But how does this come about, Master?" asks a serious young man. "I mean, what are the mechanics?"

"Well," comes the response, "the limitless intelligence we call the Self has the intrinsic ability to create; its very nature is to manifest. And so, following its own nature, it gives birth to a graduated series of beings, a hierarchy of forms of varying degrees of intelligence, power and dignity and so on, while at the same time remaining itself and quite unattached to its creations".[144]

The questioner is not yet satisfied.

"I hear what you are saying, Sir, but if the Self is unified and seamless, there can be no division in it. How then can what you describe as its inherent tendency to create multiplicity manifest itself? And once it has manifested, how can this tendency support a whole hierarchy of beings of different quality?"

"In truth, it is a divine mystery!" laughs the Master. "But, applying human reasoning, one can say that the Self contains the figments of ignorance latent within it,and thus it holds the world of name and form in potential form, but as yet unexpressed. Now, this potential is not identical with the pure Self because it is not pristine and stainless, but at the same time we cannot say it is totally different from it. This potential, then, forms the seed of the entire expanse of the phenomenal world. Now, according to the point of view taken, this ensuing creation can be described as *maya,* the great conjuring trick, or *shakti*, the divine creative power of the Goddess or *prakriti*, the implicate nature of the omniscient Lord. These are all various names for the same creative process when viewed from different perspectives. But the Lord himself, the Self that is the controlling power behind it all, remains ever hidden, unmanifest and quite distinct from his manifestation, whatever name we chose to give it. We know from the holy texts that He is unborn, undivided and without parts, so there is no transformation going on here".

"Very well. But if the Self is omnipresent, this implies that it germinates the seed of potential you describe without recourse to any outside means. So how can this be?"

"Now, we see that even limited beings who possess great power – like the gods and some saints – can materialise various objects. They create palaces, chariots and the rest, just by applying the power of their intention. And even at the humblest level, look at how the spider spins its web from threads drawn from within itself or how the lotus wanders happily from one pond to another without any means of conveyance. So even in this world we are not unfamiliar with this principle of self-generation and if all these beings naturally possess such an ability, how much more must the Self of all beings possess it?"[145]

Impurity

A devotee asks:
  "What is the cause of the mind's impurity?"
  "Its individuality" comes the unswerving reply.

Individual soul and cosmic Self

An rather earnest young monk is confused by various texts that discuss the relationship of the individual soul to the cosmic Self.

"Master, different scriptures seem to have different teachings on this point. Some say the Self can be attained through meditation, which implies that the person meditating and the object of his meditation – the Self – are different entities, as are the ruler and the ruled, for example".

He quotes some passages from the Upanishads to illustrate the point.

"Yet on the other hand" he continues, "there are those texts that avow the two are one and there is no difference between them". Again he quotes well-known passages supporting this view.

"So my question is: how can these diametrically opposing viewpoints be reconciled?"

The Master nods, evidently pleased with the young man's scriptural knowledge.

"Indeed, you are quite correct in your opinion that these texts may at first appear to be saying contrary things" he begins. "But that is because they are approaching the same question but from different angles, different levels. It is all a question of essence and appearance.

"Now, if we are going to engage in this debate between difference and non-difference, we cannot just baldly state that absolute non-difference alone is the truth, because if that were the case then we two as separate beings couldn't even be having this conversation! So there must be a reason that the texts mention both difference and non-difference and, to understand this correctly, an example that may help us is that of the snake and its coils. Now, the snake is one and undivided, no doubt, yet it has many coils. Are the coils then different from the snake? Well, the answer is both 'yes' and 'no'. Being a temporary and limited appearance of the snake, the coils can be classified as being different from it, but essentially, of course, they are one and the same. So, just this same principle applies on a more abstract level. Take the example of light. Sunlight and its source, the sun, are both luminous, both are essentially the same effulgence. They are not identical, yet we certainly cannot say they are entirely different, though that is how they are perceived and what they are commonly thought to be. So it is in the case you have brought up".

The monk smiles and nods as if to express his satisfaction with the answer but the Master is enjoying playing with the subject and is not finished yet.

"Wait a moment! We can look at it another way. Just as light appears to be diversified in relation to the activity taking place in the objects it illuminates – a moving finger, a static pot, some water or whatever – so it may be said that the one Self appears to be different because it is under the sway of limiting superimpositions. But just as we know that light is always one and undivided, in the same way, no matter what its various adjuncts may be, the essential Self is always one. And this applies not only to the world of objects, the same thing is also true as regards the individual soul and the supreme Self. Do you see the point?"

Again the monk nods in agreement.

"Now, let us take this question of appearance and reality yet one step further! It is agreed by all the wise that the bondage of the human soul results from its metaphysical ignorance. Given this, it seems to follow that spiritual knowledge is needed to dispel this ignorance, doesn't it?"

More nods.

"However, if it is accepted that the bondage of the human soul is real and that it is a particular state of the Self in the same way that a coil is a particular state of the snake or light reflected off various objects is a particular aspect of its source, then since something that is real cannot be altered, all the scriptural teachings about liberation removing bondage would be rendered useless![146] Given this absurdity, it is actually *not* the case that the Upanishads teach that difference and non-difference – coils and snake – have equal status or are equally true. On the contrary, our sacred texts emphasise that non-difference alone is the correct view. When they speak in terms of 'difference' they only do so only to refer to what conventional human experience habitually recognises to be the case. In order to be comprehensible, they take the viewpoint of the conventional and unenlightened mind, so to say. But the answer to your query is that, if we are talking about reality, there is no ultimate or essential difference between the individual soul and the cosmic Self, just as in the aforementioned examples of the light of the sun and the coils of a snake. In truth, there is only the non-dual Self as Consciousness, omnipresent and always one without a second".[147]

Those assembled are delighted at the relentless lucidity of their teacher's analysis.

Karma and enlightenment

The lake is vast and tranquil in the afternoon light, its calm surface seems to stretch forever. Around the shore a number of trees lean gracefully over the water and on a branch of one of them sits a black and white kingfisher, its long sharp beak looking almost out of proportion with the neat little body. Suddenly, without any warning, the bird drops like a stone; a second later it rises from the water with a flurry of wings and splashing. The fish speared on its beak writhes this way and that, glinting opalescent in the sunshine. As the bird heads off rapidly with its prey, silent ripples spread in slow concentric circles across the whole surface of the lake, even to the furthest shore.

One subject that frequently arises is the relationship of the enlightened being to *karma*. The Master generally emphasises two related points in dealing with this question: firstly, that the experience of the world is different in different states of consciousness and secondly that one cannot apply the reality of one level of consciousness to another level.

A sincere woman who has spent all her adult life in the spiritual search speaks up:

"One thing has long puzzled me, Maharaj-ji. To those who study the lives of saints, it is clear that the great beings often have strange things happen to them. Despite their cosmic status, they seem no less immune to mundane disease or illness or misfortune than the rest of us and sometimes they even meet an untimely death. Can you shed some light on this? It seems paradoxical to me".

The Master comments:

"Just as a well-kindled fire reduces everything to ashes, so does the fire of spiritual wisdom burn up the sense of egotism that normally accompanies the performance of an action. But spiritual wisdom can only destroy those actions that have not yet begun to produce effects. This applies whether these *karmas* were performed in the current birth before the dawning of enlightenment or in any number of previous births. Those actions from the past that resulted in the birth of a particular body in this lifetime have obviously already begun to have their effects, and therefore they will only come to an end once those effects have been fully worked out".[148]

Chuckling, he adds:

"But in this business, be careful you do not confuse the saint with his body. Rest assured, the saints themselves do not suffer from such confusion!"

Seeing her bewildered expression, he continued:

"To understand the saint's relationship to his body, see how clay pots are made. The wheel is set turning and the potter holds the raw clay on the wheel, gradually forming it into a pleasing and useful shape. Then the details are added to perfect it, however long that might take. Finally, when the pot is finished, the potter lifts it off and sets it down beside the wheel. The thing is complete, no more work needs to be done on it. Nevertheless, the wheel keeps revolving until its accumulated momentum runs down, does it not? Like that, each of us is attached to the wheel of *karma* for as long as is necessary, that is, until we are fully formed, perfected so to say. Then, when the work is completed, the Lord lifts you free of *karma* and its effects. Now, the wheel of *prarabdha*[149] must keep on turning until it has run its course but it does not touch the enlightened being, who stands aside quite unaffected, just like the pot standing beside the wheel.

"In this way, whatever appears to happen to the perfected one does not really touch him at all, for he has realised himself to be the universal Self and no longer identifies with the individual mind or body. He is established beyond all their ups and downs, comings and goings. His body roams through the world of sensations as free as a wild animal in the forest, while he himself dwells always in peace and silence, looking on, liberated from both doubt and desire".

"So from what you are saying the one who has realised the Self is not even touched by his own death?"

"Correct! How could he be? Death is an event that occurs to the body, it does not touch the ever-blissful Self. The enlightened one has already discarded his body, he is no more attached to it than a snake is attached to its sloughed-off skin! Impelled by the momentum of its past acts, his body is carried here and there automatically by the life force, like a log in a river is carried this way and that by the current. He himself is indifferent; unattached to the body he is like the still axis of the spinning potter's wheel, and when he loses that body, or mind, or life-breath, it is like a tree losing a leaf or a flower or a fruit. What does it matter to the tree if its leaf falls into a quiet stream or a running river, or lands on a common crossroads trod by one and all or on some holy ground, fenced off and consecrated for rites to Lord Shiva? Like the tree full of sap, the Self stands unaffected, replete with its own bounty".[150]

"So where does such a one go at death?"

"He is already omnipresent as the Self, so where is there for him to go? When his individual journey is done, he vanishes. Like a bird in the sky or a fish in water, he leaves no trace behind; only his name remains. Reincarnation from life to life is impelled by *karma*; the sage is liberated from *karma* and is thus immune to its effects, both during life and after what the world calls death".[151]

Laughter

Everywhere the Master goes there is a spontaneous atmosphere of celebration and joy. Such happiness is highly infectious and naturally draws all sorts of people to him, even those who might not normally have had anything in common. His wholehearted enjoyment of life evidently brings him enormous delight; sometimes his whole body will shake with merriment for minutes on end.

Question:

"Master, what is laughter?"

Answer:

"Absence of desire".

Learning is not wisdom

She is an uneducated woman who sells flowers outside the temple, and she has done so for many years as it is the tradition in her family. Over this time she has been able closely to observe the life that unfolds each day around the sacred shrine: the ebb and flow of pilgrims, the behaviour of the priests and dignitaries, the intrigues and rivalries, the hopes and dramas. Not many of those visiting the temple take much notice of her as she has long since become a part of the scenery, but few things escape her steady gaze.

"Master, how is it that some learned *pandits* who are very accomplished in their knowledge of the scriptures are still subject to the sense of 'me and mine' and seem to be as attached to their status and position just as much as any worldly person?"

"You are right in your observation, Mother. If a *pandit* displays such attachment, then all that his learning amounts to is a confusion between his little body and the unlimited Self. He who experiences the real Self as the unchanging consciousness beyond and within the world will not be attached to anything at all, whether that be pleasure, the sense of 'me' and 'mine', his own actions or whatever else. He will see all such limitations to be just the inevitable fluctuations of the world-process and nothing to do with himself".

"So you are saying that the wise and the ignorant see the world quite differently?"

"Yes, that is exactly how it is. The ignorant are attached to their own action and covet its results, whereas those who experience the unchanging Self remain free of any such attachment. Such wise beings are fundamentally different from the normal run of humanity because they do not think of themselves as 'this body' sitting here on a seat or standing here on the ground or living over there in a house. Therefore when we say of such a sage that 'he is acting' or 'he is resting', we are only speaking figuratively by referring to his body. In himself, such a being never acts because he no longer identifies with the body that goes here and there and does this and that. How is this? Because he has realised once and for all that he is the unmoving Self which is ever beyond activity. No matter what his body and mind may be doing at any one time, in his real Self he neither acts nor causes others to act.[152]

"This is what Vedanta calls Supreme Knowledge and it is not just book-learning, which to be honest, does nothing of itself to transform the way a man behaves. It is a different state of consciousness in which the transcendental Reality is directly perceived and for those who live this state, there can be no danger of intellectual knowledge masquerading as spiritual authority. As to the others ..."

The Master shrugs expressively.

"I understand what you are saying young Sir, but it all seems rather abstract to me".

"Well, you are quite correct, it is the most abstract field of life we are talking about! But, to get a more concrete idea of it, look to your own experience. When you are collecting flowers for the market each morning, you go out into the growing field and select your blooms for that day's sale, do you not? Now, are you the field or the one who knows it? Are you the roses and thorns and leaves and mud or the one who stands apart and experiences all of them?"

"I am the one who experiences it all".

"Quite so. Like that, your real Self is free of anything that may be superimposed upon it, whether it be something gross such as a body, or something subtle, like a mind with all its thoughts, opinions and the rest. The Self is the Knower and is separate from what it knows. Just as these flowers and earth are the objects of your perception each morning, so the whole universe from Lord Brahma down to a clump of earth is an object perceived by the divine consciousness that is the Self. And just as you are not affected by whether the flowers you see are open or closed or the earth is smooth or rough, so the Self is not touched by whatever qualities may be superimposed upon it, any more than the desert can be made muddy by the water perceived in a mirage.

"Any perception which muddles the Knower and the field together is just ignorance of the true situation. It is as if from a distance, you mistake a tree stump for a man. This misperception does not magically transfer the qualities of the man onto the stump, because the initial identification is itself an error, so nothing further can be inferred from it. Like that, the property of being conscious, which belongs to the divine Self, does not automatically become transferred to the body just because the two are mixed up in common misunderstanding".

"I think I understand Maharaj. But to return to our starting point, what role do those *pandits* and all their scriptures play in this?"

"The scriptures are useful for those who are ignorant of the real Self, but for those who know and live the Truth, they have no further use. Scriptural injunctions and prohibitions serve to purify the mind and behaviour and in this they have our wholehearted support, but they no longer have relevance to the one who experiences himself as forever beyond the realm of cause and effect".

"Isn't this dangerous? If people see the wise no longer needing the scriptures, won't they just abandon them themselves?"

The Master shakes his head forcibly.

"No, not least because those who know the Reality are so rare and the ignorant are so numerous! And anyway, the ignorant are unable to emulate the disinterest of the wise because they are bound to their actions by the desire to attain some result. The wise are quite different: having no such desire they are naturally unattached, both to their action and to its outcome.

"As to the *pandits*, some may indeed hold that the Self-realisation advocated by the texts applies only to the learned like themselves. Not understanding that each and every one of us is equally the Self, such *pandits* miss the truth and so will those who follow them. Only the meanest amongst the learned would twist the texts like this and in so doing they murder the Self and confound others with their own ignorance. These people are not part of the holy tradition that holds the key to the inner meaning of the scriptures, and they misinterpret the time-honoured message of texts like the Upanishads while dreaming up doctrines that have not been taught or sanctioned by tradition. No matter how well versed in the scriptures they may be, such teachers should be ignored as foolish men who spread only folly".[153]

Life too is a guru

It is a fine evening and the Master is receiving visitors on the flat roof of one of the ashram buildings. Some weather-beaten workers from the countryside have come in a large, ramshackle party. Hereditary worshippers of Vishnu, they are in Kashi on pilgrimage, wide-eyed at the big city and overawed by their chance to sit in front of such an acknowledged holy man. One plucks up courage and rather timorously asks the Master about the role of the *guru* in spiritual development.

"Could you have reached this roof without going up the stairs? Like that, the *guru* is always necessary. There are a very few who have no need of a *guru*. Trishanku was one such who did his best, but for most a *guru* is needed. Whether that *guru* takes a bodily form or operates on the inner level without the need of physical contact, *guru* there must be".

The symbolism of Trishanku is not lost on the group, who know the Ramayana story well.[154]

"But do not forget that life itself can be your *guru*, in that you can learn from anything and everything if you just use your eyes and look around you. Our scriptures tell us this. They remind us that the earth endures; it exhibits patience, acceptance, forgiveness, and it humbly supports others with no expectation of gratitude. This you can learn from the earth.

"Water is naturally pure and sweet, it has the subtlest of tastes. Just so should your conduct manifest purity and sweetness. This you can learn from water.

"The wind's nature is to move everywhere, over plants, flowers and deserts, palaces and prisons, without becoming attached to any of them. It is devoid of preference or dislike; this freedom you can learn from the wind.

"The sun is all brilliance and intelligence and gives its light with endless generosity. It absorbs water from the earth but returns it as nourishing rain. So ought you to absorb everything that comes, but transmute it and give it back in a better form. This you can learn from the sun.

"The moon is perfect, ever full in spite of its apparent waxing and waning, which come and go as appearances but do not actually exist in it. Just so, your real Self is ever full, despite the seeming ups and downs of life. This you can learn from the moon.

"And then there is space, which contains innumerable clouds, planets, stars, dust storms, but it is ever untouched by them. Just so does the Self pervade the innumerable bodies of men and animals, saints and sinners, kings, madmen and paupers, yet remains unchanged by any of them. This you can learn from space.

"And the ocean refuses no river yet it remains ever within its limits. No matter what activity there may be on its surface, it remains unshakeable and silent at its depths. Just so the mind of the realised one remains ever undisturbed, no matter what thoughts or feelings may enter into it. And this you can learn from the ocean.

"So my friends, do not feel when you are back in your village that you are far from your *guru*. Life is your *guru*, and as life is ever with you, so her teachings are all around you".[155]

Limitation and release

Question:

"Master, you often speak of our sense of limitation being the cause of suffering. Can you kindly expand on this?"

Answer:

"Expansion is precisely what is needed!"

After the laughter has died down:

"Limitation consists in the habitual and compulsive attachment of the mind and senses to their objects. This gives rise to a hankering for experience that lacks subtlety and correct proportion, causing the heart to forget the intrinsic delight of the unlimited Self, which is limitless Consciousness free of the imposition of objects. But communion with this fundamental reality is entirely natural to the human soul and very necessary for it, and, to the extent that it is overlooked or denied, there will inevitably be suffering for both the individual and society at large".

"Thank you, Maharaj".

Listen to the mahout

There is a popular story from the Master's time in Kashi that illustrates the folly of trying to impose the inner spiritual unity on the incorrigible surface variety of the material world. This event occurred at a place called Shultankeshwara, some miles south of the city. Here, at a bend of the river sits an ancient temple that is believed to mark the spot where Lord Shiva stuck his trident in the ground to make the course of the mighty river turn back north towards his home in the mighty Himalayas. Near the temple was an ancient forest, in which animals roamed freely, including a large herd of elephants.

One bright spring morning the Master was giving a discourse at the temple. His topic was the omnipresence of *brahman*, the one supreme Consciousness. Amongst the audience was a particularly impressionable young *brahmachari*. The lad was quite overwhelmed by the Master's teaching that everything is a form of the formless God. At the end of the session he prostrated in front of his teacher and, as if intoxicated by what he had just heard, wandered dreamily out into the road.

"Oh how wonderful!" he marvelled. "The trees are God, the road is God, the fields are God, and I myself am God!" He was so absorbed in his elevated thoughts that he failed to notice a magnificent elephant ridden by his *mahout* approaching down the road. When, at the last moment he did, his mood of bliss did not allow him to worry. "No matter!" he laughed as the mighty beast bore down on him, "I am God, the elephant is God; God cannot injure God, let the elephant come!"

But it was the mating season and the great beast, unpredictable and excited in his *masth*, suddenly speeded up and knocked the young man flying. Hearing the commotion, the Master came out of the temple compound to find the boy picking himself up from the ditch, much the worse for wear. "What happened?" he asked. Dusting himself down, the *brahmachari* turned angrily on his teacher.

"But Sir, you told me that everything was God – the trees, the flowers, the animals, even I myself – then how could this have happened?" he spluttered.

"Oh yes" replied the Master smiling, "everything is indeed God – the trees, the flowers, you yourself, the elephant – all are God. But the *mahout* who was shouting at you to get out of the way, he too is God!"

Luck

You can see immediately he is dejected. He holds his body like a defeated man: shoulders slumped, gaze cast downwards. As he tells his story, you can feel the sadness. He married young, very much in love, against the wishes of his parents who felt the girl was unworthy of their son. His wife died giving birth to their third child. An orphan himself by now, he was left to bring the little ones up as well as earn his meager living. Then two of the children died tragically in a boating accident. And now his health is failing and the prognosis is not good.

"All around me I see people enjoying good luck and some of them clearly don't really deserve it. They are not honest or good people, yet everything they do seems to be successful. I have done my best but nothing seems to have worked out. I guess my question is 'How can I become lucky?'"

181

The young teacher's tone is very gentle.

"Actually, what makes one person enjoy better luck than another is the good that he has done in the past. His character in this life may well not appear deserving of good rewards but fortune is on his side because in fact he has done good to others in the past. That good comes back to him in the present and now he is lucky. So what you are calling 'luck' is really the workings of *karma*. Everything that happens to us, good or bad without exception, is the appropriate result of actions we ourselves have performed in the past. Therefore, if you want to be lucky in the future, the trick is to do good to others now. Be compassionate and loving, be kind, be generous and whenever you can, do service to others – this is the way to enjoy what you call luck. It's an old story, nothing new here, the law of *karma*". The demeanor of the man shows little change.

Many problems, one solution

It has been a terrible year. The rains did not come at their usual time in early June, and as the weeks went on, the land became drier and drier. First the fields blistered and cracked, then the wells sank into putrid puddles and the rivers began to run dry, exposing beds that soon opened into gaping fissures. Topsoil turned to powdery dust that was whipped up by the hot wind into vicious, stinging clouds that penetrated everywhere, covering the houses outside and in with a gritty, cloying film. In the hottest places, birds dropped out of the desiccated trees and lay dying on the ground, soft plumage aghast.

Whole villages began to empty and move in search of water. Priority was given to the young and fit, but babies soon died, and when the men were too weak to carry the old and infirm, many were left to die also. The situation was direst for those in remote areas, far from rivers or lakes. They had to move to find water, but many did not have enough of it to make such a long journey. It seemed as if half the country was on the move, shuffling and staggering here and there in desperate groups, half-blinded by dust, thirst and exhaustion.

Then, one evening in early October, the monsoon finally breaks. As the rain lashes down in fury, rivers steadily rise, fill and flood.

The land coughs and chokes, sobbing under the sudden weight of water, but gradually begins to breathe once more. Slowly and painfully, like a patient after a long debilitating illness, life starts to pick itself up again. But terrible damage has been done and the recovery will take a long, weary time.

A group of farmers has come to Kashi on pilgrimage to the temple of Annapurna Devi, 'She who is Full of Food'. Rumour has spread that the drought and suffering were due to the Goddess' displeasure with the persistent folly of humankind, so they have come to seek her blessings on behalf of their village. The headman is there and several of the village elders. Some of the youngest members of the community have also been brought along, as it is thought that their innocence will please the Goddess and perhaps act as an insurance against her anger at some future time. After spending time at the great temple and giving all they could afford to the priests who did the necessary rituals, the group arrives at the ashram to pay their respects to the Master before they return home.

The headman pays his respects to the Master and then his wife begins to describe the horrors they have all faced during the past few months. The young *sannyasi* listens with great sympathy, nodding every so often. By the end of her tale she is in tears.

"Oh Master, how are we to cope with all these problems?"

The Master enquires as to the exact details of their circumstances and makes some practical suggestions. He instructs a couple of the ashramites to fetch supplies – rice, dried fruits, lentils – from the kitchen storehouse. While they are doing this, he addresses the group in a tone of great compassion:

"Yes, there is indeed much suffering in life, many problems. But actually, there are not many problems, for all the problems in life are in truth the various aspects of one root problem. And because there is only this one problem, there is, in the end, only one solution".

"And what is this root problem?" interjects the woman, her tone suddenly hard with suspicion.

"The erroneous superimposition of the body on the Self is the seed of all problems.[156] And therefore the solution is to gain true understanding of who and what you really are. Knowing the real Self is the end to all suffering".

Her voice full of agitation now, the woman continues:

"Young Sir, how on earth can knowing the Self prevent the drought from coming, or stop my children dying in front of me?"

Again very gently, the Master replies:

"I did not say that knowing the Self would stop these things happening. Drought can always come, children can always die; such are the inevitable ups and downs of life. Everything that happens is the working out of innumerable past *karmas*, some of which are pleasant in their effects, others unpleasant. But if one has realised the Self, which lies beyond all change, then whatever happens will no longer have the power to overshadow your innate happiness. The unshakeable stability of your own Being will remove the sting from the suffering that is inevitably part of life, and your inner kingdom will not be conquered and laid waste by the outside world".

The group is silent. After some time the woman responds, in a softer tone now:

"All this may well be true Sir, but it is scant consolation for me".

The Master nods again.

"Indeed. What is needed in the face of adversity is great fortitude and great perseverance in religious duties and spiritual practice. But rest assured, the time will certainly come when one sees that everything that happens is the expression of Divine will and, as such, it is as it must be ".

The villagers sit quietly for some time as if in acknowledgement of the limitations of words. Unintellectual folk, they wisely prefer to draw sustenance from the peaceful atmosphere that surrounds the Master, which permeates the surroundings like the unvarying *shruti* drone behind the notes that rise and fall on the surface of a *raga*. They understand intuitively that the young man in front of them has a different role in the scheme of things from others who might offer advice or comfort in such difficult circumstances and they trust that, somehow, just being in his company will help at some unseen level.

Some refreshments are served; then the villagers respectfully take leave of the ashram, their bundles on their backs.

Materialists

Of all the philosophers who come to debate with the Master, the ones he has least time for are the resolute Materialists. He refers to them jokingly as 'the body people',[157] an allusion to their basic teaching that there is no Self apart from the body and that consciousness derives only from physical interactions within that body. These Materialists deny outright the doctrine of *karma* and rebirth, claiming that a person's happiness or the lack of it is simply due to the innate nature of the person concerned, rather than their activities in a previous lifetime. They also deny the validity of the scriptures, and scorn what they see as the futility of getting lost in abstract theories of what cannot be seen or proved. On the positive side, their prescription for a happy life is to devote one's energies to such everyday concerns as agriculture and cattle breeding, or to engage wholeheartedly in trade, politics, government and similar down-to-earth occupations. Such opinions not infrequently cause the Master to remark that a Materialist does not really deserve the name of philosopher, as he possesses no more refined discrimination than does the typical uneducated man in the street.

As might be imagined, such a radical divergence of perspective yields some lively debates; what follows is a typical discussion between the supreme exponent of non-dualism and a typical Materialist.

Materialist:

"You often speak of human ignorance. How do you define the term?"

Master:

"Ignorance is the normal human experience, which is to say: lack of enlightenment. In the typical perspective, there is a mingling together of two things that are in reality quite distinct. On the one hand there is the field of perception that constitutes the objective world and on the other is the subjective consciousness of the one who perceives that field. Typically, the attributes of what is seen are erroneously superimposed on the one who sees, and thus his true nature becomes overshadowed".

"What is this 'true nature?'"

"The pure substratum of all attributes. This pristine awareness gets obscured by the attributes imposed upon it, and because of this imposition, truth gets mixed up with falsehood. A confusion of identity results, which in turn creates everyday notions such as: 'I am so and so', 'this is me', 'that is mine' and so on, none of which is in fact true.[158] So this failure to discriminate between the one who perceives and whatever is perceived gives rise to a sort of mirage; it is like seeing a snake on the path where there is really only a length of rope or imagining silver where there is only a shiny conch shell. This mirage is the cause of all human suffering".

Without any pause for reflection, the next question:

'You mentioned enlightenment. How do you define that?"

'Enlightenment is when you wake up from this illusion and realise who you really are, which is the universal Self, absolute Consciousness. Then it becomes clear that the world has no self-sufficient existence, it is a dreamlike appearance that has no abiding reality and everything is in truth a superimposition on the non-dual Self. This absolute reality can also be called the Lord and as such He exists equally in all beings, even the inanimate objects, but He stands separate from all of them and is quite unlike them. They all come into existence through being born, and therefore have no choice but to pass through all the changes of state that are necessarily subsequent upon birth.[159] But the Lord is forever unborn, and therefore He does not change and He does not die".[160]

Materialist:

"You talk of the Self as being a consciousness that is somehow independent of matter and material processes. I cannot accept this. We believe that the world is material only and it is formed from a combination of the four elements: earth, fire, water and air".

"I see. And where does consciousness fit in all this?"

"Consciousness is a faculty latent in the body and it disappears with the destruction of the body. It derives from a specific interaction between these four elements. You can say it is born spontaneously like..." here he searches for an analogy, coming up with "well, like the power of intoxication that arises spontaneously from chewing *paan*, even though such a result was not active before the chewing began"[161]

At this, the Master laughs out loud:

"You have picked a fine example Sir, indeed I think you must have been chewing *paan* yourself to have come to such a conclusion! I'm sorry, but your arguments are unacceptable. To begin with, it is simply an error to conflate consciousness with the body. And why? Because on the one hand, the body can still be intact but consciousness not present; think of the situation immediately after death, for example. On the other hand, the body may be inert while all sorts of sensations are arising in consciousness, as happens in the experience of dreaming, to name but one example.

"And as to its origin, how can consciousness which is animate arise from elements which are themselves inanimate? This is to claim that the greater emerges from the lesser. And even if consciousness could arise from those elements, being bound to them it would not be able to perceive them objectively, just as a fire cannot burn itself and not even the cleverest of acrobats can climb up on his own shoulders! No, Sir, your view is just too shot through with self-contradictions to be considered valid".[162]

Materialist:

"Well, I'm afraid I for one need to experience something in order to consider it as real. How can one experience this pure consciousness you posit?"

Master:

"Yes, this is the thing! Pure consciousness has no attribute and as such it cannot be known in the way that any other object of knowledge can be known. It depends on nothing outside of itself, and being the very essence of the mind, it cannot therefore become an object of the mind's scrutiny. This is what the sacred texts mean when they say that one cannot see that which is itself the essence of seeing or think that which is the essence of thinking.[163] And as it is itself devoid of any identifying characteristic – whether name, form, action, kind or qualities – in order for this pure consciousness to shine forth, everything that habitually obscures it must be removed. This is precisely why, when the texts are pressed for a description of the Self, they reject all limiting qualities, and answer instead 'not this, not this'".[164]

Materialist:

"This is all getting a bit too abstract for me. I can only believe what I can see in front of me, what is here and now, tangible in some way".

Master:

"Yes, and this is your difficulty: you confine your investigations to what you can gather from direct sense perception. But sense perception refers only to the realm of phenomenal experience, it cannot apprehend the Self, because the Self is beyond the material and transcends the sensible realm. Moreover, all phenomena come and go, whereas the Self persists unchanging. So if one is dealing with something that lies beyond both the objective world of relations and the limited perceiving subject, then sense-perception, and indeed any other conventional means of knowledge, is of no further use".

Materialist:

"Well, what about reason? Reason is a conventional means of knowledge and you yourself are a renowned thinker. How can you then deny the value of reasoning?"

Master:

"I do not deny the value of reasoning; I only say that reason is limited. Even the greatest rationalists using all their intellectual powers can well come to different conclusions on the very same topic, because the human intellect is always various. Moreover, even though reason is valid in many spheres, in what we are discussing now it is unreliable, because only a type of knowing that is supra-rational can allow one to experience that which, as the hidden nature of everything, lies beyond the range of the limited mind. And this is precisely why the Vedas are so important, because they describe realities – such as *karma*, rebirth and enlightenment – that transcend ordinary human understanding.[165] This is why a person who discusses *brahman* and wishes to investigate the essence of the cause of the world, must base himself on sacred scripture as well as using his own reason. By doing so he is freed from the boundaries of always having to accept the conclusions of conventional perception. After all there is no point in remaining a fool just because one's forefathers were so! Recourse to scripture also saves a seeker from relying on his own imagination, which is always restricted and partial. On the other hand, the person who does persist in basing his arguments only on conventional perception and experience has no way to transcend the limitations inherent in those ways of knowing".[166]

Materialist, after a pause for thought:

"Well, as I say, I for one have to deny the reality of something I do not experience directly".

Master:

"Actually, it is impossible for you to deny the Self, because you yourself are, in truth, that very Self! The Self is the basis of everything. All the modifications in the material world, all the innumerable fluctuations of time, space and causation exist only because prior to them exists that which is their own foundation, their own inner nature. This foundation of the universe, lying beyond the senses, is what I call the Self, Consciousness itself, untrammelled".[167]

The debate has reached an impasse. After sitting for a few minutes while the discussion moves on elsewhere, the Materialist leaves the *darshan* hall, deep in thought.

Maya

Of all the Master's formal teachings, the doctrine of *maya* is probably the single most controversial one. He is often questioned on this subject and on each occasion answers in a manner appropriate to the needs and capacity of his audience. Thus while he is always delighted to expound *maya* as a subtle metaphysical concept when with philosophers and monks, he will also explain it in simpler ways to the common people.

One day towards the end of the monsoon, a party of villagers on pilgrimage comes to see him, troubled by the fact they have heard he teaches that the world is unreal. After each of them has touched the Master's feet respectfully, they gather together on the veranda outside the ashram shrine, wrapped in shawls as the evening has suddenly turned cool. Colourful rugs have been laid down for visitors but no refreshments are served as it is a time of fasting.

"Now," begins the Master energetically "let us be clear about one thing: our Vedanta does not teach that the world is an illusion as some people may misrepresent it. The world is certainly real, it exists of course and this is everyone's common experience – how can that be denied?"

So saying, he strikes the ground forcibly with his open palm and the sound cuts through the crisp air.

"Yet, at the same time, we know the world can be deceptive. Just look to your own life. You all hold opinions about the world that are coloured by your own experiences, your own emotional attachments and aversions. But these opinions are very unreliable. One year the king raises taxes and you think he is a rogue and hate him; the next he lowers them and you think he is the most marvellous fellow and love him. When you are feeling good your wife is the source of all comfort and joy in your life, but on a bad day she is the source of all your problems!"

There are rueful smiles in the audience.

"These fickle feelings may have nothing at all to do with the actual character of the king or the wife, but they shape your thoughts and actions towards them. Like that, you hold all sorts of opinions about life that are really not based on anything substantial, just whims and fancies muddled up with how you have interpreted various events, how you happen to be feeling at the time. This goes on all through our life, and these fancies have no stable continuity. When we are young we see the world in one way, when middle-aged in another, when old in yet another. All people are the same in this. Their minds are swayed by rumours that blow through the village like a wind through the paddy fields, bending the ears of rice this way and that, and their hearts are poisoned by gossip that moves through the market like a flea, biting this person and then jumping on to the next, with everyone left itching and scratching and no one knowing where the bite has come from!"

Again, many smiles.

"Very well, we can see that our normal understanding of the world is a partial, biased affair and this is why it is necessary to purify the mind and heart so that we can begin to see more clearly the truth of any situation as it arises. So this is the first thing, the starting point of the spiritual life: to purify ourselves through devotion and worship and the practice of the virtues, so that we can at least begin to see life a little more clearly and more as it really is. And in our attempts to see more of the picture we have the scriptures to guide us; later on there will be meditation and the practice of discrimination. But unless we develop that deep inner stability that comes from following all these practices, we will continue to be caught up in false views both about ourselves and the world at large. Life will toss us up and down as a dry leaf is tossed by the wind and our short time here will be full of suffering. So the upshot is: if we want to know about *maya*, let us understand it as a name for that mesh of false views and illusions that so often makes our world a deluded, frustrating and unhappy place".

The party leaves the ashram in a quiet but contented mood, pleased that they too can now understand spiritual philosophy.

Meditation

One topic that is frequently discussed is meditation. This is a word everyone has heard and there is a general agreement that its practice is indispensable to the spiritual life. But in fact there is a great deal of confusion about the subject. Some people think meditation involves concentration on sounds or images, others a more reflective use of the intellect, while yet others construe it as the attempt to empty the mind of everything whatsoever. As a result, most have very little idea of how to proceed.

The Master always insists that meditation is a practical discipline and not a theoretical consideration. Accordingly, he rarely speaks publicly in any detail on the subject, preferring to instruct those who are interested individually or in small, or family, groups. This he does according to the Vedic guidelines of what is appropriate to each caste and stage of life. Moreover, all his teaching in this area is couched in the context of the three-fold division of spiritual paths according to the Vedic *kandas* – those scriptural passages that lay down the regulations for an ordered, progressive and successful life for each individual according to his level of evolution.

The first of these paths is the Way of Ritual Action (*Karma Kanda)* that details the religious rituals that purify the participant and bring him success in the world, the attainment of a felicitous state after death and an advantageous rebirth. For many people, the attainment of these religious ends marks the limit of their abilities and aspirations. The Master will encourage the adoption of this path by those for whom he feels it to be relevant.

More evolved souls are referred to the Way of Worship and Meditation (*Upasana Kanda).* By worship is meant the various types of sacrifices to please the gods – those subtle powers operating at the causal level of life – and win their blessings in daily life. On a more interior level, *upasana* also covers numerous meditation techniques. These aim to invoke the name and form of a particular deity, or some other apt symbol of the Absolute, and thereby bring about a direct communion and eventual merging with it. The result of the uniform flow of thought that characterises the deeper levels of *upasana* is support in the fulfilment of worldly desires leading to a more advanced state of material benefit, and the attainment of an enjoyable state after death.

These *upasana* meditations are cumulative practices, 'like pounding paddy to produce the rice' as the Master likes to say. They must be pursued, not only until their particular fruits are realised but even until death, for it is the individual's state of mind at death that determines his future direction and quality of rebirth. Thus the Master teaches this path to the more spiritually advanced householders, as a means of gradual release that allows them to lead a life that recognises the importance of both material and spiritual advancement.

From the point of view of Advaita, however, the main benefit of both these paths is to purify and concentrate the mind to make it fit

191

for eventual Self-realisation. Although they may serve to avert calamity, enhance power and provide the means of a gradual release, they are limited. Dealing only with the manifested or relative phases of living they are motivated by an attachment to material results and generally ignore the transcendental Self as the spiritual basis of life.

It is only the Way of Direct Knowing (*Jnana Kanda*) that leads unerringly to the Self. This knowledge is self-sufficient, requiring no other accessory for its illumination, any more than the sun requires another light to shine. Unlike the fruits of religious ritual or meditation, Self-realisation is not the result of any action of the hand or mind, but is a direct revelation of the transcendental pure Being that lies beyond time and causation. A student must be suitably prepared for, and deserving of, this revelation, which is effected by a process of hearing and deep reflection on certain statements that most pithily encapsulate the Truth.[168] Amongst these is the great saying 'You are That' (*Tat tvam asi*). It is this process of growing spiritual insight that leads, through a refined process of analysis and discrimination, to a destruction of all that veils the true nature of the Self, the transcendental field of life that is quite separate from all activity. The Self is the Truth all of us seek, and Truth is that which is always the same, never-changing, indestructible, that which neither improves nor decays.

This discriminative practice, which the Master called *parisamkhyana* is not a meditation in the conventional sense of the word; far less is it the facile adoption in the waking state of ideas such as 'I am the Self' or 'All is Consciousness' and trying to maintain these concepts on the superficial thinking level of the mind. It is, rather, a process of continual subtle discrimination between what is real and what is not. Guided by the enlightened teacher, this process of discernment destroys once and for all the pupil's illusion of being a separate individual who acts in and on the world, and through its application is brought to an end what the world falsely imagines to be the distinction between the one who experiences, the process of experiencing and the object of experience. Through *parisamkhyana* the three become one; what remains is the unity of the Self, forever shining in its own glory.

Though the Master's teaching of Advaita allows and utilises all lesser paths as provisional and purifying approaches to ultimate truth, it is essentially the Way of Direct Knowing. By virtue of its radical nature, this path is traditionally considered more suited to the reclusive way of life, as it uncompromisingly affirms that humanity's ancient longings can only ultimately be satisfied by Self-realisation, rather than any external circumstance. This being the case, it is to Self-realisation that all serious spiritual effort must eventually be directed, whether in this lifetime or a future one. This fact necessitates acting on the realisation that humankind finds its true happiness neither by attempting to fulfil endless material aspirations, nor through the consolations offered by conventional religion, but only through complete self-transcendence in Enlightenment.[169]

Memory

Question:

"Do the enlightened beings retain the memory of their life prior to realisation?"

Answer:

"It is like waking up from a dream. When you regain waking consciousness each morning, you rapidly forget whatever dream you have just had. Now, if the dream has been particularly dramatic or powerful it may linger for a while and there may even be some initial confusion as you readjust to the reality of the waking state, as if you are in both states at once, so to speak. But it will not be long until you are fully engaged in the waking state and the dream has gone, quite faded from memory and you just get on with enjoying your waking life. It is like that".

Q:

"Are you saying that the enlightened has absolutely no memory of what happened prior to his enlightenment?"

A:

"All the functional memories of how to act and speak and all the rest of it remain, of course. On a psychological or emotional level, if it is really necessary one could certainly recall something from the prior life. But in general there is no point to it. The past is past, so why should it persist in the present? It has no useful function to perform in the new situation, no current reality; it has gone and that's that".

Q:

"But surely we need to retain personal memory so that there is some continuity of our individual personality before and after enlightenment".

A:

"Why are you so keen to maintain this little personality and all its memories? In fact, it is the weight of unnecessary memories that keeps you confined to an unenlightened life of suffering and limitation! Moreover, all these memories are themselves just a type of forgetting, because everything to do with ignorance is a forgetting of who you really are, which is the universal Self. That level of life is always free of the past and its endless histories. So losing the memories of the previous life of ignorance amounts to remembering what is actually and has always been the case: Enlightenment".

Q:

"But memories are such a source of pleasure..."

A:

"Relative to what? Consider the butterfly. Does it remember what it was like to live as a caterpillar, crawling along, always searching for food and always in fear of being eaten? Does it think about the days it spent hanging as a chrysalis, bound up tight, restricted by the threads it has spun itself? No, the butterfly enjoys flying and fluttering freely, caressed by the warm sunlight and sporting its glorious colours as it drinks the nectar from one flower after another. Those other stages in its growth belong to the past and it is surely happy to leave them behind like the dried up case".

Q:

"But isn't the present caused by the past?"

A:

"In truth, the present is always uncaused, ever fresh. The conventional perspective sees cause and effect progressing through time and working themselves out through material conditions, but beyond the conventional perspective stands That which is motionless, beyond matter and causation, the one pure Consciousness, unborn and undying. In that eternal peace, all limitations of time and space stand revealed as being devoid of any real substance, recognised as mere appearances".[170]

Memory is the best medicine

It is high summer now. No rains have yet come and everywhere the roads are very dusty. A woman in the *darshan* hall has red swollen eyes that are weeping and evidently causing her much discomfort. She has travelled a long way to see the Master and is naturally upset to miss this precious opportunity. Noticing the situation, the Master makes arrangements for her to be put up in the pilgrim rest house down the road from the ashram and has one of the *brahmacharis* bring a special ayurvedic medicine made from clarified butter for her to rub in the eyes.

The next evening she reappears in the hall.

"And how are the eyes now?" enquires the Master kindly.

"Much better, Maharaj shri, thanks to your grace. I feel very happy".

He smiles. "Well, I think it was the medicine that did the trick! But the interesting point here is a question that arises out of your recovery of clear sight. Is it a new happiness you are now experiencing or is it actually the return of your previous happiness that you had temporarily lost?"

"Well," she considers for a second "it feels like a new happiness, but if I think about it, I guess it is my normal state that has returned".

"Correct! Just like that, when our present ignorance goes, we remember who we really are and who we always have been. What we call enlightenment is not the addition of anything new, but the recovery of our natural state that we have temporarily forgotten".

Mindfulness

A serious young follower of Buddhism is keen to discuss his practice of meditation which he has recently learned from a monk. It is the Theravadin technique of *vipassana;* he refers to it as 'mindfulness'.

The Master receives him cordially, but gently admonishes him saying:

"Our teaching is not about being 'mindful'. Actually, here we prefer to be mindless! Lose the limited mind and find the universal Self, then everything will be perfectly alright".

Natural bliss

A wealthy local merchant who deals in cotton comes to *darshan* several days running without saying anything. Then one evening he finally asks:

"Maharaj-shri, you often talk of bliss and you say that life is in essence bliss and the enlightened ones experience this bliss as a perpetual state. I have never had this bliss, but I think I understand a little of what you mean from my own experience. Sometimes, when I look at my children or see a beautiful flower or enjoy a lovely sunset, I feel an intense, profound happiness. I suppose this is the bliss you are speaking about?"

The Master gently shakes his head:

"Yes, but... much greater, much greater" he begins.

"Actually, it is not possible to imagine what this wholeness of life is by comparing it with any normal experience. To tell the truth, any normal experience is but a tiny part of life, a thorny little fragment of life, whereas the bliss of the Self is the ultimate reality of life. It is the state of wholeness, the ever-undiminished Divine, *brahman*. Wholeness is felt as a loving bliss that is not isolated in space and time or located in any particular experience. This bliss is available to everyone, in every space and every time, as it is the nature of their very own Self. What you are describing – a smile, a beautiful scene – that little, concrete bliss", and here the Master chuckles, "is fine, of course, but it is a small kind of nothing to tell the truth, it's not the real bliss. It's as if you are searching for bliss in little isolated drops of rain, whereas the bliss of the Self is an ocean made up of innumerable drops, innumerable. That is the real bliss, not some single, isolated drop of bliss".

The questioner looks bemused. The Master continues:

"You are calling bliss what you can see, some nice thing; what you can hear, some nice melody. What you can touch. These are isolated values of happiness derived through the senses, and they are very, very fragmented, little unstable fields of sensation transmitted by the senses or the mind. Normal life knows these tiny little waves of temporary happiness, but the Self is a different realm, a very different realm. It is the essence of life itself ".

Another questioner asks:

"You say this bliss is the ultimate level of life but on other occasions I have heard you describe that transcendental area of ultimate reality as a field of nothingness".

The Master smiles.

"No contradiction here, but to understand this you must dive deep within yourself and find the unbounded Self. And with regular practice, you will see that that which appears as emptiness because it contains no thing, that nothingness – hollow, unmanifest – is simultaneously and always the fullness of everything. It is the Self, which is the all. It is bliss, pure loving bliss. When this realisation is naturally established, the whole of life swings in the waves of bliss, the waves of loving bliss ..."

Just to speak of this state clearly transports the Master, and so strong is the feeling that descends in the room that those present feel their questions evaporate. All sit quietly now, overcome by the thrilling power of the atmosphere.

Nine nights

It is now the autumn festival of the Nine Nights, that time when the energy of Mother Divine is closest to the earth plane and Her blessings are most easily enjoyed. There are many *pujas* and celebrations going on all over the town. Each district has erected its own image to be worshipped and people are moving from one to the other, enjoying the different forms of the Mother and the company and hospitality of friends and neighbours. It is a very happy and sociable time. At the end of the festival all these local images will be immersed in the holy river, but tonight is the eighth night and the climax of the festival is to be the procession of the moveable deities from the temple of Mother Annapurna, the goddess who protects the city, down to the waterside for *puja* and then back again.

A local *raja* has invited the Master and some companions to watch the festivities from the roof of his palace overlooking the procession route. The cavalcade duly passes by: the images of the various forms of Annapurna and her attendant deities are made from gold, silver and copper and dressed in gorgeous silks and covered with flowers. Carried head-high on decorated platforms by temple priests, the splendid figures are accompanied by music and enthusiastic *bhajans*.[171] A feeling of devotion saturates the air.

"These deities are indeed beautiful", comments the Master who is evidently enjoying the proceedings, "and it is very good that everyone has a chance to see them. But do not forget that the main deity, Mother Divine herself, remains fixed and stable in the temple, She never moves. And when the festivities are over, all these deities will return to Her and sit quietly there by her side. Like that, the mind and senses are but the agents of the Self. Roaming around, they give us experience of the world and everyone enjoys, but the Self remains ever stable, never moving. And when their activity is spent, the mind and senses retire to rest quietly at their home in the Self".

"Do you mean in sleep?"

"Yes, in sleep or in *samadhi*".

"What then is the difference between sleep and *samadhi*?"

"*Samadhi* is sleep in the waking state!"

No coming and no going

An aristocratic woman from a well-known Shaiva family down south is visiting Kashi during the Nine Nights, specifically on pilgrimage to the Vishvanath temple. She is accompanied by her daughter, several members of her family and servants. When not attending *pujas* in the temple or associated functions, the family members are spending their time seeing the sights of the city, but the woman, who is very devout and a keen seeker, has spent all her spare time at the ashram having the Master's *darshan*. Now the time has come for her to leave and so she is paying a last visit. She explains that due to family commitments she has to return home and, thanking him for all the time he has graciously put at her disposal, adds that she will be returning to Kashi as soon as possible, probably for the Shivaratri festival the following spring.

"Very good", responds the Master. Then, as she is about to leave the hall, he adds a little mischievously:

"And do not forget that you don't really go anywhere – there is no coming and going for you".

The woman replies that she doesn't understand what he means and asks for an explanation.

More seriously now, he continues:

"You say you are leaving this place and going home. To do this you will travel in a cart from here to your lodgings, where you will transfer to your carriage and then proceed back home to your place?"

She nods in agreement.

"And on the way you will doubtless pass all sorts of beautiful houses, trees, fields and so on?"

"Yes, I shall".

"But let's look at the situation a little more closely. In fact, you will not move at all! You will sit without motion while the various conveyances do all the moving, not you. And you will not really pass those trees and houses and so on; they will approach you, pass and recede behind you while you just stay sitting immobile, calmly enjoying the changing scene around you. Like that, the Self is ever still. It is the world, not the Self that comes and goes. Nevertheless, everyone says: 'I went here'; 'I travelled there' and so on, even though the Self remains unmoving, a silent witness to whatever comes and goes. Moreover, it is just this confusion between the body and the Self that is the seed of all our problems. The Self is your real nature. This being so, you are the unmoving one – here, there and everywhere. So how could there be any coming or going for you?"[172]

The Master's eyes twinkle with humour. He smiles graciously and gives her a flower; the woman respectfully makes her *pranaams* and departs.

Nothing is ever lost

One day during a rather dry discussion on the concluding verses of the Isha Upanishad, which are to do with the departure of the subtle body from its physical vehicle at the moment of dying,[173] the question arises as to the importance of the last thought at the time of death. Bored, the Master deftly changes the mood with the following story:

"You know", he begins, "nothing is ever lost. There was once a man who did penance for a hundred years in his worship of Lord Shiva. Nothing seemed to come of it, and as he lay dying he thought miserably to himself, 'What was the point of all my efforts? I have got nowhere'. He died and was reborn as a bee, no longer thinking of Lord Shiva, his rituals or his penances. But no spiritual gain ever goes astray; at the very depth of the mind sitting in its new body lingered the devotee's persistent desire to reach his Lord.

"One afternoon the bee flew here to this holy city of Kashi, quite unaware in his new form that he had arrived at the very place on earth where the object of his aspirations is graciously pleased to reside. Naturally drawn into the well-kept garden of a wealthy merchant, the bee alighted on a beautiful flower, intent on drinking its nectar. So absorbed was he in enjoying the delicious ambrosia that he quite forgot the passing of time and when night fell, the flower closed up and trapped him inside.

"The next morning the merchant came out into the garden looking for flowers to offer in his morning worship. He happened to pluck the flower that contained the bee and carrying it inside, duly offered it to the image of his chosen deity: Lord Shiva. As the sun rose, its warm rays fell on the flower, opening its petals up and allowing the bee to crawl out.

"Lord Shiva was delighted and said to himself: 'Oho! So here comes one who worshipped me for so many years when a man and now takes the form of a bee to come even closer to me!' He offered the faithful little creature the boon of whatever he wished. The bee asked to stay united with his Lord for ever. And so, indeed, he was".

Play of maya

Some monks are gathered for a recitation. After lengthy excerpts from the Rig and Sama Veda come passages from the Upanishads. The sonorous rumble of the ancient Sanskrit, like thunder from the very dawn of time, is thrilling:

> All the sacred texts, all the holy offerings, all the ceremonies, and all the rituals; the past, the present, and the future; all the Vedas speak of and this whole universe – all are projections of the imperishable *brahman*, conjured up by *maya*, the Mother of illusion. And through the art of *maya*, we are charmed by her creations. Know that all of Nature is but a magic theatre, that the great Mother is the master magician, and that this whole universe is peopled by her many parts.[174]

The Master comments:

"What this particular text is telling us, O. forest of ascetics, is that to live the reality of life you must first be educated in its unreality. Then when this discrimination has taken you to the Real, firmly established in That, you can live life as it really is – the spotless mirror of the Divine".

Personality

A devotee makes the honest confession:

"I suppose what I do not like about enlightenment is the idea of losing my personality".

"What do you mean by your 'personality'?"

"I suppose I mean that which makes me '*me*', my personal self which has created its own unique history, makes its own choices and so on".

"Fine, but this unique self has been exercising its choices all through your life, yet it still has not brought you real happiness, has it?"

"Well...I suppose that is true", he admits somewhat grudgingly. "But I still cannot reconcile my desire to find truth with this idea of transcendence, with no longer being a 'somebody'".

"Actually", laughs the Master "anybody can be a 'somebody', for to do so is to merely live out our karmic inheritance. And the passage of time will accomplish that anyway, whatever your life may be! But if it is real happiness you are after, then the trick is for this 'somebody' to evolve into a 'nobody' and then that 'nobody' will be free to become 'everybody'".

The Master's wit is lost on the questioner.

"What do you mean, Sir?"

"I mean that your clinging to the idea of the little 'self' is the barrier to realising the universal Self".

The man frowns, says nothing and sits thinking for some time before touching the Master's feet and leaving.

Past lives

To spend time in the company of the Master is to sojourn in that blessed land where only the infinite present exists. A young man from a good family has come for *darshan*. It transpires he is very keen on finding out about his past lives. He has undertaken some yogic practices to this end, feels he has experienced a number of episodes from previous births and wants to know what the Master thinks about all this.

"Your past lives belong to an earlier and therefore less evolved state of life, so why spend precious time and effort examining the funeral processions of long ago? The relevant result of all those accumulated lives is manifesting right here and now, so if you really want to know about the import of your past lives, look to your present life. There is really no point spending time with past lives".

"But some people claim to have clear memories of their past lives", persists the questioner.

"They do indeed. But unless the mind is quite exceptionally clear, such so-called memories are very unreliable. All sorts of mental impressions may be muddled up together and wishful thinking born of unconscious needs and desires will also play its part in the mix".

"Then how can we gauge the validity of these memories?"

"How do you know who you are each morning when you wake up from sleep? You remember who it was who went to sleep the previous night and so there is a clear thread of continuity isn't there? Otherwise, the consciousness born each morning would be totally new and if that were the case, how could there be any continuity of memory? Just so, to have truly unambiguous knowledge of a previous life, you would have to remember it as clearly as that. So, the practical thing is: first direct your time and effort to perfecting the art of being fully here in the present and then see whether you are still concerned with all those lives that occurred in the past".

Politics

A local Raja has come to the Master to seek his advice as there have been troubles on the borders of his kingdom. A very pious Jain who has always believed in non-violence, he is by nature more of an aesthete than a warrior and so is feeling very conflicted as to how to deal with the situation. To date, his rule has been uneventful and his religious principles have not been tested in this way; the kingdom is small and prosperous and its people have been happy to let him and his ministers conduct the business of daily governance while they get on with their lives. Recently however, troublesome elements have arisen and the situation is fraught.

The Master listens sympathetically to the details of the man's dilemma, and then tells the following story:

"There was once a fierce cobra who lived under an ancient banyan tree in the heart of a village. All the people respected him and fearfully kept their distance. Unbeknownst to them, however, this snake was also a great devotee of God and did much penance serving a great *guru*. Eventually he achieved enlightenment. When the villagers realised he was now no longer dangerous but always peaceful and content, they began to mock him, throwing stones and jeering. Confused, the cobra went back to his *guru* for help.

"'Just raise your hood and hiss!' was the advice".

Power of attention

A long queue is shuffling past the Master for *darshan*. One by one, individuals or small groups stop in front of him for blessing. He smiles or nods, accepts the flowers or salutations offered him and, from time to time, engages in conversation with whoever is before him. Far back in the line a young man waits patiently, an aspiring musician. He has no questions, but is keenly hoping for direct eye contact with the Master, as he has heard that such a connection with a saint can bring great benefits to a seeker. Finally, his turn comes. He looks intently at the Master's face, but the look is not returned and no words are exchanged. Instead, the sage glances for a moment at the young man's neck, and then, almost before it has begun, the *darshan* is over. The young man follows those ahead of him on their way out of the hall, deeply disappointed and wondering if the whole event has been a waste of time.

Some four decades later, the man long since acknowledged as the foremost classical vocalist in the Land of the Veda, will recall the incident.

"I did not realise it at the time, of course, but the whole thing was to do with purifying the *vishuddhi chakra,* the subtle centre that governs communication. That look opened my throat to sing."

Practice

The Master always sets great store by personal experience; in fact he places it above scriptural knowledge and ritualistic performance in the journey to enlightenment, as the following exchange shows.

The Master has been invited to oversee a *yajna* performed on the Dashashvamedha *ghat,* the most celebrated part of the waterfront, built by Lord Brahma himself to welcome Lord Shiva to the city. After the ceremony is over and people are seated around, quietly enjoying the serene atmosphere such rituals always engender, a sincere seeker after liberation approaches. Middle-aged, he is from a good family and well-educated in Vedic lore, but remains dissatisfied.

"Young Sir, you speak most eloquently about Vedanta, the realisation of unicity. I have heard the same teaching in the various Vedic texts I have studied for many years so I have no theoretical doubts on that score. But my question is a practical one: how do we make Vedanta a way of life, a living experience?"

"Reflect continually on your personal experience. How do I experience? What do I experience? And who is it that is engaged in experiencing? Like that, things will gradually become clear to you. This is what the yoga texts call *svadhyaya* ".

Then:

"Moreover, paying close attention to the experiences of others also will help you greatly in this regard. Understanding the mechanics of experience is an essential part of the enquiry that leads to Self-knowledge".

Purpose of the scriptures

A senior government official from the western desert lands comes to offer his respects. A pious and intelligent man with a keen intellect, he has been feeling disturbed ever since a wandering *sadhu* who visited his home-town preached very convincingly that the enlightened no longer have need of the scriptures. This has created some confusion amongst his local people, most of whom have hitherto been devout followers of religious authority. Arriving in Kashi on pilgrimage, the official hears of the Master's reputation and he has decided to come and see if he can get some guidance on the matter.

One of the *brahmacharis* shows him up to the ashram roof terrace, where he finds the master Vedantin sitting on an elevated ledge gazing peacefully out over the broad river. Seeing the visitor, the monk descends to the terrace. He moves spontaneously like a child, utterly free of tension; his skin has an extraordinary lustre. The visitor tells his story while the Master listens carefully, then frames his reply:

"The purpose of the scriptures" he begins, speaking slowly and carefully, "is to regulate the behaviour of the ignorant – by which I mean those who identify themselves with the non-Self, those who take themselves to be the limited personality that operates in the relative field of cause and effect. The wise, on the other hand, do not suffer from this identification, because they experience the Self as quite separate from, and different to, the realm of cause and effect.[175] And they experience this separation as clearly as the difference between fire and water, or light and darkness, which not even the dullest of minds would ever claim were identical. Now, that direct, continuous experience that you are yourself the Absolute takes you beyond the realms covered by the Veda. Indeed, the scriptures themselves state clearly that to an enlightened being, the Vedas are as much use as a small well in a place already flooded by water.[176] Therefore, it can legitimately be said that the prohibitions and injunctions of the scriptures do not apply to those who are liberated".

On hearing these words, the official is clearly torn between respect for the measured reply of the young man in front of him and his own turbulent emotions.

"I find this hard to understand", is all he could muster by way of reply.

"Well, imagine you are standing in the street talking to a friend, let us call him Devadatta. All of a sudden, someone else appears and calls this Devadatta by name, commanding him to do something. You hear the command clearly but you would not think that it refers to you, would you? You might perhaps think that you had not heard the command properly, but as it is, you know it is the person standing in front of you who has been addressed and not you yourself. Like that, he who directly experiences himself to be the transcendental Self realises without any doubt that the commands of the scriptures no longer pertain to him".

"Alright, Swamigal, I understand that the sage experiences the transcendental Self as separate from the relative world of cause and effect. But even such a wise man has a long history of identifying with his body in the past. Due to this ingrained habit, can he not still consider himself bound by the injunctions of scriptures when they advocate a certain action for desirable ends or prohibit another action because it would lead to evil? To adapt your previous example: what I am talking about would be like a father and his sons who, notwithstanding their differences of maturity and seniority, continue to regard themselves as part of one family in which each of the family members is equally bound by the same injunctions, despite their obvious differences as individuals".

Smiling, the Master shakes his head.

"I appreciate your reasoning, Sir, but the fact is that once one has become the Self, it is simply no longer possible to identify with the limited selfhood that is part of the world of cause and effect. However – and this is the practical point here – it is certainly the case that this freedom comes only after one has scrupulously obeyed the injunctions and prohibitions laid down in the scriptures and not before. Fulfilling such duties is undoubtedly of help in the emergence and acquiring of Supreme Knowledge, even though these obligations have nothing to do with the fruit of such knowledge, which is eternal liberation".[177]

After a pause, the Master adds:

"And of course, to become a student deserving of Supreme Knowledge is no casual undertaking.[178] Nevertheless, from whichever side we approach the matter, the conclusion is that the injunctions of the scriptures refer only to the unenlightened".

The official seemed rather crestfallen.

"In that case, if the non-believer disregards the scriptures out of ignorance and the enlightened do so out of wisdom, then what is the point of having them at all?"

The Master smiles broadly:

"Ha! Well, it is certainly true that neither the enlightened who know the Absolute nor the ignorant who deny the spiritual side of life perform Vedic rites! But there is yet another category – those who know about the Absolute through the scriptures but do not yet live it as their own essential nature. These people still follow scriptural advice as to what is allowed or what is forbidden and, because they still cherish a longing for the results of Vedic rites, they perform them devoutly. Wherever you look in society, this is quite evidently the case, so it cannot be said that the scriptures serve no purpose".

"I am happy to hear that", continues the official. "But the followers of the sage, seeing that he does not bother to perform the rites, may decide to follow his example. Surely in that case the scriptures would serve no purpose?"

"Not so, and for several reasons. For one thing, the man who attains Self-knowledge is a very rare being. Only one among many does so, so there is no likelihood of large numbers of people following such an example. Secondly, the ignorant, by definition, do not actually follow the example of the wise – that is why they remain ignorant! They are as if blinded by their own selfhood, so they ignore good advice and may even fall from the spiritual path by practising black magic and so on. And when all is said and done, sacred rites will always be performed because it is the very nature of man to be active in the world and to strive to avoid suffering and improve his lot. And because such rites will always be performed, it follows that the scriptures which prescribe them will always serve a purpose".

This seems to satisfy the visitor, but nevertheless, the Master would not let him leave without making a final point:

"Nevertheless, the fact remains that the world of cause and effect is based on the misperception that it is actually what it appears to be. Such illusory understanding does not touch the pure intelligence that is the Self any more than the water in a mirage can wet the dry salty earth on which it rests".[179]

Reason, scripture and Truth

A philosopher:

"Maharaj shri, you obviously have a very clear intellect and always present your arguments rationally, but in the end you seem to be saying that reason is not much use in the search for Truth. I do not understand your position on this".

The Master:

"Conventional reason is certainly useful as far as it goes, but the intellect cannot help you to know what is beyond itself. It is the instrument by which you learn about things objectively but not about that which is its own source, the pure subjectivity of the Self. You can see clearly the limitation of reason by the fact that it demonstrably leads to conflicting conclusions. Just imagine if all the logicians of the past, present and future were assembled here in front of us now, they would be quite unable to agree on anything! This lack of congruity is not only because each separate mind has a different perspective and therefore a different opinion. More importantly, the essential fact is that Truth lies in the transcendental field of pure Being, beyond thought. This is why the sacred texts are so important in the search for That which is the very cause of the universe. It is only with their help that we can become familiar with this transcendental level and thereby terminate the endless conflict of relative, partial opinions. Reason is the operation of the mind and the mind itself stems from Being, but Being is beyond reason just as it is beyond the senses. So in order to be truly reasonable, reason must serve that which transcends it, which is beyond individuality and is supra-rational".[180]

"How is reason best employed in the quest for Truth then?"

"It is a question of stages. Authoritative sacred tradition first presents the thesis that the world of duality is illusory, whereas Truth is non-dual. This thesis is then supported by examples, reasoning and logical reflection. In this way, scriptural authority is combined with reason in order to establish the validity of the original thesis. And in this whole process, the status of scripture, as mediated through the line of realised teachers, is crucial. Now, if scripture is regarded only as revealed and unassailable truth, then the non-believer can just reject it out of hand and nothing is accomplished. But even though it is, in fact, revealed and unassailable truth, scripture should also be treated as a means of knowledge and as such be subject to the scrutiny of reason. Only in this way can the teacher bring the normal mind gradually to understand the true import of scripture, and thereby transcend conventional rationality and gain liberation".[181]

Relative and Absolute

Question: "As I understand it, Advaitin non-dualism teaches that everything is in reality the one pure Consciousness?"

Answer: "It does".

Q: "If this is so, how can we understand the world?"

A: "It is like a city reflected in a mirror. However magnificent and variegated this city may be, it has no existence apart from the medium in which it inheres. If the mirror is withdrawn, the city will no longer be there. However, if the city itself were somehow to be withdrawn, the mirror would continue, quite unaffected. Indeed, it was also quite unaffected even when bearing the reflection, because the superimposition of the city did nothing whatsoever to the surface of the mirror. Like that, the relative, ever-changing world is superimposed upon the eternal, unmoving Absolute".[182]

Sitting is best for meditation

A Buddhist monk from the distant island of Shri Lanka has a question:

"Sir, in my order we practise various walking meditations, yet you recommend sitting to meditate. Surely, as meditation is something mental there can be no restriction as to the attitude of the body? It can be as well practised whether you are standing, sitting, or lying down and not only while sitting".

"Not so" replies the Master. "By the term 'meditation' we understand a continued mental focus, and this is not possible when you are walking or running, since the act of moving naturally activates the body and this movement in turn tends to distract the mind. Even when the body is standing, the mind is occupied in maintaining the body in an erect position and is therefore incapable of entering into the subtle strata of thinking. And when lying down, we tend to be overcome by sleep, for that is our lifelong habit when the body is supine and deeply relaxed. A sitting person, on the other hand, is not bothered by any of this. Thus sitting is the best position in which to practise meditation".[183]

A lay person speaks up:

"What do you mean by mental focus?"

"Mental focus means a person's mind is absorbed in one and the same object. While their attention is thus fixed, their limbs will move only very slightly, if at all". "But surely this in an unnatural state?" comes the objection. "Not at all", replies the Master. "It is entirely natural and therefore it is not unique to the state of meditation. Think of how a crane is effortlessly focussed as it stands motionless waiting for a fish, or how a woman sits absorbed, naturally preoccupied, while thinking of her man who is away from home on a journey. Now as regards meditation, this sort of absorption comes easily to those who sit. Thus, as I say, meditation is best practised while sitting".[184]

Sankhya made simple

Several learned *pandits* are discussing the Sankhya system, the philosophical sister of yoga, both of which belong to what are known as the Six Right Perspectives.[185] Sankhya is attributed to the Vedic sage Kapila, and it teaches a basic dualism. One side of life is comprised of the various material realms, gross and subtle, which taken together comprise the relative field of *prakriti*. The ceaseless activity of *prakriti* is carried on by the interactions of its three constituent elements, known as *gunas*,[186] On the other hand is the absolute phase of life or *purusha*, which is pure spirit, and exists quite separate from the worlds of matter.

The discussion is becoming rather abstruse and dry. The Master makes the point that the eternal separation of spirit and matter is not just a philosophical idea to be accepted or rejected in the waking state, but the actual lived experience of the enlightened. This realisation is the fruit of prolonged and sustained spiritual practice, the best use a human being can make of their time and energy. To emphasise that the theoretical understanding of Sankhya is brought alive by the purifying practice of yoga, and that they are mutually reinforcing, he concludes:

"The wisdom of Sankhya arises only when the practice of yoga attains maturity".[187]

One of today's visitors, a robust and moustachioed farmer from the Jat caste who is in Kashi to carry out the cremation of his father, suddenly speaks up from the back of the hall:

"Honoured *pandits*! This may be all very well, but I'm an uneducated man and to tell the truth I find this discussion too intellectual and too abstract to have much practical value".

Some of the *pandits* look askance and would probably have liked to rebuke him for lowering the tone of the discussion, but the Master is quite unfazed by the interruption; indeed, he seems to welcome it.

"Fair enough, Sir! Let's look at it this way. There was once a traveller on his way to a mighty city that everyone talked about but nobody seemed to have visited. He was passing through a thick forest when he was ambushed by three *dacoits*. One bound him with a rope, while another pulled out a knife to stab him. At this point the third robber relented and pleaded with the other two not to kill their captive. After some time he persuaded them to set him free and the two rapidly quit the scene.

"On learning that the traveller was on his way to the famous city, the remaining robber offered to escort him there. When they reached the outskirts, the man excused himself saying that he could go no further, as he was well known in the area and would be running the risk of capture by the authorities if he did. So saying, he turned back and the traveller entered the city alone.

"Like that, our pilgrim soul has been overpowered by the three *gunas*. *Tamas* binds the soul down to the world, while *rajas* keeps ceaselessly prodding it into action. The role of *sattva* is to liberate the bound soul from the clutches of the other two. But *sattva* is itself a *guna*, and as such, can only take you to the limit of relative life; it cannot enter the realm of the Absolute. So all three qualities must eventually be left behind before you can dissolve into the boundless expanse that is your own Self. And he who enters that divine city never returns, because he has become one with the eternal".

Some of the *pandits* look nonplussed; the farmer is evidently satisfied.

Sat-chit-ananda

A young seeker, who has been following the Master for several months, asks:

"Maharaj-ji, I am rather bewildered by the different terms used to describe the Absolute. Some call it 'the Self', others 'pure awareness' or 'Being'. Religious people refer to it as 'God' or 'the Divine' and so on. Do these terms denote separate things or are they all just synonyms? Can you clarify all this confusing vocabulary?"

The master Vedantin laughs.

"Indeed! The thing is, in itself the Absolute is indefinable, so in truth we can say nothing about it. But, on the other hand, as it is omnipresent, we can say everything about it!"

Again, his body rocks with laughter.

Then in a more serious vein he answers:

"Either way, all attributes or no attributes, the Absolute cannot be the object of conventional, sensory knowledge, like any other mundane object. So, how then can we describe the indescribable? Well, at the least we can say that it exists, it *is*, it is pure existence, existence to the ultimate degree. As such, it is the essential constituent of everything that comes into existence, while in itself never becoming limited by any particular form of existence. Sooner or later, without exception, every single form will change, but *existence* itself – that abstract something of which any specific form is but the temporary manifestation – that quality of existing continues. So from this point of view we can describe the Absolute as Being (*sat*), the eternal and static Being which is beyond any becoming, and yet is the source of all, beyond all the changing expressions of itself. All right so far?"

"Yes, I understand".

"Now, although abstract and unmanifest, this Being is obviously not inert, dead or devoid of vitality. How could it be? It is lively and creative, no doubt, and in and through this endless creativity it exhibits above all the quality of intelligence – so we can call it Consciousness. Not an individual consciousness, limited or defined by a particular object or taking the form of some localised sensation, but Consciousness in its own nature, unbounded and without any object, Consciousness as such, simply aware of itself – *pure* Consciousness (*chit*). Now, this boundless Consciousness is in its nature pristine and unalloyed, but for most people it is continuously obscured by the changing states of their mind – the cycle of waking, dreaming and sleeping that is experienced by everyone. If it were not so obscured, everyone would be enlightened just by virtue of being conscious, being alive! So we can also call it transcendental, because it lies beyond the three relative states of waking, dreaming and dreamless sleep, and it continues unbroken, witnessing everything that arises in those three relative states, while itself remaining serene, motionless and undisturbed.

"Moreover, the living experience of this transcendental Consciousness is not devoid of feeling. It is a state of loving happiness that thrills the entire body and overflows into activity, irrepressible. It cannot but be expressed through the one who knows it. This happiness is intrinsic; it has no cause external to itself and therefore it does not diminish when circumstances in the outer world change. It is self-sufficient and quite uncaused. So if we are describing it, we must differentiate it from what is normally called 'happiness', because that is a temporary state which is always liable to turn into its opposite, which we call 'unhappiness'. This state has no opposite and so we call it 'bliss', 'loving-bliss' (ananda). So, to return to your question, and for the purposes of understanding, the Absolute is unqualified, yet it can be said to have these qualities: Being, Consciousness and Bliss".[188]

The Master ends by making the point that this is not just another consoling theory.

"Mark well, this Absolute is not something outside us and far away, like some heaven or celestial region, to be attained after death by the fortunate. It is our very own nature, our Self, here and now in the midst of life. At his deepest level, every single limited individual is this unlimited cosmic Self. I am That, and you are That and everything without exception is That, and That alone endures".[189]

Seeing God

An elderly man who has travelled the length and breadth of the country on numerous pilgrimages asks:

"Can God really be seen?"

The Master smiles serenely: "Indeed, God can be seen, just as I am talking to you".

"So what does He look like?"
The Master indicates the audience. "These are all His forms".

Shiva as Self

It is Maha Shivaratri, 'the Night of the Great Lord Shiva'. This festival, held each year on the night of no moon between the death of February and the birth of her younger sister March, is celebrated as the time when the energy of the Lord is most vibrant for us who inhabit the earth plane. While for some devotees this festival celebrates the occasion when Shiva saved the world from being engulfed by poison by drinking it himself, for others it marks the anniversary of Shiva's wedding to Goddess Parvati. On an esoteric level, as the moon is the presiding deity of the mind, when it has waned for fourteen days, it remains just the merest slither. As such, it emulates the reduction of mental activity to almost complete quiescence, which is the state of freedom. Among the *yogis*, Shiva's company is always sought as an aid to cultivate this inner silence and his help is believed to be especially available to them. The Lord's assistance is also there for the common people absorbed in the world. At midnight on Shivaratri, when the divine vibrations descend close to every human heart, it is believed that if people are engaged in holy tasks, they will become suffused with the Divine. As Kashi is the earthly dwelling place of the Lord, the ancient city is naturally filled with tens of thousands of pilgrims. The bustle, clamour and sense of expectation are intense.

The Master and a group of his people have retired beyond the northern outskirts of the city, a mile or so past Raj Ghat, and are camping out in an ancient Shiva temple there, close to the banks of the river. The place is somewhat dilapidated but has a very serene atmosphere. The shrine's isolated position is emphasised by the venerable *banyan* trees with their long roots straggling down to the ground like the unkempt tresses of some primordial ascetic, and it provides a welcome respite from the noisy festivities further downriver. The distance from the town also serves to filter out casual visitors, as only those with a serious spiritual interest would take the trouble to come this far for *darshan* when so much is going on in the town.

The Master, who seems in particularly scintillating mood today, is seated with a group on the sandy riverbank. The conversation turns to the origins of the Shivaratri festival. A visiting *sadhu* from Nepal ventures that at this time each year the forces of negativity are particularly intense, and yet, despite the shrouding ignorance, Shiva remains eternally awake, shining forth in all his glory. It is to emulate and encourage this wakefulness that devotees celebrate the festival by abandoning sleep and food and staying up all night, singing *bhajans* and celebrating their Lord.

Someone else asks the Master if this is not rather like the enlightened man, who retains his spiritual lustre even in the midst of the darkness all around him.

"Yes, yes!" he replies forcefully. "That is exactly it. You have seen something very beautiful, absolutely beautiful. See, it is like this", he reaches for his staff and draws a short line in the sand. "This is the world – ignorance, suffering, the three *gunas* – all that inevitable nuisance! Now, how can we minimise this situation, how can we draw its sting without getting embroiled in it, without even touching it?"

No one has an answer.

"Like this!" laughs the Master delightedly, drawing a much longer line under the first one. "Now the first line fades into insignificance, doesn't it?"

Everyone laughs too, enjoying yet again the childlike brilliance of their teacher.

"Like that, without ever getting entangled in the misery of the world, one can reduce its impact to nothing, simply by establishing the mind in the Self, in pure Being. And what we can do on an individual level is just what Lord Shiva is always doing on a cosmic level. The two are one. That is the real meaning of our Shivaratri: the one unbroken pure Consciousness shining eternally in the midst of the surrounding darkness. It's so beautiful, so very beautiful".

Sleep

A psychic healer visits the ashram. He believes that dreams are a way to understand the past and foresee the future and therefore considers dreaming to be in some sense a superior state of awareness to normal waking consciousness. A lively debate ensues on the relative merits of the waking, dreaming and sleeping states.

The Master agrees that dreams can sometimes act as omens about the future, but points out that from the point of view of what the texts call 'the fourth' – the unchanging, transcendental awareness that lies beyond the sates of waking, dreaming and sleeping – there is very little to choose between the three. They all obscure the pure awareness, are all limited by the conditions of time and space and are all mutually exclusive. Moreover, on these counts, none of them can be said to have an abiding reality.

"But if one had to choose, sleep is definitely the superior state".

Everyone is surprised by this.

He explains:

"Pure awareness is our real nature, but normally obscured. In the waking state gross names and forms are registered, in the dreaming state solely mental creations are perceived and in sleep, the mind rests in the causal level. In this suspended state the individual soul is as if absolute because all limitations fade away and what remains is a tranquillity undisturbed by differences. There is a complete absence of any body-awareness and any limiting perceptions, problems or suffering have disappeared. This tells us two things. Firstly, that all problems and suffering are consequent on body-awareness and its associated mental activity. Secondly, that sleep has an enjoyable nature that approximates to our real nature, the Self. And this is clearly stated in the Upanishads. It is because of this enjoyment that the mind voluntarily renounces all external awareness in sleep, and why everyone enjoys being asleep. That state beyond mental activity gives a taste of the inherent happiness of the Self. So, on this analysis, there can be no doubt that sleep is superior to waking and dreaming!"

Some of those who are present look perplexed as they try to assimilate the implications of what they have just heard.

With a rather conspiratorial smile, the Master continues:

"Well, do you doubt this? Look how people prepare for sleep so as to experience the happiness it brings. They pile up soft cushions, lay down silk sheets and shawls and dim the lamps, all to put an end to the state of wakefulness! Yet once they are asleep, all those efforts are useless, they have served their purpose".

"Alright," comes an objection "but there is no positive pleasure in sleep; it just gets rid of fatigue, that's all".

"Yes, it does indeed get rid of fatigue, but the point here is that the one who enjoys that freedom from fatigue continues to exist. That is why on waking everyone says 'I slept well', 'I had a wonderful sleep and feel good' and so on. So there is some continuity between sleeping and waking, on the basis of which the pleasure of the former is remembered in the latter. This continuity is the state of pure Being".

The questioner still looks sceptical, unable to grasp the argument. Seeing this, the Master continues once more:

"Well, do you deny that you continue to exist in your sleep also?"

After a moment's thought the other replies:

"No, I suppose I do continue to exist, but the thing is I am not aware in my sleep, so it is as if I don't exist, and I might just as well not".

"Now, look closely at that 'as if'! In sleep, as we have just agreed, there is no awareness of the body and the world, and so it appears to be a state of dullness because there was not the individual there with a mind to conjure up images, thoughts and the like. But the fact remains that there *is* a continuity, otherwise, how would you know who you were when you woke up the next morning? So despite there not being the subjective experience of being an individual perceiving objects, a continuity is there. This continuity is what endures and it is opposed to what is discontinuous and transitory, which is the experience of the outside world fed us by the mind's activity. This is because the state of Being is permanent and the body, mind and world are not".

"But if the experience of deep sleep is bliss as you say, why do I not recollect it more clearly?"

"It is like those fishermen who dive for jewels. They locate pearls at the bottom of the sea, but cannot make their finds known to the merchant who is waiting expectantly on the shore until they emerge from the water. Like that, the sleeper cannot express his experience because withdrawn deep within he has no contact with the outer organs of expression until, in due course, he is woken up by the re-emergence of his mind, and the waking state takes over once more. Still, the lingering recollection 'I slept well' persists, at least, just as the diver remembers the pearls he has seen".

"If sleep is really so enjoyable, why does the mind return to waking?"

"Due to the force of its latent impressions, unfinished actions, the pull of memory and so on".

"So your point Master is that, relatively speaking, the experience – if we can use that word – of the sleep state is nearer to pure awareness than the experience of the waking or dreaming states?"

"Certainly it is, yes."

After a moment's pause, the *sannyasi* continues:

"And there is yet another way that sleep can been seen as similar to pure awareness. It is your daily experience that when you pass from the peace of deep sleep to waking, the 'I' thought comes back and with it the body and the world. Now, if you want to be clearer about this, train yourself to be aware of the waking-up process. If you do, you will see there are stages in it. First there is sleep. Then, just before waking fully, comes a state of just being, free of thoughts, a junction point between the state of sleep and the waking state, as it were. Associated with that junction point is a native happiness. Next comes the first stirring of the latent mental impressions that give rise to the sense of 'I', and these stirrings develop into complete wakefulness along with the awareness of the outside world and all the rest of it".

"Should we then stay asleep as much as possible?"

"Oh no!" The Master rocks with laughter. "To begin with, to do so is impossible, because waking, dreaming and sleeping come and go automatically of their own accord, beyond our control. And even though sleep can in some sense be called enjoyable, as we have just seen, because it comes and goes, the enjoyment it offers is nowhere near the bliss experienced by those who are liberated. Those sages enjoy a happiness that is unbroken. And whereas sleep is for most people a blank, devoid of awareness, liberation is a direct consciousness that persists continuously, no matter which of the three transitory states may be superimposed on it. Pure Being is not dull, but lively, a happiness in which stillness and awareness are balanced. As such, it can be said to lie between sleep and waking and also between the rising of two thoughts. It should never be confused with sleep.

"Now, in practical terms, the thing is to stop worrying unduly about sleep, and start valuing the waking state! Use it to make every effort to transcend the changing modes of the mind altogether. That way you will find the pure Being in your own case and then all these things will be self-evident".[190]

As so often, all present are delighted by the Master's ability to enter a discussion from a fresh and unexpected angle and thereby shed a radically new light on the topic under consideration.

Soul and God

"Master, what is the difference between the soul and God?"

"Paddy and rice. Remove the skin of the paddy and it is rice. Like that, remove the covering of *maya*, and the soul will reveal its pure inner nature, which is God".

Soul and Self

A teacher called Ashmarathya came to the ashram to promote his teaching. He was well-known as an opponent of Vedantic non-dualism, preferring instead a doctrine that taught the individual soul constitutes a paradox: both different, yet not different, from the universal Self.[191]

Having saluted the Master respectfully, he begins to put his case: "As I see it, the relationship between the individual soul and the universal Self is like the sparks and the fire they arise from. The sparks are not absolutely different from the fire, because they are made of fire, yet on the other hand they cannot be said to be absolutely non-different from it, because if they were, they could not be distinguished from it nor, indeed, from each other. Similarly, individual souls, which are a reflection of the Self, are neither absolutely different from the Self – for that would mean that they are not made of pure intelligence – nor can they be said to be absolutely non-different from the Self, because in that case they could not be distinguished from each other and they would all be omniscient, as is the Self. And if that were true, apart from anything else, it would be useless to give them any instruction! Therefore, to be accurate, we have to say that the individual soul is an ontological paradox; it is somehow different from the Self yet also somehow non-different".

Despite the acuity of this visitor's argument, today the Master is in no mood to humour him. Shaking his head vigorously he replies: "According to Vedanta, which is acknowledged by the wise to be the culmination of knowledge[192], the individual soul and the cosmic Self differ in name only. The perfect oneness of the two is proven by the experience of the fully enlightened on the one hand and countless

219

textual authorities on the other.[193] So it is senseless to insist on a plurality of selves or to claim that the individual soul and the universal Self are different from one another. Certainly, the Self is called by many different names, but it is always and only singular and non-dual. Whatever differences may appear to exist are solely due to the impositions of conditioning factors, such as the body and mind, which have no ultimate or enduring reality. These differences are therefore the imaginings of ignorance, no matter how real they may appear to the conventional or unawakened intelligence.

"Likewise, the conceptual divisions and boundaries that spring from such false imaginings have themselves no enduring validity. In short those teachers, such as that fellow Audulomi, who insist there is a distinction between the individual soul and the supreme Self violate correct logic and imagine that liberation is something that is somehow produced by the mind. They also oppose themselves to the true meaning of the sacred texts and by so doing they act as obstructions to perfect knowledge, which is the open door to supreme beatitude".[194]

Realising there is to be no agreement, Ashmarathya makes no reply and sits quietly for the rest of the *darshan*.

Speech and silence

Although the Master spends much of his time in verbal teaching and instruction, there are many occasions when he gives silent *darshan*, saying nothing, just radiating the ineffable peace and happiness he always carries with him. All who come into this atmosphere feel its effect; for many it can be a life-changing experience. The subtle instruction being imparted here is that the Self is omnipresent in the midst of everyday activities, without there having to be any discussion or cogitation about it. A questioner asks:

"Maharaj shri, how can silence be so powerful?'

"A realised being naturally emits waves of spiritual influence which can draw many people towards him. He may sit in a cave and maintain complete silence, yet just to come into contact with such a soul, even if he says nothing, will certainly have its effect".

Then:

"Words are limited. After all, how does speech arise? First there is the abstract consciousness, out of which the ego, the limited sense of 'I' arises. This 'I' in turn gives rise to thought and from thought is born the spoken word. So the word is but the great-grandson of the original silent source. If the word can produce an effect, then you can see for yourself how much more powerful a teaching through silence could be".

Spiritual experiences

Question:

"I have been doing yoga, meditation and service of the poor for many years, yet I have not been granted any of the spiritual experiences that everyone says accompany the journey to enlightenment. What am I doing wrong, Sir?"

Reply:

"This is a beautiful question. Note well, what are commonly called 'spiritual experiences' are in fact temporary modifications of the mind, alterations to the limited sense of 'I'. Such inner experiences may be glamorous or exotic, distracting or consoling, but they are still just modes of the ego. There is an 'I', a limited self somewhere that is seeking respite from fear or suffering or boredom by enjoying these exalted experiences. And no such experience, whether we label it spiritual or worldly, can last, no matter how much we may wish it to. So the real meaning of experience lies not in itself, but in its role as a means to understand the one who experiences. It is only when the experiencing ego is fully transcended that the beauty which lies eternally behind it will shine forth in all its glory".

"And what is it that lies behind the ego, Sir?"

"The transcendental Self".

Stages on the path

It is early one morning in January and, as happens each morning at this time of year, the mighty Ganges is hidden by a heavy mist. All along its bank people are beginning to go about their daily routines, shadowy figures swathed in heavy blankets and shawls, spectres in the cold half-light. The whole scene has an unreal, dreamlike quality to it.

A group of pilgrims arrives at the ashram. They are from the Great Desert to the West; tall, good-looking people, the men with full beards and huge white turbans, their women wearing voluminous heavy skirts beautifully embroidered in bright colours and intricate patterns. Camel and goat-herders by trade, their tribe has a tradition of taking a keen interest in spiritual teachings ever since, generations earlier, some of the early followers of the Buddha set up monastic communities in their remote lands. The group is in a celebratory mood today, on their way to visit the birthplace of Lord Buddha in the Himalayan foothills, while stopping off to see the sights and take the *darshan* of holy men along the way. Yesterday they went to the Deer Park, the site of the Buddha's first discourse, which is situated some miles beyond the walls of the holy city that is Kashi.

For his part, the Master seems in a particularly playful mood as well. One of the pilgrims asks him:

"Maharaj-ji, you have a great reputation all over the Land of the Veda and we are seekers after Truth. Can you tell us how many stages are there on the path to Enlightenment?"

"There are two stages" comes the reply. "The first is to realise who you really are; the second to realise what the world really is".

"And that is it? This is strange to my ears, Sir, because we have always been taught there are many stages on the way".

"Actually," continues the Master, "there is only one stage. You are the Self and the world is the Self and there is nothing but the Self, so there is only one stage to accomplish and that is to realise the Self".

"Now you say there is only one stage?"

"Strictly speaking," confides the Master, chuckling now, "there are no stages at all! The Self always is and the Self always has been and the Self always will be, so how can there be any question of realising it in stages? Actually, all that can happen is that whatever appears to be obscuring this ever-present Self has to be removed, that's all.

It is just this process of removal that gives rise to ideas of a path and stages and all that rigmarole".

"Oh Maharaj! Now I am completely confused! First you said there are two stages, then one, then none – which of these positions is true?"

The answer comes in a more serious tone now.

"To tell the truth, they are all true. As with everything else in life, it just depends on your point of view".

The Master gestures beyond the window.

"It is like the beginning of the day. Everything starts off dark, covered in mist, but as soon as the sun begins to rise, the darkness retreats and the mist starts gradually to thin out and eventually, as the sun rises higher, darkness and mist vanish without a trace and there is the full sunlight. Like that, ignorance takes a little time to thin out and disappear, and this is why we follow the path, practice our meditations, visit the temple with devotion and so on.

"Ultimately, the Truth will stand revealed in its full glory as That which has always been the case. And once you are enjoying the warm caress of the sun, who cares to remember the darkness or think about the mist, analysing how thick it was at one time and how much thinner at another time and so on? It has vanished, that's all, like the mirage it always was, and all that remains is the enjoyment of the sunshine".

The party feels energised by the Master's robust and uncomplicated exposition. Fruits and *prasad*[195] are distributed and the pilgrims go on their way in a cheerful mood, buoyed up by the encounter.

Stay in one boat

An elderly woman comes for *darshan*. She was initiated into meditation by a highly-respected yogi in the Himalayan foothills and practised under his guidance for some time. Then she met another teacher who taught her a different method. She tried that. Then, unsatisfied, she tried combining the two systems. Now she is confused.

"The spiritual path is like crossing a river. If you want to cross a river, you stay in one boat don't you? You don't keep jumping from one to another; to do so creates a lot of fuss that just delays your journey, and you could even fall into the water! No, generally, it is advisable to stay in one boat".

"Well, I did that for some time with my first technique, Sir, and it didn't seem to be getting me anywhere, it didn't seem to be working".

"Were you following the instructions correctly?"

A momentary hesitation.

"Yes".

"Then it *was* working but its effects were just not what you had imagined they would be. It is a question of correct understanding. Perhaps the fault lay not so much in the teaching as in your erroneous expectations of what would be its effects".

A longer pause. Then:

"So what is the yardstick of a valid teaching, Sir? How can we judge if we are using the appropriate method?"

"Its efficacy when practised correctly".

"And what is the test of a teaching's origin?"

"The authentic tradition of transmission behind it".

Then, after another pause:

"Of course, we do see that when a child reaches the limit of a particular class in school, he moves up to the next one. To do so is a natural and necessary progression. Like that, it may happen that the seeker needs to move on from one teacher to another, but there are limits in this also. If one is fortunate enough to have been exposed to the authentic Vedic tradition, there is no higher level. Our Vedanta teaches non-duality, the oneness of all life. What could surpass that?"

Stories

People who come to the Master are often charmed by the stories that he tells to illustrate various points of the teaching. He is a natural raconteur with an unerring sense of timing and humour.

One day a woman asks:

"Maharaj-ji, you speak so eloquently! Please tell us one of your beautiful stories".

But the Master shakes his head.

"Lecturing is not my profession! My profession is to produce the effect of expansion in the awareness of everyone who comes into my contact. It is not a matter of telling stories, no. My profession is to help the drop expand into the dignity of the ocean. This has nothing to do with telling stories".

Strange darshan

For some weeks now the Master has enjoyed visiting an ancient Shiva shrine known as the Tilbhandeshwar Temple. The *lingam* in the holy of holies is kept under worship by a dedicated old priest and people consider it to be especially powerful, though due to the shift in the financial circumstances of the family that has traditionally been the patron of the temple, the place is not well kept up. The grounds have reverted to nature and become overgrown with huge, brooding trees and tangled with creepers, while the walled compound is littered with pieces of masonry that have fallen off the building due to the heavy rains of successive monsoons. Some of these stones are quite large and assume strange shapes in the half-light. The whole place has a powerful, haunting atmosphere. Tantrik sadhus with their matted hair and atavistic energy camp in the surrounding woods, especially at festival times, but most of the common people give the place a wide berth, fearing it to be full of spirits.

At dusk one evening the Master is sitting here serenely, with a group of followers around him. Suddenly a large king cobra appears, seemingly from nowhere and only three or four feet in front of him. Nobody noticed it enter the circle and there is sudden consternation. One of the *brahmacharis* leaps up and grabs a stick but the Master motions him to stay where he is.

He stares intently at the snake, which has risen up, opened out its magnificent hood and is swaying from side to side in a hypnotic sort of dance. The communication between man and beast seems to be direct and mutual. This play continues for some minutes, until the creature finally lies down again, slithers right up to touch the feet of the Master and then slowly moves around to go behind him. It disappears into a pile of overgrown rubble at the edge of the compound.

The Master immediately orders the shrine be prepared for the ritual of *abhishekam*, despite the fact that it is the custom in this place to perform *puja* only once daily in the early morning. Still, the Master insists that the priest be summoned and all preparations made. He asks the group to leave the temple; he alone will stay for the ritual. His followers carry out his instructions, dimly aware that something momentous has occurred but unable to say exactly what.

Supernormal powers

The Master generally demonstrates little interest in supernormal *siddhi* powers, although they are frequently attributed to him. On the other hand, many who come into his orbit are fascinated by the topic. When questioned on the subject, he often replies that the value of supernormal powers is limited, because they result from the operation of a mind that is still confined to its own individual activity, albeit at an extraordinarily refined level. Thus while such powers can be considered to be the perfections of an awareness that is still extraverted, they remain antagonistic to that inner consciousness – the pure Self – which resides forever unattached to each and every movement of the mind.[196]

Given this, *siddhis* in themselves count for little in the spiritual life. In fact, because they confer power on the aspirant, such abilities can actually constitute a diversion, or even a danger, on the path of complete self-transcendence. Nevertheless, the Master is happy to discuss *siddhis* if and when the question arises usefully in the context of instruction about the path to enlightenment and the application of higher consciousness to the world structured within the boundaries of time and space.

The starting point for the following discussion is the ability of enlightened beings to project their consciousness into other bodies.

"Certainly, the accomplished *siddha* can enter into multiple bodies! And how can he do such a thing? Because his mind is not as firmly anchored to his individual body as is the case with those whose karmic residues are dense and heavy. See, in the normal person, their large mass of unresolved *karmas* ties the mind firmly to a particular body but, due to the repeated experience of *samadhi*, this mass becomes thinned out and loosened up, as it were. This attenuation of karmic ties first gives the *yogi* knowledge of how his own mind moves – what thrills it, what deludes it, what disturbs it and so on – and then, when he knows his own mind with clarity and dispassion, he can draw it out of his body and install it in other bodies. And as his mind goes, so the senses follow it, like the bees follow the queen when she leaves the nest. If his subtle life-energy is successfully installed in another body, then that body becomes animated by it and the senses are distributed throughout it. In this way it is possible for the accomplished *yogi* to enjoy awareness and experience through the body his mind has assumed.[197]

"This is extraordinary Sir! How can a limited individual exhibit such an almost unlimited power?"

"They are the fruit of his limited mind enjoying a prolonged sojourn in the unlimited Absolute. In the whole scale of things, this process of attaining *siddhi* powers is comparable to reaching a heavenly realm or realising an identity with a particular deity. But let us be clear here: all these accomplishments are not the result of full and direct liberation into the Absolute".

On another occasion a question arises about the status of a *siddha*:

"It is taught in the scriptures that a *siddha* attains spiritual sovereignty and all the gods bring him tributes. Does this mean that such a one is omniscient?"

"No", is the firm reply. "The enlightened being is intimately familiar with everything that arises, for he himself is the omnipresent Self and the Self is everything. So he sees himself in everything – from Lord Brahma the creator of the universe right down to the dullest inanimate objects – and by the same token, he knows all things as the one Self.[198] So because he knows the essence of everything that exists, and this knowledge is unfailing, in that general sense it can be said that he 'knows everything'. But in specific terms he does not know everything, every detail, no. He does not know the number of grains of sand on the banks of the Ganges – how could he and why should he? Even if such a thing were possible, what would be the point?

"Having said which, when it is focussed, such a mind has powers far beyond the normal. The usual mind has to gain its knowledge through the senses or the intellect, but the purified mind can attain knowledge directly, through a kind of intuitive perception that has no need to utilise any cumbersome senses or reasoning. It just bypasses them. This situation is like an expert goldsmith who can tell the weight of a lump of gold instinctively by looking at it, without having to use the scales. He just knows, whereas others who do not have his expertise have to go through a lengthy process before they can come to a conclusion: picking up the gold, putting it on the scales to weigh it, then reading how far the needle has moved and so on. But we cannot call this intuitive way of knowing 'omniscience' in the sense that the word is usually understood".

"That sounds more like a supernormal power ..."

"Not really", continues the Master. "After all, the principle of possessing a different ability that enables one to go straight to the point is readily observable in daily life. We have just heard about the goldsmith. If you need another example, imagine a heavy rock with several men working together to lift it. Then along comes one fellow who is exceptionally strong and he can lift it easily on his own without needing the help of all the others. Job done! Like that, the pure mind can cognise objects directly due to its inherent clarity of awareness, without needing the co-operation of the body and senses in the way the typical impure mind does".[199]

"Are the great *siddhas* omnipotent, then?" persists the same questioner.

"Again, the answer is 'no' and for the same reason. As the Self, the realised man becomes the vital energy of all beings; he is the mind of all beings and the actions of all beings and nothing can obstruct this sense of essential unicity. Through it, so to speak, he becomes the doer of everything. This is because being himself infinite, he is the wholeness, the totality that is manifesting itself through innumerable various pieces and parts. But it is not that he is identified with each and every one of these finite parts itself. So when he becomes all bodies by virtue of being one with their essence, of course he is not thereby subject to the pains and pleasures that each separate and particular body may be feeling".

"Can you explain further, Sir?"

"Alright, let us now imagine there is an argument in which one man insults another. Now, a realised being who saw this argument would feel himself to be the Self of the insulter, but equally he is the Self of the insulted. Therefore he would feel no pain on account of it; having no partiality, you see, he is perfectly unattached to both parties. Or, to take another example, it is like a person who is grieving at the death of a family member. Some onlooker to the scene who is not a member of the dead person's family or one of their friends will not feel any personal bereavement or sense of loss.

"Like that, although he sees his own Self to be the doer of everything, the realised man does not feel himself to be connected to, or indeed separated from, anything in particular. He is infinite and so he remains perfectly unattached".[200]

After a pause, the Master continues pensively:

"There is also another reason why the word 'omnipotent' cannot be applied to a person who has *siddhis*. Omnipotence must imply the ability to govern the universe, must it not? Now, this power belongs only to the ever-perfect Lord, the Self; only that One can create, maintain and dissolve the universe. It is to emphasise this unique stature that the sacred texts describe him as 'eternal'. No *siddha* can justly be termed eternal, because his abilities result from a gradual process of perfection that takes place through time, they are not innate or present there all at once. So even the most accomplished *siddha* is dependent on the will of the Lord, he does not enjoy that omnipotent status himself, though he certainly has divine powers.

"And anyway", he chuckles "just imagine if all those *siddhas* actually *were* omnipotent! Each one still has a different mind and all those different minds could have conflicting desires. One might want to dissolve the universe, another to preserve it and a third one something else again. What on earth would happen then?"[201]

The room sparkles with laughter, knots of thought are loosened.

The topic clearly continues to fascinate those present and another question follows immediately:

"Then if a *siddha* chooses to indulge in these divine powers, can we say he is thereby limited in some way?"

The Master nods.

"And does this then mean that he will have to return to this earth after death?"

"Ah, this is a beautiful question. On this point our great Master, Badarayana,[202] liked to refer to those texts that teach that *siddhas* do not return to the whirlpool of human life after death, but go instead to the celestial world of Brahma, the Creator. Once they have reached that level, their ignorance becomes finally destroyed by right knowledge and their vestigial individuality becomes dissolved in the Eternal. And this is also how all those who commune directly with the Absolute through its finite manifestations can themselves avoid returning to earth".

With these words the Master becomes quite abstracted, his awareness seeming to retreat within. A great silence falls on the gathering. Time seems to hang suspended; when he returns he remarks, almost inaudibly but with immense peace and conviction:

"They do not return, because this is what the Upanishads teach us. No return; this is what the Upanishads teach us".[203]

Textual consistency

"It seems to me, Sir, that you base your arguments on cleverly selecting only certain verses from the scriptures and rejecting others".

"Fine!" beams the Master, quite unfazed by the provocative tone of the question, which comes from a scholarly young priest.

"Let us look at these scriptures together. Now, the Vedic texts teach us about the nature of the Absolute. Indeed, it is clearly stated that those scholars of the Veda who do not know about the Absolute deserve to have their cattle taken away from them! And in fact there are many well-known tales of such ignorant teachers meeting bad ends. I'm sure you know about Yajnavalkya and Shakalya?"[204]

"Yes, Sir, I do".

"Good. Now, of all the Vedic texts, it is the Upanishads which describe that Reality most clearly; all the various verses of the Upanishads taken together form one coherent whole, which is oriented only and always towards celebrating the Absolute and realising the Absolute. This being so, no saying of the sacred scriptures may be rejected but, once heard, it should certainly be added to the rest, even though these already form a consistent whole. Moreover, the omission of something in one place in the scriptures cannot override its inclusion in another".[205]

"Well, I have no doubt that you are always emphasising the formless Absolute, but what about those passages that clearly reiterate the necessity of performing rites?"

"The first thing we have to understand is that the only way the sacred texts can speak about an entity that is not yet known, which is wholly abstract and transcendental, is by resorting to ordinary, familiar words with ordinary, familiar meanings. We approach the unknown through the known. There is a story that the great Vedantin teacher Dravidacharya used to tell:

> There was once a prince who was discarded by his parents at birth and brought up in the family of a fowler. Unaware of his true descent, he grew up imagining himself to be a fowler and pursued that occupation when he grew up. But it chanced that a very compassionate man, who knew the real situation, came by the fowler's house one day and told the young prince the true state of affairs. Appraised of the reality, the young fowler immediately abandoned his hut and moved into the palace to take up his real duties as a monarch. Like that, when a man living in ignorance and suffering is told by a teacher that he is in reality nothing but the Absolute, but has been living in exile so to speak, like a spark separated from a fire, then he realises his true status and abandons identification with the limited self and all its miseries.[206]

"So, like that humble fowler discovering his royal identity, Self-realisation involves a complete turn-around in consciousness on the part of the seeker. If the true state of affairs is to be described to a man in ignorance, the only way to make it comprehensible is to use examples that he is already familiar with".

The questioner nods; he has got the point.

"Now, to return to your question. The concrete world of religious rites is concerned with improving man's material lot and such an endeavour is certainly more familiar and comprehensible to most people than the abstract spiritual reality of the Absolute. But this does not mean that the Upanishadic passages on the Absolute must clash with the authority of ritualistic texts and their injunctions. It is just that they have a different meaning and a different end, that is all.

"Nevertheless, it is also the case that there are indeed certain absolutist passages in the scriptures whose sole purpose is to inculcate a detachment from the objects of the senses that everyone is habitually attracted to. When the mind is weaned off its usual tendencies, there arises the non-attachment that culminates in the direct experience that you yourself are the Absolute. And rest assured, once it dawns, this glorious realisation will take you far beyond the realm of the Vedic rites".[207]

Texts, rules and meditation

A yoga teacher speaks up.

"Surely Swami-ji, it is said clearly in the holy texts that certain conditions are necessary for meditation: you must sit in a certain place, face a particular direction, practice at a certain time and so on. Yet I have heard that you are relaxed about such things".

The Master replies evenly:

"Actually, all that really matters as regards the time, place and direction is that they are conducive to focussing the mind without effort. The scriptures do certainly prescribe detailed rules of procedure, but these apply only to certain fire offerings to the deities. No such specific regulations are recorded for meditation. In fact, mental focus may be attained anywhere".

The questioner is not convinced.

"But with respect, Sir, some passages *do* mention specific rules. For example, it is said in the scriptures:

> Let a man apply himself to meditation in a level and clean place like a windless cave, free from pebbles, fire, dust and noise, far from public places full of people, a place favourable to the mind and eye.[208]

"Well, yes", admits the Master, "such instances can indeed be found but these are only ideals. The teacher who is a real friend to his students is always pragmatic about strict rules such as these. And notice the phrase you just quoted: *'favourable to the mind'*. Surely, this implies that meditation may be carried on wherever it is easy for the mind to settle".[209]

Textual contradictions

A learned scholar from an academy of philosophy comes forward with a direct challenge:

"Sir, you teach Vedanta which is based on the Upanishads, but I find that particular system to be baseless!"

"Oh, do you now? How so?"

"Because its principal texts all contradict one another! For example, when describing creation, they disagree on its successive stages. One says the Absolute *brahman* gave rise to space from which emerged matter, another claims that creation began with fire, another with light. Then one teaches that creation originated from 'Non-existence', another says from 'Pure Existence', while yet another offers the theory that the world arose spontaneously. In practice, it seems they are really describing many different creations and therefore they cannot be accepted as authorities for determining an ultimate cause. If we wish to find the Truth, our only hope is to ignore the muddle of the texts and have recourse to human reason. That way at least there will be some consistency".

"You are correct in so far as Vedantic texts such as the various Upanishads may well conflict with each other when they describe the stages by which creation unfolds, but they are always in agreement when describing its first cause. In every case they concur that this cause is the Absolute. It may sometimes be personified as the omniscient Lord of all, but the non-dual Absolute is always said to be the creator of everything. Mark well: conflicting descriptions of how creation manifests once it has been initiated in no way affect the statements concerning its ultimate cause".[210]

There is a pause while a *brahmachari* brings some query about ashram business to the Master's attention and he deals with it. Then:

"And anyway, a conflict of statements regarding the world doesn't really matter greatly, since the creation of the world and similar topics are not really what these scriptures wish to teach. As they themselves point out, and as we ourselves can easily observe, a person's happiness has nothing to do with his being conversant with such abstract theories. Such things are therefore of secondary importance. All the passages dealing with them serve a single and greater purpose, which is to teach about the Self. So the analogies and hierarchical categories and complex lists that describe the manifestation of the world are there to show, from various points of view, one thing and one thing only: that the effects, no matter how various, derive from a single ultimate cause.

"Every teacher who follows the true tradition agrees on this. Gaudapada the Great said it very clearly: if creation of the many from the One is represented by means of various similes – pots formed from clay, tools made of iron, sparks springing up from a fire and so on – that is only a means for making it understood that in reality, everything

233

is a manifestation of one sole unifying cause, the infinite Consciousness we call the Self.[211]

"And as to human reason", the Master continues, "the scriptures expressly mention that the fruit of knowing this Self is 'obtaining the highest and overcoming grief'. Such an exalted gain can never be the result of laborious reasoning, but stems from direct spiritual intuition and insight into the ultimate nature of things. And what is more, this immediate Self-knowing is the only way that one can go beyond death and achieve immortality".

This is stretching things for the scholar.

"Immortality? How can this be?"

"As soon as a man directly experiences the truth of the phrase 'You are That', he becomes one with the Absolute which is simultaneously his immortal Self and the undying essence of all."

"But overcoming death...?"

"As the Self does not die, it cannot reincarnate. And anyway, as it is already omnipresent, how could it leave wherever it was and where could it go that it was not already present? Therefore it is also taught that the whole edifice of death and reincarnation vanishes for him who becomes one with the Self".[212]

The Absolute is uncaused

In all he does and teaches, the Master is one-pointedly concerned with communicating the Absolute. For him, all forms celebrate the Formless, and his unceasing joy is to be and live and radiate that undying essence of life. While he is adamant that the Absolute has to be a direct experience and not just a dry intellectual concept to be discussed, much of the time he is called upon to refute the theories of philosophical opponents on the subject. This he does with gusto and evident enjoyment, utilising a combination of rational argument and pragmatic examples in a manner that proves irrefutable. The following exchange is typical.

A highly educated man asks:

"How can the supreme Reality be described?"

"Nothing can really be said about the nature of the Absolute", comes the answer. "To tell the truth, it is beyond words, indescribable. This is because the absolute Totality we call *brahman* has two aspects which are logically opposed. One aspect appears full of limitation, due to the various attributes of the universe produced by the superimposition of innumerable names and forms; the other aspect is devoid of all attributes and appears to stand apart, quite opposed to them.[213] Many sacred texts reiterate this paradoxical fact. Nevertheless, for the sake of better understanding and to give us a means of approach, we can provisionally assign attributes to the Absolute. So, we can describe it as that pure Being, unqualified Existence, from which the entire universe of time and space originates. Or, if you prefer, we can look on it as the supreme Lord, who creates, ordains and guides the empirical world".[214]

"You use the word 'creator', Maharaj. How do we know that the Absolute itself did not spring from something else?"

"In the sequence of cause and effect, the cause is always prior, and therefore senior, to the effect. If we look at the world, we see that anything particular or concrete is the effect of something that is subtler, more general or more abstract. For example, it is clear that jars and pots are produced from clay, not the other way around. But there is nothing prior or senior to the Absolute. And why not? Because as we have seen, the Absolute is omnipresent Being or pure Existence and there can be nothing subtler, more abstract or more general than that. Therefore, we can conclude that just as the greater cannot emerge from the lesser, the Absolute cannot spring from anything particular, nothing could have caused it, nor is it the effect of anything else. Any other opinion defies logic. This is irrefutable, is it not?"

The Master is clearly enjoying himself. The opponent retorts:

"But some authorities say Being arose from non-being".

"Oh no, that is impossible! A cause is the self of its effects to be sure, but 'non-being' is mere absence. As such it has no self-nature to enable or empower it to be a cause of anything. Everywhere throughout the universe, effects in turn become causes themselves and thus give birth to other effects, but the Absolute is not the effect of something other than itself, as we have just seen. So in this case we must admit the Absolute to be the ultimate causal substance which is itself uncaused, otherwise we would fall into an infinite regression of causes, which is nonsensical".[215]

235

The bliss of liberation

Few things are more thrilling to those around him than when the Master speaks of enlightenment. At such times his joy and vitality seem to know no bounds, and it becomes obvious that what is being offered in his teaching is not just some modification of the tired old patterns of human behaviour and development, but an order of existence that is a radical departure from the past, yet simultaneously our ancient birthright. A new evolutionary possibility for humankind is being displayed and such ecstatic glimpses serve to motivate his followers to pay renewed attention to the process of their own spiritual growth.

"Maharaj-ji, how would you describe the enlightened being?"

"Above all he is *happy*. But his happiness is not the usual human happiness, dependent on a transient object or circumstance – such happiness always lives in the shadow of its opposite, for the object or circumstance can always change. The sage's happiness is a continuous loving bliss that has no specific cause and therefore no opposite. It derives from the Self, which is one without a second, and as loving bliss is the nature of this non-dual Self, so he who knows the Self is by nature loving and blissful. This bliss depends on nothing external, it is just the joy of Being, the ecstasy of fully-enlivened Consciousness, which is naturally and spontaneously happy under all circumstances".

"How can we understand such bliss in terms of our normal experience?"

"Ha! It is as if the enlightened being enjoys all pleasures. And he enjoys them not one by one or sequentially, as a normal man might, but all together instantaneously, in one cognition that is as swift as the light of the sun. Now, how can such a state exist? It is possible because such a one is always enjoying the goal of all desires, which is the Absolute. Because he has realised his identity with the Absolute, in that capacity it is as if he enjoys all pleasures at once, and as his very own Self. His sport and delight are in the Self alone; for him, all is just loving bliss, always and in every way, occasioned solely by the Self and independent of all limiting external objects such as a body, or senses, or a life of *karmas* or any mere physical enjoyment depending on another. He has been crowned an independent spiritual monarch in his own lifetime and he rules without effort over a kingdom that is infinite and undivided, far transcending any kingdom in the mundane world. He has become the supreme Spirit, utterly serene, forever established in its own nature as the Self of all.

"As such then, he roams free, playing his way through the world and singing the ecstatic song of non-difference wherever he goes. He is always enunciating the unicity and sole reality of the Self for the benefit of all beings and he is also continuously astonished and delighted by the freshness of his own realisation that he himself is everything he comes across. He is the food and the eater and the eating that unites them! He is the entire world because he is the Self of the entire world, and he simultaneously engulfs the entire world with his true nature, which is the Self, the unsurpassed Lord of all. The light of his infinite awareness is as eternal as the sun and in him alone rests the immortality of all beings. Truly, my dear friends, this state is utterly glorious and as such it lies far beyond normal comprehension".[216]

The body is not what you are

The Master frequently cites identification with the body as the prime criterion of metaphysical ignorance and worldly suffering. Conversely, freedom from this attachment is central to the enlightened state. He teaches that limiting one's sense of identity to the body is an erroneous perception – a hallucination in effect – that is universal, operating just as much in those who are learned in the scriptures as in the unschooled. Lack of identification with the body is not just an intellectual position, however, it is a living experience. The enlightened being rests free of body-identification, not because he doggedly holds onto the idea 'I am not the body', but because he has naturally woken up to the fact that he is the transcendental, non-physical Self. Non-dualism teaches that the Self is that boundless consciousness which endures as the essence of all transitory phenomena, the bodiless spirit in all bodies and the unstained, unattached awareness that persists through all the changing modes of the mind.[217]

Such fine distinctions are not always easily grasped by many of his listeners, as the following exchange makes clear.

A merchant comments:

"I must say I find it hard to conceive of living and acting without being attached to your own body. Forgive me for saying so, Maharaj, but to be honest, such a state sounds almost deranged to me. What am I if I am not the body?"

The Master laughs heartily for a long time.

"Yes, strange though it may sound, the majestic glory of the liberated one is precisely the realisation that he is bodiless. But you are right, from the conventional point of view it is not easy to understand such a state. So, let us imagine a wealthy householder who is very attached to his possessions. It is obvious that if he loses them, he will suffer pain. But one cannot then go on to say that when that same householder has renounced all those possessions and gone on the road as a wandering ascetic that he will continue to experience pain at being parted from them. Like that, when one is established in a natural state of renunciation from the body, one is automatically no longer affected by the pleasant or unpleasant events which that body may undergo. The scriptures are very clear on this", he adds, quoting a text to the effect that 'the Self suffers no running eyes or nose, decrepitude or death'[218]

A monk speaks up:

"I have heard that text myself, Maharaj, but I have always assumed it referred to the state after death".

"Oh no", replies the Master. "Identifying with the body is simply the result of wrong knowledge in life. It is a misperception that comes from erroneously conflating the Self and the body, as we discussed yesterday when we were talking about action and attachment".

The merchant again:

"This lack of identification you extol sounds a rather negative benefit to me, Sir. I can see it may well save one from physical hardship and discomfort, but it doesn't seem to provide anything really positive or pleasurable".

"Actually, the situation is quite the contrary! To be bodiless is to swim in bliss, because in this state there can be no recoil from anything. All feelings of dislike or difficulty come from experiencing something to be other than oneself, which means other than, and separate from, one's limited body-self. But for one who sees only his pure Self everywhere and in everything, there is nothing outside of himself to cause antagonism or revulsion. For one who has developed such all-comprehensive vision, what delusion or pain could remain? Delusion, suffering and their manifold consequences do not touch the one who lives as the pure, transcendental Self. For such a being, all is everywhere the non-dual and loving bliss".[219]

After a few moments of silence, the merchant picks up the thread again:

"May we come back to this question of identity, Sir? If I am not the body, as you say, then what on earth am I? This Self sounds all too abstract to grasp".

The Master laughs again at this, clearly pleased by the man's lack of pretension and his sincere desire to understand.

"A very good question. The truth is you are nothing on earth and nothing in the heavens either, come to that! Your true nature is transcendent, unborn, omnipresent and without a taint. You extend in all directions infinitely and have no relationship with any object whatsoever, including, strange though it may sound, your own body! You are immortal, self-luminous and always perfectly satisfied. Each and every change of circumstance that impinges on the body or mind is in truth nothing to do with you, since you are changeless. Seen in this light, all such mutations are really no more real than a dream. You are the supreme Consciousness, one without a second, immaculate. The simple fact is that you are the Lord of all who is ever the same, present in all beings and motionless as the heart of the ever-moving world".

The force of the Master's words charges the atmosphere with an awesome power. It is as if some other being has entered the room, an invisible but clearly palpable presence.

After some time the monk speaks up once more:

"If this is the case, Maharaj-ji, how then is such a one reborn?"

The Master shakes his head.

"Whoever is consciously established in their identity as the Absolute cannot be reborn. Again, our scriptures are very clear on this. Once the seed of mistaken attachment to the body has been transcended, the fruit of future embodiment cannot exist. People caught up in the 'body-delusion' run around here and there claiming 'this is mine' 'that is yours', 'this is who I uniquely am', and so on and so forth. The great ones, on the other hand, suffer no such delusion and are therefore free of its consequences. Awakened to the essential nature of consciousness as quite unconditioned, perceiving only itself through all the apparent configurations of manifestation, the sages are no longer attached to an individual and limited centre of awareness. Therefore they are free from any limiting sense of desire or agency consequent on that limitation, and they remain unattached to whatever action such an agent may perform. This being so, they are also free from the consequence of all such action, which is what fuels rebirth".

"So they do not reincarnate...?"

"How could they? As the Self, they already exist beyond all boundaries and so can have no other state to reach; being already omnipresent they can have no other place to go to".

The Master chuckles:

"As the Mahabharata tells us, even the gods would be driven mad by trying to locate where such liberated ones go after death! All true knowers of the Veda agree on this".

"But we see sages acting ..."

"Oh yes! Certainly, such great beings live and function in the everyday world of duality, but doing so does not for one moment blind them to the unity that pervades everything. They act in the world but experience themselves to be unlimited and beyond all sense of agency or ownership. Such are the knowers of Reality, and it is these great beings who have upheld our noble tradition of non-duality throughout the ages".[220]

The efficacy of ritual

An expert in Vedic ritual arrives seeking a debate with the Master. A devotee of Lord Rama, he is attached to the ancient temple, deep in the old city, where the faithful Hanuman-ji pleases his devotees to reside.[221] This man is a specialist in the performance of 'yajnas for heaven', a specific class of fire-offering that brings enjoyable experiences to the soul while it is residing in the subtle levels of creation after the death of the physical body. He is a subtle thinker, greatly respected by the common people and enjoys a reputation as something of an orator.

His opening words are ones the Master is very well used to hearing from the defenders of orthodoxy who seek him out.

"I have heard, young sage, that you teach knowledge of the Self to be of greater value than the performance of Vedic sacrificial ritual, because such rituals do not lead to final liberation?"

"That is so".

"Can you explain your position on this?"

"I can. We know that the life of the orthodox is ordered by numerous rites and injunctions as laid down by the sacred texts. These rites serve a valuable purpose in regulating the behaviour of those people who are prone to the usual human shortcomings – passion, hatred, spiritual dullness and the like. Such people are habitually driven to seek their own advantage in visible, material ways, and this tendency is what disinclines them to follow the teachings of the scriptures. Though they may be unaware of it, their very senses and organs are under dark influences and therefore the scriptures and rites serve a beneficial purpose in redirecting such people's natural impulses to higher ends. In this way, correct meditation and understanding can gradually dawn.[222]

"But none of these rites has anything to do with realising one's unity with the Self. And in this respect, it is legitimate to say that there is no difference between the ordinary religious rites that mark various stages in the life-cycle, such as the taking of the sacred thread, and those more specialised procedures that are ordained for particular occasions and specific results, such as the acquiring of cattle, children, wealth and so on. All such rituals apply only to those who live in the world of differences; none of them can lead to liberation".[223]

"And why not, Sir?"

"Because liberation is not an effect that is caused by something else. Liberation arises spontaneously with the destruction of bondage and bondage itself cannot be destroyed by any work or any action, because work can function only in the visible realms. Work can modify, purify and create conducive conditions, but this process is not in itself liberation; at best it acts as a preparation. Liberation, however, is the direct spiritual knowledge of the Self. And as the Self is eternally pure, it cannot be modified or purified or effected by something else, because all of these operations imply change and time and causality, none of which obtain in this case".[224]

The priest considers the answer carefully for some moments. Then:

"Very well, Sir, I understand your position. But surely you cannot deny that a soul can certainly enjoy the effects of its *karma* after shedding the gross body at death? We know from the scriptures that it continues to exist in the celestial levels of existence and while sojourning there it reaps the rewards of its actions".

"Yes", the Master nods his agreement.

"So, if rituals do not win a soul final liberation, are you implying that after it has enjoyed the fruits of the '*yajna* for heaven' in the celestial realms, it returns to Earth to take up a new body?"

"I am, yes".

"But how can this be Swami-ji?" continues the priest. "What is it that could draw the soul back to the bonds of earthly rebirth once it has tasted that celestial happiness?"

"The unresolved *karmas*".

"Ah, so you mean some residual effect of 'the *yajna* for heaven' is left over to draw the soul back into rebirth? This is similar to, let us say, the residual coating of oil that sticks to the inside of an oil jar, even after it has been emptied?"

At this point a large crow flaps noisily into the room and perches on the back of the Master's couch, eyeing the two men quizzically. Both laugh at the interruption, but the priest, keen to press his point, continues immediately:

"So, you are saying that a soul can no longer stay in the celestial levels once it has experienced almost all the effects of the '*yajna* for heaven'. To use another analogy, we could liken this to a man who has joined the king's service equipped with all the things which such service demands, but after being at court for a long time, he can no longer remain there because most of his things have become worn out. All he has left is, say... a pair of shoes and an umbrella!"

The Master smiles at the image.

"Ha! These are all nice arguments but I'm afraid they do not hold water, any more than your friend's worn-out umbrella does! Look, your reasoning is altogether unfounded because it ignores the fact that the effects of any action follow only that particular action. So, if rituals are performed to gain advantage in the heavenly worlds, it is only in those worlds that their effects will be manifested. Moreover, they will continue manifesting for only so long as that soul stays in that particular heaven. In this matter we firmly take our stand on scripture, which denies that rituals for heaven produce even a particle of an effect for a soul after it has once again descended to earth.

"And, as to your analogies: you are right when you say that some part of the oil does indeed continue to remain in the jar and some parts of the courtier's equipment do remain with him. This we can commonly see. But I'm afraid such metaphors are invalid in this case simply because, as I have just pointed out, the scriptures are clear that rituals performed to influence the soul's experience in the heavenly realms have their effects in those realms only. So with such rites, nothing remains over to influence life on Earth.

"What is more, once a soul is located back in an earthly body subsequent to its return from heaven, it will inevitably undergo both pleasant and unpleasant experiences, as we know well from common experience. Such mixed effects cannot be due to the residual consequences of the 'yajna for heaven' because if some effects of that yajna did in fact carry over to the earthly plane, those effects would always be beneficial because of the benign character of that particular ritual. From this we can see that the 'remainder' which draws the soul back to another body on earth is the residue of those actions performed in this world previous to the yajna, along with their appropriate fruits. This is nothing to do with the heavenly realms".

The priest looks thoughtful, unable to find a way around the young sannyasi's logic. After some consideration he picks up the thread once more:

"Hmm. Well, I see what you are saying Sir, but just how does all this operate? What are the mechanics?"

"Well, it operates in the same manner as karmas normally operate. In this life, the consequences of any action cannot begin to manifest if they are obstructed by the consequences of another action that are already in the process of manifesting. Just so, at the time of death, karmic consequences of less force will be obstructed in their operation by other karmic consequences that are of greater force. As in life, so in death: the more powerful take preference, as it were.

"And let us not forget, just because a body dies does not mean that all the various karmic fruits it has yet to experience have to be manifested together all at once. On the other hand, we cannot say that because only some of a person's karmas manifest with death, it means that the others are altogether extinguished. To say so would contradict the well-known fact that all actions must inevitably have their appropriate consequences; whether these consequences are manifested sooner or later in the scheme of things is beside the point.

"So, given all this, we have to understand that having enjoyed the fruits of 'the yajna for heaven', a soul descends once more to earthly life to reap its earthly karmas. You see, there is nothing random here. It is as the scriptures say: people belonging to the various castes and stages of life who sincerely perform their duties experience the appropriate fruits of their actions after death. Then, according to their residual karmas, they get born once more on earth in a certain environment and an appropriate family. In that new birth they duly enjoy varying amounts of beauty, longevity, knowledge, good conduct, wealth, happiness, intelligence and all the rest of it. Rituals for heaven on the other hand, along with their specific fruits, are only concerned with enjoyment in the celestial worlds experienced in between these successive earthly lives".[225]

The Master turns to stroke the crow that has been sitting quietly behind him all this time, its head on one side as if straining to catch each word. The bird stretches its glossy neck out and is obviously enjoying the attention.

After a few moments he turns back to the priest and easily picks up the discussion again:

"So, to return to our starting point: from the transcendental perspective of the enlightened state, scriptural injunctions and prohibitions are erroneous concepts, in the sense that they only apply to someone who cannot see that their Self is no more connected to their body than empty space is bound to an earthen pot that appears to enclose it".

"Then, you *are* saying that the scriptural injunctions are useless!"

Patiently, the Master continues:

"No, I am not saying that. Listen carefully. What I am saying is that scriptural injunctions are of use for those who take themselves to be the body. Such people certainly have need of them. Fine. But someone who has gone beyond the falsely-imagined identification with the body and has become the bodiless Self that inheres in all bodies, *that person*" – here he emphasises the words – "that person has no use for these injunctions and prohibitions, because he has become the Totality. And in this enlightened, all-encompassing state he already possesses, as it were, everything that could be gained or achieved".[226]

After the priest had made his obeisance and left, one of the monks quotes a curious passage from the Brahma Sutra to the effect that one who does not know the Self is 'the food of the gods'. He wonders if this is relevant to the debate in some way.

The Master nods his approval and launches the following radical analysis:

"Indeed it is, well seen! Now, the word 'food' here is used metaphorically to mean the cause of enjoyment. It doesn't refer to physical food as the gods do not eat as we humans do, chewing and swallowing. The Veda is clear on this when it says: 'The gods do not eat or drink; it is by merely *seeing* the nectar that they are satisfied'.

"So, the image of 'eating' here refers to the pleasure enjoyed by the gods, the nourishing gratification they derive subtly from the performances of sacrifices and the devotion of those who perform them. Just as a king is nourished by his subjects and a man by the feelings of those who love him – his wife, his children, his friends and so on – so the gods 'eat' the performers of ritual. However, in this process of enjoyment, the performers of the ritual are the subordinate partners. Both the gods who receive the sacrifice and the humans who perform it enjoy their mutual relationship and both gain benefit from it, but the performers are clearly in the inferior position. They live in debt, as it were, like the servants of a king who are subordinate to him, while at the same time living off his largesse.

"Now, this state of affairs all follows from the fact that those who sacrifice are ignorant of the Self. Again, scripture makes it very clear that someone who worships a deity – which, because he is ignorant of the Self, he thinks is separate from him – is in fact in thrall to that deity. In other words, by propitiating the gods with oblations and offerings, a man puts himself in their service. He becomes like a beast that works for its master. Whether these rites are performed here on earth or elsewhere in the celestial worlds, the person who performs them remains dependent on the gods; moreover he enjoys only those benefits that they choose to assign to him.

"For their part the gods are very happy with this unequal relationship, and they have no wish for it to end. Why would they? However, deities can thwart a man as well as help him, for if his knowledge of identity with the Self puts an end to a man's offering sacrifices, why would the gods like him having such knowledge? To extend our previous analogy, they would then become like a man who has had his useful domestic animals stolen from him!

"On the other hand, the sacred texts on liberation in no case serve to bind people, nor do they ever force them to act like slaves. So rest assured, monks, the upshot of all this is that knowledge of the Self renders all these sacrificial rituals a secondary affair, very limited when all is said and done".[227]

The enlightened being and action

Many sacred texts describe the enlightened sage as being 'beyond action'. Because of this description, there is a philosophy that advocates quietism being put around by some deluded teachers. This doctrine seeks to reduce all actions to an absolute minimum in an attempt to emulate the liberated state. The Master is vigorously opposed to all such so-called teachings and warns that they are dangerous misinterpretations that confuse the seeker by falsely conflating the inner state of awareness and the outer world of activity.

In a discussion on this topic, someone asks:

"What, then, Master, is the relationship of an enlightened being to action?"

Answer:

"In the case of the enlightened sage, everything that needs to be done gets done, yet such a one is always established beyond action. How is this? Because he is awake to his own identity with the unborn Absolute, which is always inactive, unmoving. The Absolute is his own Self and as his Self is intrinsically devoid of movement, so he has spontaneously renounced all activity. Ever-fulfilled in himself, he experiences the inaction of his Self in the midst of the world's activity. In fact, in the light of this transcendental awareness he sees that even what the world calls 'inaction' is, in fact, still action".

"Can you explain further, Sir?"

"Well, people in the world habitually superimpose the idea that they are an individual body and an individual mind onto the unmoving stability of their own Self. In so doing, they attribute action to what is in fact always beyond it. This is like a man rowing a boat, who erroneously thinks that the trees on the river bank are moving past him; he sees movement where there is, in fact, none. Labouring under this limiting identification, not only do they assume themselves to be acting but when their body is resting or staying quiet, by the same token they think that they are enjoying inaction. Unaware that they are really the ever-stable Self, they continue to be hoodwinked by error and so remain constantly in thrall to action, whatever their body may or may not be doing at any particular moment. This is a very deeply ingrained misperception, even amongst the intelligent, and much repetition of the true state of affairs is needed to overcome it.

"So much for the ignorant. The sage, on the other hand, sees clearly that the realm of non-Self, in both its active and passive modes, is always permeated by the inactive Self. And as he is that Self, he realises himself to be essentially quite free of the boundaries of intention and action, whatever may be happening on the surface of life. And being free of action, he is also free from all its consequences".[228]

The questioner still does not grasp the distinction between inner and outer.

"So does this mean he just does nothing?"

"Not at all! Certainly, once he is free of the idea of being an individual self, the wise one rests perfectly content, unconcerned with obtaining objects or satisfying individual wants – either in this world or in any other. But while being in this state *internally*, he might very well be highly active in the outside world. Nevertheless, however active he may be, his apparent action is in reality always inaction, because whether he acts for the good of others or to set an example to the world, having on the level of consciousness become the Self that is beyond all action, he in fact does nothing at all!

"And because of this non-attachment, he is always content with what arises and enjoys a buoyancy of spirit that nothing can diminish. Living without personal desire, jealousy or enmity, he is always balanced within himself, whether, on the outside, he undergoes what the world praises as success or what it condemns as failure. So even though he may well appear very active to those around him, the enlightened being's outer action is the expression of his inner silence and peace; indeed, his very action *is* silence, it *is* peace. Whatever the world may see him doing, subjectively and in his own direct experience, he feels 'I am doing nothing' and so he is quite free of the burden of being an acting agent".

The questioner continues to press his point:

"Very well, Sir, I understand your answer, but could it not be said that technically the Self is in fact the indirect agent of action, due to its intimate proximity to the individual body, the mind and so on? Its position could perhaps be understood through the example of a king, who in effect acts through his ministers and servants, even though he sits in his castle and does not actually carry out the actions himself".

"Not so! In the case of the Self, there is simply no relationship with the body and its organs such as you suggest in your example. Their imagined connection is, once again, just the result of false identification. As I said, the Self is forever and always unattached to the material world. This is why the scriptures tell us that, once he has become the Self, the liberated man is as unattached to his body and the world as is a snake to the cast-off skin it leaves lying on an anthill. He shines forth as the Self, the bodiless Absolute, even as light itself. There are many such passages that refer to the sage as having transcended all attachment to the body, and once he is free of the mortal frame and all its endless wants – children, money, power and all the rest - he becomes immortal, liberated from all the self-interest and the limiting sense of agency inherent in bodily attachment".[229]

"You have graciously explained the enlightened being's relationship to worldly action, Maharaj-ji, and I thank you for that. But what about sacred action? How does the sage relate to that?"

"You mean religious ritual? No different from any other kind of action. In that case, while performing *yajna*, the enlightened being sees the ladle with which he pours clarified butter into the sacrificial fire to be the Absolute. He sees the oblation itself to be the Absolute and the sacrificial fire likewise to be the Absolute. And as the Absolute is offered with the Absolute into the Absolute, so the one who performs the offering is also the Absolute, and the very act of oblation itself is the Absolute too! And likewise, the goal of the sacrifice is the Absolute and he who has undertaken that action is also the Absolute and he has the Absolute as his final destiny. Thus to such a blissful seer, always and everywhere, there is only the Absolute and he himself is That".[230]

There is nothing left to say.

The enlightened being and duty

A pious merchant enquires:

"I have heard it said that the scriptures teach that anyone who has realised everything as the Absolute, no longer needs to abide by sacred injunctions of duty as laid down by the Vedas. Can this be true?"

"It is so. The knowledge that you are yourself the Absolute takes you beyond the realm of the Veda. The ritual actions enjoined by the Vedas are rules designed to safeguard the evolution of the individual bodily self, but they no longer impinge on the enlightened who stands free of any such identification with the body. Such a one perceives everywhere only the unity and sole existence of the Self, and thus he has completed his journey of evolution".

"But Sir, such a total sense of freedom sounds dangerous to me", opines a woman. "Could it not lead to irresponsible behaviour?"

"One cannot judge the actions of the enlightened", smiled the Master. "But in general we see that irresponsible behaviour comes from ignorance and a lack of discrimination, and both of these are born of the false sense of self that is predicated on identification with the limited body and mind. All beings labour under the binding power of this erroneous self-conception, but in the case of the enlightened, as I have said, it has vanished. So it in no way follows that because the sage is beyond ritual injunctions, he just behaves irresponsibly, any old how. If a man is truly beyond the necessity of performing sacred rituals, he is certainly beyond the possibility of aberrant behaviour. In his state of total renunciation, free of the mistaken identification with the limited self that thinks it acts, he stands equally beyond both rules and the follies they seek to forestall".[231]

"As we are talking about behaviour, Master, I have heard that the scriptures recommend that an enlightened being should not bother with appearing wise, but just act spontaneously, like a child. But all the children I know are very uninhibited; they say what they feel, eat whatever they like, run around here and there, answer the calls of nature as and where they please, and so on. How does this fit with a man of knowledge such as you describe?"

"Yes, this *shloka* comes from the Brihadaranyaka Upanishad. But, be very careful when you quote scripture", the Master chuckles. "It is not enough just to obey a text, one must first understand it correctly. Now, such a verse obviously does not recommend that the wise man emulates a child in everything, and anyway, even if he wanted to, no one can summon up the nature of a child at will. No, the scriptures here are not advocating childishness. What they mean is that the enlightened being is naturally childlike: he is innocent, untainted by sensuality and he is naturally devoid of pride, hypocrisy and other vices. And like a child, such a one exhibits a certain diffidence; he does not show off his learning or his knowledge, nor does he parade his righteousness. Rather, he exhibits the qualities of simplicity, purity, naturalness and spontaneity, roaming around here and there, contentedly, innocently and without ostentation – that is the point being made here".[232]

The familiar question

"I hear that you teach the world is unreal".

"I do not teach the world is unreal; this is a misunderstanding. I teach that the world is commonly misperceived. This world of apparent duality exists, it has a surface, provisional existence of course, which no common-sensical person would deny. But it has no ultimate reality in and of itself; it is not self-sufficient. Why? Because it is in fact nothing but the temporary and wholly contingent superimposition on the supreme and unified Consciousness, that eternal vastness the scriptures call *brahman*. And this is not just my fancy! It is the ancient wisdom of life. Let us listen to what our sacred scriptures have been proclaiming since time immemorial".

The Master signals to the red-shawled Vedic pandits who are sitting near his couch; they begin to recite in vibrant, mellifluous Sanskrit:

> *'All this that exists is nothing but the immortal brahman. In front, in back, on the left, on the right, up above, down below – this world is everywhere brahman, the supreme non-dual Reality, the ever-undivided Oneness!'*[233]

The highest form of yoga is samadhi

A group of *sadhus* from the eastern reaches of the Land of the Veda has arrived to pay respects. Itinerant yogis, they are a wild bunch and carry with them a strongly charged collective energy. Wearing only black cotton loin cloths and large colourful turbans, they have ears pierced with huge rings made of bone, ivory, and for the senior members, gold. Their talk is animated and a technical discussion full of the intricacies of *karma yoga, kundalini yoga, hatha yoga* and so on soon ensues. There is much quotation from various tantric texts, for these renunciates are scholars as well as adepts.

The Master remains serene without speaking as the discussion goes back and forth. Finally, one of the *sadhus* asks him directly:

"Maharaj, there are so many different forms of yoga and each has its venerable lineage of transmission from guru to disciple and its own devoted followers. As a highly respected *sannyasi* and lover of the Veda, can you help us find which is the highest?"

"The highest form of yoga? To let the mind gradually transcend thought, and abide steadily established in the Self".[234]

Somewhat surprised by the simplicity of the answer, the group remains silent for some time. Then one of their company speaks up. He explains how he has worked for many years, manipulating the body and mind and practising sexual continence in an effort to experience the 'supreme light' mentioned in the scriptures, but without success.

The Master shakes his head slowly.

"When the scriptures refer to the supreme light, they are not talking about some limited individual experience of inner radiance. Certainly, this radiance comes with the very settled level of the individual mind, when the discriminating intellect is purified and it brings with it a pleasurably increased steadiness in meditation. At this level, the mind has gone beyond subtle experiences of the senses and enters a sorrowless state, but the stability of this radiance is not yet fixed. This is one level, a station on the path. What is then needed is that the meditator penetrates the essence of 'I-am', the pure nature of his own being. This is another level of inner radiance, where the perceiving consciousness is like a crystal that stands quite apart from any coloured object that may hitherto have been reflected in it and clouded its true clear nature.[235]

"But by using the word 'supreme' the scriptures are here referring to the pure intelligence of the Self alone, which passages such as 'You yourself are That' clearly show to be the essence of the individual soul, the substratum of 'I-am'.[236] Now, as long as this individual soul is identified with the body, senses and mind, and as long as it fails to realise the Absolute, so long he remains confined within the limits of individuality and is bound by what he experiences. But when he rises above this limited individuality he understands that he is, in fact, unlimited and universal. Then he directly experiences himself to be the immortal Self and so discards the habitual error of identification with the reincarnating body.

"Such a one becomes free of suffering and aberration; the knots of the heart are severed and he becomes conscious he has always been one with the Self, the universal Consciousness. Even the gods cannot object, for he has become their very own Self! All this is pointed out in such scriptural passages as 'He who knows the Absolute becomes the Absolute'".[237]

The *sadhu* is confused:

"But if we already are the Self, how does this come about? How can the Self attain its own nature if it is always that anyway?"

The Master smiles in acknowledgement of the question's validity.

"Yes. Now, before Self-realisation the consciousness of the soul is mixed up with the body, the senses and the mind along with all the fluctuating experiences they undergo. As has just been indicated, it is like a pure crystal that appears to lose its intrinsic clarity and becomes totally overshadowed by the colour and form of any object that is placed next to it. When that object is red, the crystal becomes red, when blue, it turns blue and so on. But when the situation is examined more closely, it becomes clear that the crystal never really lost its original transparency, it just appeared to have done so. Like that, acute mental discrimination will reveal that the soul is not in fact one with the limitations of the world presented to it by the mind, but on the contrary, it is united with the absolute Self. The individual soul that witnesses the inner and outer world is in truth the universal Self. This radical change of perspective is what, from a conventional point of view, we can describe as the soul's 'attaining' its essential nature, even though, in reality, that nature was never lost. Without such radical discrimination, the real nature of the soul remains hidden, so to say, but when there is such discrimination, it is clearly manifested".[238]

"And what brings about such fine discrimination?"

"*Samadhi*, repeated experience of the deep levels of *samadhi*. *Samadhi* is the heart of yoga because it serves to purify the acting agent and its necessity goes without saying. *Samadhi*, along with appropriate disciplines, sacred rites, sacrifices and purification of the body and mind, all these will help to clarify the mind and relieve the feeling of being an acting agent, which is an unconscious and chronic sort of misery. When the mind becomes pure like a mirror, then true knowledge shines forth. No doubt about it".

"And how would you define 'true knowledge' in this context, Maharaj?"

"True knowledge is the realisation that you are not, and never have been, the little acting agent; you are the undisturbed Self that witnesses everything".[239]

The logic of the Self

The Master always emphasises that Truth is a state of being and not just some philosophical theory. Yet at the same time he is unequalled as an exegetist, bringing out subtle layers of meaning from the texts with dazzling displays of logic and reasoning that have become famous throughout the city and never cease to delight those of his followers who hear them. A saying is now circulating around the bazaars: 'You'll never win an argument with that *sannyasi* from the South'.

An example follows in which the Master defines the Self by means of an analysis of everyday perception. As it will soon be Janmashtami, the annual festival celebrating the birthday of Lord Krishna, the text under discussion is the celebrated passage from the Bhagavad Gita in which the Lord is instructing Arjuna about the different levels of reality. One of the monks recites the relevant verse in well-articulated Sanskrit:

> *The unreal has no being; the Real never ceases to be. The final truth about them both has thus been perceived by the seers of ultimate Reality. Know that to be indestructible by which all this is pervaded. None can work the destruction of this immutable Being.*[240]

"Now," begins the Master, relishing the prospect of the inevitable debate, "the Lord here is clearly saying that the unreal – by which he means the realm of opposites perceived through the sense organs, the everyday world of heat and cold and so on – has no self-sufficiency, no abiding existence.[241] And why would He make such a claim? Because everything in the relative world of time, space and causation is the effect of something else; it is contingent and dependent on its cause, whether that cause is seen or whether it is hidden. Moreover, all these caused effects are constantly changing. They are temporary, impermanent, fugitive. So, each and every form can be likened to ..." looking around for an analogy, he points to a water jug nearby, "let us say, that clay pot. Now, a clay pot cannot be said to have an absolute reality, because it has no existence apart from its constituent material, which is the clay. The pot is but the temporary form of clay, the provisional effect of its essential cause. What is more, just like that clay pot, no form or phenomenon can be perceived before its production, nor can it be perceived after its destruction. Therefore, we are fully justified in concluding that it has no substantial or abiding reality".[242]

"Then what you are really saying, Sir, is that nothing exists!"

"No, not at all! What I am saying is that if there is something we can justifiably call temporary, we must in logic admit that there is something we can call permanent, against which the temporary can be measured. We cannot have one without the other, by definition.

And in fact, when one sees clearly from the level of the Self, every experience involves two simultaneous levels of awareness: there is the abiding awareness of what is real, which is that which never fails, and then superimposed on that, so to speak, there is also the awareness of what, relative to the Self, can be called 'unreal' because it is always changing. They are like a background awareness and a foreground awareness, but taken together; the changing and the changeless form the one total reality. This reality is what the Sages call *brahman,* 'The Totality'. Or, we can use the simple, comprehensive pronoun 'That'. So when we see something, whatever it is – a pot, a piece of cloth, an elephant – we have the consciousness of the existence of a temporary form, but we also have the consciousness of the Reality that is the essential constituent of that form. That abiding reality is existence itself, pure Being".

"But surely, to take your example, when the consciousness of the pot ends, so also the consciousness of existence must end too?"

"Not so! The consciousness of existence that was previously associated with the pot continues, but now with reference to some other object – the piece of cloth or the elephant or whatever. There is a continuity. Moreover, even when we say 'there is no pot', meaning there is now only an empty space that was previously occupied by the pot, the words 'there is' can be seen to signify continued existence – by referring to the place and state in which the pot previously existed and from which it is now absent. Now, this consciousness of pure existence, independent of any particular limited object or condition, is nothing but the eternal matrix of Consciousness in which all objects come and go, what our Upanishads call the Self".

"So, Master, what you are saying is that, at the same time, one of the aspects of this, as it were, two-fold consciousness is real and the other is unreal? How can such a contradiction exist? Surely both must be real or both must be unreal?"

"Well, it is like a mirage. When we see a mirage, our awareness tells us 'there is some water over there'. Now that is not really the case, there is no water, objectively, but there was a substratum – a field or a road – on which our unreal perception of water was superimposed. Like that mirage, the entire world of opposites, being impermanent, is in itself unreal, whereas the Self, the pure awareness on which the whole paraphernalia of cause and effect is superimposed, never ceases to exist. The Self remains quite separate from any cause and effect and it persists unbroken. Therefore we are justified in calling it the Real. In this way, the enlightened see the world as composed of the Self, which is eternal and abiding, together with the non-Self, which is transitory and contingent. To experience these two together is to know the non-dual *brahman.*

"Bear in mind, our tradition is always to follow the view of those that see the Truth. Transcend ignorance and suffering, and, being assured that all phenomena are like a mirage, calmly abide in the midst of the opposites as they arise, whether they are pleasant or unpleasant, whether they last for a long or a short time".

"If this is a way to live with the unreal, what about the Real?"

With eyes full of light, the Master is like a lion in his response: majestic, immoveable and full of a fierce joy:

"Unlike the unreal, the Real – whether we call it Truth, the Absolute, pure Being, Self or *brahman* – persists beyond change. Just as pots and all other changeable objects are pervaded by space, so That pervades the entire world, even space itself. It does not undergo increase or loss because, being a unified field of Consciousness, it has no parts. It is inexhaustible and cannot be diminished by losing anything, because nothing belongs to it anyway! A man may be ruined by losing all his money, but the Absolute does not suffer any loss in that way. No one can bring about its disappearance or its destruction, not even the Lord, for the Lord is himself the Self, and the Self is the Absolute, and the Absolute is pure Being, and how could pure Being destroy itself?"[243]

The power of the discourse renders all further questions irrelevant. All present are thrilled by its force.

The maker of arrows

The following day, the discussion is still about the Bhagavad Gita, but has moved on to Arjuna, the warrior hero of the epic.

"Oh yes, he was the greatest archer of his time," comments the Master, as if he had known him personally, "and even before he met Lord Krishna, he had learned a very great lesson from the man who made his arrows".

People are surprised. They have never heard about this.

The Master tells the following story:

"That craftsman was utterly devoted to his occupation. One day while he was beating out an arrow, the King and his entourage went past in the street. So attentive was he to his work that he didn't even notice the extravagant procession. Later someone asked him how he had enjoyed the fanfare, and he replied: 'What are you talking about? I heard nothing!' Just so, you should focus your mind on the Truth and let nothing distract you from your quest for enlightenment. One-pointedness, that is what Arjuna learnt from the man who made his arrows and it is the most valuable of qualities".[244]

The nature of pain

A respectful and dignified middle-aged woman asks the Master about pain.

"Revered young Sir," she begins "When our bodies are cut or burnt, we have the direct experience of pain and it is very real. And, speaking personally, I notice that bodily aches and pains are getting worse as I grow older, and this is also the common experience amongst all of my age. Yet the holy texts tell us that the Self is ever free from pain or suffering and it not only remains unaffected by such ordinary bodily conditions as hunger or thirst but is even free from old age and death.[245] This is my problem: I have the direct and actual experience of pain and suffering, undeniable, and yet you teach that I am the Self that is beyond pain and can never suffer. To be honest, however hard I try, I just cannot square these two positions".

The Master replies in a kindly tone:

"Now, Mataji, you say that when you are cut or burnt you have the direct experience of pain?"

"Yes".

"Actually, that is not the case! Let us look carefully at what happens. When you have the feeling of pain, that sensation is felt as belonging to the body, is it not?"

After a moment's thought: "It is, yes".

"Now, the body is not the Self, it is an object perceived in that matrix of consciousness which is the Self. The body is an object to the

Self just as much as a tree is to you, and you would not feel pain if a tree were burnt or cut, would you?"

The woman shakes her head, wondering what is coming next.

"So, the pain occurs in the same place as the act of burning or cutting which give rise to it – and that place is the body, not the perceiver of the body".

The woman nods, a little uncertainly now.

The Master continues:

"We know this situation very well from everyday experience. When a person says that they have a pain, they point to their stomach or their chest or wherever the pain is occurring. They don't point to themselves as the perceiver of the pain. But if the pain were really taking place in themselves, they wouldn't point to the body but to themselves when they wanted to locate the sensation and the act of burning or cutting that was causing it. And if the pain was actually arising in themselves as the perceiver, they would not be able to register it anyway, any more than the eye can see its own colour and shape! So the pain is perceived in the same place as the burning or the cutting, and both the act and its consequence are objects in, and of, the consciousness that perceives them".

The Master pauses to let the import of what he has said sink in. Then:

"Now, as we have seen, these physical processes must have a physical location, just as rice must be placed in the pot to boil. The location of pain itself is in the body, but the location of the *impression* of that pain, and the memory of it, these are retained in the mind. And it is this memory-impression of past experience that will give rise to feelings of fear and aversion in similar situations in the future".

After another moment's pause:

"So, what we can see from this analysis is that the body and mind are both objects witnessed by the Self. And, as you rightly say, the holy texts teach that the Self is pure consciousness, ever beyond the experiences of body and mind, prior to feelings of fear, desire and all the rest. Therefore, the fact that you experience feelings such as pain in no way contradicts the fact that you are in fact the Self beyond all grief. In truth, you are that all-pervasive oneness which the texts call 'the bodiless one present in all bodies'.[246] The error here lies in identifying yourself with an individual body and mind that continually undergo changes of state. In truth you are nothing to do with the impure body or the changeable mind or its impressions, you are that absolute Self, the unchanging consciousness in which everything else, including the body and mind, arises".[247]

Later the woman leaves the *darshan* hall, her expression a mixture of relief and confusion.

The palace of Indra

A famous astrologer wants the Master's opinion on various competing theories about time, concerning the age of the universe, the relative length of the Four Ages[248] and so on. The Master replies that he is not an expert in this matter, but that there is much in the Vedangas[249] on the subject. The astrologer presses his point strongly and will not give up. He seems to assume the Master is merely being diffident but, to those who know the sage better, it is evident that he has no real interest in pursuing the matter.

Pressed again, he shakes his head and then laughs:

"You should know one thing. The mighty Indra, King of the Gods, once determined to have a new palace. He wanted it to be the most splendid building ever seen and so he hired Vishvakarma, the patron deity of all craftsmen and a being of great wisdom, to be the chief architect. Work went on for months, and gradually a fantastic building came up, more splendid than anything ever seen before. Eventually it was finished and the day the *jyotishis*[250] deemed auspicious for the grand opening ceremony arrived. All the gods and goddesses were invited to attend and tremendous work was put in motion preparing all the grand festivities.

"When the sumptuous affair began, Indra was seated on his throne at one end of the great hall of public audience, raised up on a dais above the assembled gathering, with Vishvakarma occupying the seat of honour at his right hand. In the middle of a long and rather tedious congratulatory speech from one of the many guests, Vishvakarma suddenly began to laugh. Offended by such frivolity, Indra turned to him demanding: 'And just what, may I ask, is so funny as to make you interrupt such an important and solemn occasion?' 'I do apologise, Your Majesty', replied the architect, stifling his giggles, 'but I have just noticed those ants'. So saying, he pointed to a long line of ants that stretched from one of the plates of sweetmeats that covered the banquet table all the way back across the lengthy hall to the doorway.

'So, there are some ants', replied Indra, 'what of it?' 'Well, Your Majesty', came the reply, 'I have just had the insight that each and every one of those ants has already been an Indra in the past, or is destined to become an Indra in the future'. At this, the mighty Indra lowered his head and said nothing".

The paradox of seeking

Seeker:

"I am confused, Maharaj. You say that our true nature is the Self, and always has been, and therefore the one who 'achieves' cannot himself be the one 'achieved'".

Master:

"Correct!"

Seeker:

"Then why do the sacred texts clearly differentiate between the individual soul and the Self, and why are they always advising us to make every effort to seek the Self and to strive ceaselessly to attain the Self and so on, as if it were something existing separately from us?"

Master:

"This is a beautiful question. Now listen carefully, because a beautiful question deserves a beautiful answer!

"The thing is that, being ignorant of the Self, a person mistakenly identifies with his limited body and his individual mind. These are *not* the Self, and while such false identification does nothing to diminish the universal and unlimited status of the Self, the minute it has taken place, it is inevitably followed by the mind's perception: 'Oh, the Self is separate from me, and therefore I have to seek it' or 'The Self is unattained and has yet to be attained' or 'The Self is unknown and has got to be known', and so forth. Now, the limitless Self is indeed different from that limited little 'self' who thinks it is a body experiencing the world and labours under the sense of being 'the doer', but from the perspective of Truth, there is only ever the non-dual Self, the Blissful One".

Seeker:

"Could you explain further, sir?"

Master:

"Well, it is like the clever magician. By his art he makes himself appear to be different from the person who climbs up a rope into the sky, waving his sword and shield. In reality, the magician who stands still on the ground is the very essence of the one who climbs, but the audience is somehow hypnotised into seeing the two as separate. Like that, the normal person is as if hypnotised as to who and what he really is. Similarly, the unlocalised Self is quite unaffected by the hypnotic displays of sensory experience that hold the limited mind in thrall". [251]

The rope trick

The next day, by a strange coincidence, an event occurs which serves to reinforce this teaching.

The Master and a group of disciples were invited to preside over a function in a grand aristocratic house by the river. There had been a *homa* sacrifice to bless the building of a new structure on the site. Recitation of the Veda was followed by a short informal discourse from the Master, then came the ritual feeding of *brahmins* and presentation of shawls and robes to the religious. Everyone enjoyed the event: patrons, priests, family members and visitors.

On their way back to the ashram, the Master's party comes into a square where a fair-sized crowd has gathered. The centre of attention is a magician. He stands in front of a patched cloth screen, next to which is an old wooden hand cart hung with feathers, faded coloured ribbons and what look like painted bones. The cart is piled up with old straw boxes of various sizes; one of which must surely contain a toothless cobra, dozing in its warm, dark prison awaiting the summons of the magician's flute. On the ground next to the cart sits a bamboo cage containing a green parakeet that from time to time, to the delight of the crowd, screeches out the lines from popular *bhajans* it has been taught. The man himself wears a faded orange *lungi* but his thin shoulders are covered by a fine shawl of shot silk that glistens gold and turquoise in the afternoon sun and he sports a large red turban tied in the flamboyant style of a tribesman from the mountains of the north-west. In one thin hand he holds a brightly painted hand-drum that he uses to summon the crowd and add dramatic emphasis to his presentation. Alongside the magician stands a dusky boy with wild hair, perhaps his son. The lad must be six or eight years old but is small for his age. The crowd is hushed and expectant; the magician certainly has the knack of holding their attention. Several of the younger monks in the Master's party lower their gaze to avoid polluting their senses with such a vulgar entertainment, but the Master himself appears as interested in the proceedings as anyone else.

The turbaned man produces a large coil of oiled black rope and with a dramatic flourish throws it up in the air. Somehow, it seems to stay there suspended for a moment and then, under its own force, starts to snake upwards towards the sky. The crowd is captivated. When the rope extends perhaps twenty feet straight above the ground, the little boy approaches it with exaggeratedly cautious steps and then begins to climb up. Miraculously, the rope takes his weight and he continues climbing right to the top. The crowd is transfixed now, not a single eye strays from the astonishing spectacle. The magician beats his drum furiously and then – all of a sudden – the boy disappears! A huge gasp goes up from the crowd, the rope hangs in mid-air for a second then collapses down in a heap, more drum beating, the boy reappears from behind the screen and before the stunned crowd can gather its wits, he is darting nimbly among them, holding out a wooden bowl for money. People seem dazed, looking incredulously at each other and laughing while they try to work out how it all happened.

That evening, the Master is in a very joyous mood.

"Wasn't that a fine instruction we had in the bazaar this afternoon? Did you notice how everyone's attention was captivated by the rope and the boy? They were transfixed, following every move. Now, the unfurling of the rope was like the procession of the three normal states of mind – waking, dreaming and sleeping – while the boy was like all the experiences that take place in those states. Everyone took him to be the clever one, but the real artist was the magician who orchestrated the whole performance. He stood quite apart from it, silently uninvolved and so no one paid him any attention at all. That magician was like the fourth state, pure consciousness. It too, is unseen, obscured by its own magical creation, yet it is the supreme Reality from which everything comes. And the crowd? Well, the worldly man is completely absorbed in the passing show and looks no deeper, whereas the noble ones, the seekers of liberation, are only interested in its source. And one advantage they enjoy by being focussed on the ultimate is that they are thereby saved from wasting time in endless and unprofitable speculations about the ever-mysterious nature of creation!"[252]

The sage's activity

A well-dressed visitor approaches the Master's couch in a humble manner.

"Swamigal, I have been here in the ashram many times now and from the way you are and the things you say, it seems clear to me that you have achieved the goal of life, the state of mind the sages call enlightenment. So I bow down to you as a great Master and consider myself lucky to be able to come and see you like this. But, if what I say is correct and you have indeed reached that state of bliss, then may I ask why is it that you are still so active, going around here and there and seemingly always so busy? Why not just sit back, enjoy your peace and be done with everything?"

The Master smiles.

"There is no contradiction here! Look at the mighty Mother Ganga. Long ago she reached the ocean and yet, even while fast united with her goal, she still continues going forward, never stopping. Why should she behave like this? Because by so doing she continuously gives life and nourishment to all along her banks; this is her nature and so she loves to do. Like that, this body keeps on working in the world and it will do so as long as such work profits those it comes into contact with. But rest assured, however active it may be in the eyes of the world, from its own perspective this body has already done with everything long since and is always just sitting back and enjoying the peace".

The real Self and the false self

Very many people come before the Master full of intellectual doubts about the Self. Sometimes he will cite the sacred texts that teach about such topics, but at other times he just refers them back to the simple fact of their own awareness, pointing out that consciousness, when understood in its profundity, is their real Self. Thus, the Self is already established simply because we are conscious; all that is needed is fully to understand what it is to be conscious. Nothing else is required.

An intellectual who has studied Buddhism for many years attacks the very concept of the Self, saying:

"You speak of the Self's being eternal, blissful and so on, but the teaching of the Lord Buddha is quite clear and quite contrary, for he teaches that no such self exists".

"Whatever the Buddha may actually have taught, and whatever his various followers may claim he taught, let us leave all that to one side for the moment.[253] First of all, let's start where we are. Just look at yourself. Are you saying that you do not exist? If so, who then is taking part in this debate?"

Falling back on a classical Buddhist formula, the intellectual counters:

"Well, of course, in the usual way of speaking I could say 'I' exist. But looking at it more deeply, I would say, from my side, that this debate is being conducted by a conglomeration of perception, intellect, concepts and so on, but there is no 'self' there behind the scenes in charge of it all. The illusion of such an orchestrating self is due to the rapid succession of these mental phenomena, each of which is but momentary".[254]

"Alright, but the awareness that recognises these various momentary means of knowledge presupposes the existence of a continuing consciousness; one cannot refute the existence of such a thread of continuity, whatever we may call it. To do so would be absurd, would it not?"

"How do you mean?" asks the other, warily.

"Well, look", here the Master picks up a water jar from the table beside his couch, "if I ask you 'What are you seeing now?', to remain true to your theory, you would have to say 'I am not seeing anything'. Why so? Because for there to be the experience of actually seeing something now, and for there to be the memory of what a jar is from one second to another, there has to be a continuity of 'I', a single subject that has perceptions from moment to moment and also has a memory – in this case, the memory that this object I am holding is what we call 'a jar'. According to your theory, however, which claims that no continuing self exists to serve as a link between experiences, the perception of this jar and the memory of what it actually is must belong to another person who just happens, quite uncannily, to resemble you! According to your theory, your honest answer to my question would have to be along the lines of: 'What someone who resembled me in the past once saw is what 'I'– by which is meant a different being that I have to admit somehow appears remarkably similar to him – am now seeing'. This is just complete nonsense, is it not?

"And it is ludicrous because it is simply contrary to our common everyday experience. It is like saying that because dung and milk both come from a cow, you can make a delicious milk pudding out of cow dung! You cannot make pudding out of dung, any more than you can make memory out of a mind that consists only of a succession of discrete and unconnected moments.

"No, there has to be the continuing idea of 'I' as a single and identical subject of perception, memory and ideas, and the present possessor of the 'I' notion is not separate from the past and future possessor of it. This has nothing to do with philosophy, it is just common sense based on direct perception, which is actually the weightiest of all proofs. We don't need any other complex intellectual evidence to prove this, any more than we need a mirror to see a mark etched right there on the palm of the hand".[255]

The questioner remains silent.

"However," the Master continues, "let us look a little more closely at the status of that continuing idea of 'I'. What your Master always denied was any ultimate status to the common concept of a 'self', and in this he was quite correct, because the usual sense of being a 'self' is contingent on the possessor's identifying with his own limited body separated from other objects in space, his reactive mind, his transient sense perceptions and so on. But the Self that our Vedantic tradition celebrates is not dependent on anything whatsoever. If it were an effect of some other cause, if it were in some way adventitious or contingent, then its ultimate reality could certainly be denied, but it is none of these. Being self-established, unlike any other separate entity in the world – be it jar, pot or pitcher; a bracelet, armlet or earring, a needle, an arrow, a sword or whatever else you care to name – the Self is *uncaused*. And not only is it uncaused, but it is itself the cause of all causes! Moreover, as pure Consciousness, it stands prior to time and senior to mind and all the other secondary means of knowledge – perceptions, intellect, verbal concepts and so on – that you mentioned just now.

"So we can see that the Self, as the basis of everything, thereby constitutes the very nature of even the one who would deny it. Something external to oneself can always be doubted, but one cannot doubt the existence of the doubter, any more than the heat of the fire can be denied by the fire itself. The Self may have various objects of knowledge in the past, present and future and the particulars of these objects of knowledge may change, but the essence of the knower himself does not change, for that is ever-present. And as it is ever-present, one cannot conceive of any change in its nature. Even if the body is reduced to ashes, the Self remains untouched. Whatever else may happen in the world, the Self remains. And how so? Simply because it is not an effect or a product of anything else, whereas every other thing in the universe, even down to the subtlest stratum of space, is an effect or a product of something other than itself".[256]

No answer.

There will always be many beliefs

Question:
"You frequently talk of *brahman*, which you define as the one and sole Reality. But if there is indeed only one, why are there so many different religions and sects claiming to reach it? And what have you to say about those who insist that only their religion is the right one?"

Answer:
"Because *brahman* is infinite, there is an infinite variety of conceptions of it. *Brahman* is everything, every kind of belief, which includes even the disbelief of the atheist."

Then, with a chuckle:
"The belief in non-belief is itself a belief, is it not? To disbelieve implies that you admit belief! Just so, *brahman* is in all forms and also in the formless that transcends all forms."

The sense of 'I'

In a discussion on the status of the sage, the question arises: "We are always taught that enlightenment involves transcendence of the ego. Does, then, the enlightened man have a sense of 'I'?"

"Why not?" replies the Master, to many peoples' surprise. "He is the unlimited and immaculate Consciousness. Consciousness is conscious, so it is awareness, and this awareness can be designated 'I', no harm in it".

"But if the unenlightened thinks of himself as 'I', and the enlightened does so as well, then what is the difference between them?"

"Infinite! The unenlightened limits his sense of 'I' to the body and thereby thinks himself to be separate from the rest of the world. The enlightened man sees everything as 'I', he experiences directly the unmediated truth of the Vedic verse *Aham brahmasmi*: 'I am the Totality'. Such a being sees the Self in everything and everything in the Self. At one with everything, from Brahma the Creator god down to a clump of grass, he is established beyond fear and always filled with the bliss that comes from contact with this Totality. Everything is as dear to him as his own Self and he is thereby eternally free. Nothing can shake that liberation".[257]

"Then what is the relationship of the limited 'I' to that unlimited Self?"

"As a spark to a fire. The conscious ego has, as it were, split itself off from its own source, the pure Consciousness. As the limited sense of 'I' confines itself to a body, it imagines it undergoes birth and death, changes, suffers, reincarnates and all the rest of it. The Self, on the other hand, being immaculate, unlocalised and independent, remains ever blissful and free, quite beyond birth and death".

"So the goal of life is to reunite with the source?" comes the question. The Master smiles, but says nothing.

The silence

Thursday, being the Guru's day, is traditionally a day of silence in the ashram. The day's routine begins with an early morning *puja* to Dakshinamurti, Lord Shiva in his form as the supreme guru and patron of *yogis*, who sits under the evergreen Tree of Knowledge and teaches through silence. (The Master refers to this embodiment of the Divine as having been his personal inspiration at one stage in his early life). Activities continue as usual throughout the day, but with no talking until after the evening *puja* and *satsang* session that follows it.

Many of the ashramites, as well as those who visit, like the system so much that a number of monks go to the Master to ask if the practice can be extended in some way.

"Do as you wish", comes the reply. "Disciplining the habit of speech is certainly a useful exercise for those who need it. Too much talking is the result of too much thinking, and both dissipate time and energy. But the real value of silence is internal. That silence is also the deepest communication, unhindered by ordinary speech".

"How is that so, Master?"

"Silence is the natural state of the Self. As such, it is not increased by any practice; nothing can be added to it or taken away from it. Being the transcendental field of life, it outstrips all barriers and can contain all sounds, whilst simultaneously lying ever beyond them. And when that great inclusive silence has become your own being, whatever your mind may be engaged in – whether you are talking, laughing, crying or even shouting out loud – it will not leave you. It is your eternal companion, whether the mind is awake or dreaming or suspended in deep sleep. This has nothing to do with keeping your mouth closed!"[258]

The Soul

The Master seldom launches into discourse on his own initiative. As he is always open to whatever arises, he is unburdened by the need to impose a personal agenda on events, but simply abides in a continuously present state, alert and receptive to the emerging evolutionary necessity. As regards teaching, this means that much of his time is spent responding to questions, as these express others' perceived need of the moment. His answers, however, not only deal with the topic in hand but are simultaneously a clear and accurate appeal to the deepest inner nature of the questioner as, when all is said and done, it is ignorance of this nature that has prompted the question in the first place.

One day a group of four seekers comes for the morning *darshan*. Friends since boyhood, they are now in late middle age, all intelligent and successful in the world. Throughout their lives they have taken a keen interest in philosophical and religious subjects and now, having done well in their professional lives, they are devoting their time to trying to find answers to the ultimate questions that they feel might make some sense of all they have gone through over the years. Despite their sincerity, they remain confused by the many different views held by the various saints they have visited. In fact, to a man, they had all but decided to give up their quest but, on hearing of the Master's reputation as a teacher of Advaita Vedanta, they resolved to come and visit him in the hope that he might be able to clarify their confusions.

Hearing the story of their lifelong quest, the Master nods slowly:

"Certainly, these metaphysical questions can be confusing and that is basically because the normal waking state can never really understand the reality of the enlightened. The words may be recognised, intellectually, but the experience to which they refer can never be grasped second-hand. So there will never be fulfilment to the spiritual quest and all the intellectual doubts associated with it unless and until the actual experience of enlightenment is gained. And what is more, everyone understands the world according to his capacity, and capacities vary enormously. This is why, amongst a group of pupils being instructed, some will understand the teacher correctly and some incorrectly, while others will understand the opposite of what is being taught and still others will understand nothing at all! This is the case even with secular topics, so how much more must it be the case when we are discussing the Self that transcends the senses and outstrips the mind with all its concepts?[259]

"So, the lesson from this is that knowledge is different in different states of consciousness; the world is always as you are. Nevertheless, bearing this in mind, it is good to discuss these matters, even if only from a distance. At least one can have some intellectual clarity from a theoretical point of view and this will help one's progress towards the time when what is under discussion becomes a living experience. So, let us proceed together step by step. Is there a particular topic you wish to discuss today?"

"Sir", begins one of the men, a retired government worker, "we have recently been told by one teacher", he mentions the name of a famous *yogi* resident in Allahabad, "that the individual soul is separate from the Absolute, yet others we have visited teach that it is one with the Absolute. Can you clear up our confusion on this point?"

"What we call the individual soul is nothing but consciousness or pure cognition and as such, is solely the reflection of the higher Self, the eternal and immutable Consciousness", replied the Master. "But because this absolute intelligence is mediated through the individual nervous system and apprehended through the individual intellect, its universal character is obscured and it appears to be a limited and individualised awareness. It is like the sun shining on pots of water. We cannot say the reflection of light in the pot *is* the sun itself but nor can we say it is something completely different. And if one pot is shaken and the reflection in it moves, that does not mean that the reflections in the other pots nearby move as well. Like that, due to its adjuncts of mind and body, each soul is individualised like the water in the pot, and then it becomes associated with, or shaken by, the results of its previous *karmas*. But when this happens, no other soul is likewise affected. Of this you can be sure: the *karmas* of different souls do not get mixed up together".[260]

"Does this mean that the soul is subject to birth and death?"

"No, the soul is not born and it does not die. Again, it is the superimposed individual attributes – the body, intellect, mind and senses – that come and go, not the soul itself. This is clearly stated in the Vedic text: 'In truth, this body dies when deprived of the soul, but the soul itself does not die'.[261]

"Now in common parlance we say that the soul comes into association with a body, and after some time, when that individual body and nervous system ceases to function, that soul is parted from them. But in fact, the movement is not in the soul. Similarly, although we may talk of a soul's having distinct characteristics, in fact these characteristics are only in terms of the limiting adjuncts of mind and body associated with that soul, its medium. These adjuncts are superimpositions, external to the soul and they do not reflect its true, essential nature which is a mass of pure intelligence – endless, unfathomable and pellucid".

The questioner continues:

"But if, through our individual soul, we are in fact the Self, which is always blissful, why do we experience the world of limitations and feel 'I am mortal', 'I am miserable' and so on?"

"As I have said, we suffer because the soul is unaware of its immortal status and therefore it identifies with the individualised limitations of the body, the organs, the individual mind and its impressions. But all these are like the foam and bubbles on the limpid waters of the supreme Self. And just as a river entering the immeasurable ocean no longer has a sense of being an individual river, so when the individual soul returns to its cause and realises its true identity in the universal Self, it no longer entertains notions such as 'I am so-and-so', 'This is my land and these are all my possessions', 'I am happy or miserable' and all the rest of it. Those identifications are due to ignorance, and, when ignorance has been transcended, all limiting sense of individuality vanishes".[262]

The second of the men, a respected school teacher, then takes up the debate:

"Well then, Sir, let us agree that, as you say, the soul is in its essence the absolute Self. If this is indeed the case, what I don't understand is why the Self, which as the supreme Lord suffers no necessity to undergo birth and death, would willingly choose to enter into the limited mortal body. Why would He expose himself to the pain and suffering that are inevitably associated with embodiment?"

"Yes, the logic of your doubt is correct," replies the Master, "but here you must consider the way in which it can be said that the Lord 'enters' the limitations of the human form. The thing is, the Lord cannot be compared to any normal human being. He is immaterial and contentment itself, free of the unfulfilled desires that plague ordinary beings. [263] This being so, the Lord has not 'entered' into the body in order to attain or suffer anything. If we wish to use that word, He has 'entered' it solely as a reflection and it is this reflection of the universal in the individual that we call the soul, as I have just explained. But due to his ignorance, the usual man is quite unaware of this state of affairs and does not realise that his true nature is the divine Self. On the contrary, he considers himself to be a limited ego in a mortal body, and in this state of limitation thinks: 'Now I am happy', 'Now I am miserable', 'I am mortal', 'I suffer' and all the ensuing paraphernalia. This is like a pure crystal taking on the colour of a piece of red cloth placed in front of it. In fact, the crystal remains quite unstained by the colour, and in the same way the divine Self remains quite untouched by any thoughts and feelings pertaining to a limited selfhood or its associations".

"I think I see what you mean, Sir ..."

The man is hesitant and so the Master switches to another analogy.

"Consider this then: it is as if you are looking at your reflection in a mirror. You appear to have 'entered' the mirror, but there is no real connection between you and the mirror, is there? Moreover, whatever blemishes the mirror may have, or whatever dirt may be sticking to it, they do not touch you, even though these imperfections may spoil the clarity of the reflection. Like that, the Self who is the Lord, remains ever unaffected by the limitations of the localised material in which it is reflected".

The third member of the party, who is a professor of philosophy, has been listening intently. Now he breaks in:

"But Maharaj, if the soul is only a reflection, as you seem to be saying, then it must by your definition be unreal."

"Well said! But in fact, the individual soul is real because it is essentially one with the divine Self; it is a reflection of the divine intelligence, pure and limitless. Nonetheless, this reflection, being ignorant of its own essential nature, consequently labours under all sorts of misapprehensions, as we have discussed just now. In that state of ignorance, the soul is just like anything else in the world: unreal when considered as self-sufficient in itself, but real when seen for what it actually is – which is a form of the Self".[264]

At this point, the government official, who began the debate and is now having some difficulty following the twists of the argument, bursts in exasperatedly:

"So it is real and unreal at the same time? Is it all just one great paradox then?"

The Master smiles graciously:

"On the level of language it may indeed sound paradoxical, but this is just the limit of language. Words cannot designate that Reality directly because it transcends all mundane categories and reconciles all apparently opposed positions. But on the level of experience, it becomes self-evident and unambiguous, quite perfect in fact!"

Quizzical looks.

"Well, gentlemen, let us go back to our example of the mirror. The reflection of the face in the mirror is different from the face itself, because there may be some blemishes in the mirror that are not there in the face."

Nods all round.

"In addition, the reflection is also different from the reflecting medium, the mirror. If it were not different from both the face and the mirror, it would continue to exist when either of them were removed, which is clearly not the case! Just because the reflection is called 'a face' doesn't mean it is the same as the actual face, because once the mirror is removed, even though the actual face remains, the reflected face vanishes. Like that, the Self is the ultimate and persisting reality, while its individualised reflection and the medium that gives rise to that reflection are temporary and have only a contingent reality".[265]

A lengthy pause follows, allowing the men to digest the import of what has been said.

Finally the oldest of the four, a wealthy landowner, makes his contribution:

"If what you have said is so, young Sir, what are the implications for reincarnation? Who, or what, reincarnates?"

The Master laughs, delighted that an unconscious and unvoiced concern about family inheritance has prompted a profound metaphysical question.

"Well, it certainly cannot be the Self, because, as an omnipresent mass of Consciousness, how could it go anywhere that it is not already present? To do so would be an absurdity. As it does not move, the Self is necessarily ever beyond birth and death. Nor can it be the individual reflection that reincarnates, because, as we have just seen, that limitation does not really exist apart from the temporary juxtaposition of those conditions that give rise to it. To say it does would be like claiming we can trace the footprints of the birds in the sky. So our conclusion must be that, strictly speaking, there is nothing that undergoes reincarnation!"

This was too much for the men, who look at each other in bemusement. Laughing, the Master continues:

"Now, we must be very careful here! You must understand that this is the truth described from the absolute viewpoint by those who live the experience of liberation, which is that they are the one Self that rests unmoving beyond birth and death. But, for all practical purposes, as long as a person is identified with the limitations of the body, mind and so on, they will consider themselves to be a discrete individual self. And as such, they will be attached to their desires and the outcome of those desires and thus they will continue to create and suffer *karmas*. And therefore, it will be necessary for them to reincarnate in order to fulfil those desires. This is a law applying to all those who are unenlightened at the time of death, even if they have studied this matter theoretically during their lives. So for all those people who labour under the delusion of a separate selfhood, reincarnation is a reality, an undeniable fact of their experience".[266]

At this point one of the *brahmacharis* brings in refreshments, and after a short time the four visitors rise and, each in turn thanking the Master with genuine politeness, quietly leave the ashram together.[267]

The true yoga is without strain

A large band of naked Natha Panthis[268] has arrived in the city from the forests further upriver, taking over a part of the *ghats* not far from the main *dhobi* area. Followers of Lord Shiva and rigorous practitioners of both *tantra* and *hatha yoga*, they are a wild, anarchic bunch, arrogant and often irascible, chasing off anyone who comes near them. As a result, the women who traditionally do their washing at the *ghat* have been frightened off going down to the water. No one knows what to do about the situation.

The topic comes up one afternoon in the *darshan* hall. Someone comments it is giving the whole field of yoga a bad name.

"Yes", agrees the Master, "Just because you practice yoga doesn't mean you are a true *yogi*. Our holy tradition derives from the Upanishads and the yoga it teaches is characterised above all by supreme non-attachment. This only comes when the *yogi* has realised his essential identity with the Absolute, and the outside world is seen to have a merely contingent existence. Mistakenly considered to be separate from its essence, which is also the Absolute, such a world has little reality.

"Now, such a state of realisation, in which there is unity with that which stands beyond the mind's partiality, cannot give rise to acceptance or rejection. The non-dual state enjoyed by such Knowers of Reality is hard for many so-called *yogis* to understand, because they assume it involves disintegration of their individual personalities and this fills them with fear. In fact, knowledge of the Absolute is, on the contrary, a state of utter fearlessness, a freedom that depends on nothing outside itself. Not being caused by anything, it is spontaneously maintained without any laborious procedure, that is to say, it is what we call *sahaja* - natural and effortless. Moreover, nothing without exception can be excluded when the non-dual Truth is revealed in its purity, because that *brahman* is always total, complete and whole.

"Now, those who are ignorant of the true Upanishadic tradition and are yet still seeking the peace and liberation of the Absolute, believe the removal of suffering depends on trying to control the mind. For them, the waking mind must be kept disciplined and constantly restrained, lest it becomes dispersed amidst outer objects. But such a strategy requires as much persistence as is needed to empty the ocean drop by drop using a blade of grass! The aspirant has to tell himself that even his natural happiness is false and nothing but a type of ignorance, and therefore he must strive to withdraw his attention away from it. This effort has to be maintained continuously; even the sleeping mind has to be controlled in the same way. It is a long, long difficult path involving constant strain; no wonder so many fall off the edge whilst trying to follow it".[269]

The use of religion

Q:
"The texts tell us that the gods are always standing at the threshold of our life, waiting to bless us".
A:
"And so it is".
Q:
"Why then do so many people feel their lives are anything but blessed?"
A:
"Such people have too many *karmas* piled up blocking the doorway!"
Q:
"What part does religion play in all this?"
A:
"What we call religion is just the means to remove those obstructing *karmas*".

274

The washerman and his donkeys

In answer to a question on spiritual ignorance, the Master makes the following observation:

"Your trouble is that you confuse what happens with what is true. As any storyteller will remind you, plenty of things are true that have never happened, and plenty of things have happened that are not true".

Chuckling, he goes on to tell the following story:

"You should know there was once a *dhobi wallah*[270] who used many donkeys to carry his customers' washing back and forth. One day he fell ill and asked his son to load up the beasts and take the washing down to the river as usual. The boy loaded each one and tried to get them moving, but they stood firm and refused to budge, despite not being tied up. The boy was perplexed and went back to his father to get help. The *dhobi wallah* laughed and said: 'I'm sorry, I forgot to tell you that in the evening I always run my hand over their hooves, as if I am tying them up with a rope, and each morning I do the same, as if I were untying them. That way they stay quiet all night'. The boy went back and ran his hands over the donkey's hooves, and, lo and behold, each one started to move!

"Now", he continues, "This is just the condition of the normal man: he thinks himself to be bound and so acts as such, like the donkey that cannot walk. This ignorance is the universal illusion and it has the entire world in its thrall. The truth is that each one of us is really the Absolute – free, blissful and unbounded – and this whole creation is the manifestation of the Absolute also.

"Nevertheless, just to repeat this intellectually is not enough. Whether we like it or not, the fact is that the illusion of being unenlightened is there and it has been kept in place for many lifetimes by the long force of habit. So just adopting a new concept, such as: 'I am really enlightened' or 'I am not really unenlightened' will do nothing whatsoever to alter the situation. Once the donkeys have had the evening touch, they must also have the morning touch. The evening touch is universal ignorance, kept in place by the circumstances of our birth and the general social agreement as to what constitutes reality, a fiction that has been maintained over countless generations. The morning touch is following the spiritual path under a teacher. This is the process by which the existing illusion is removed. And be assured, it must be administered, because if it is not, no one will ever have clean clothes!"

Transcend the opposites

Devotees are discussing an important verse in the Gita that describes the illumined sage as being: 'beyond the pairs of opposites; balanced in success and failure'. [271]

The Master concurs with the sentiment of the verse, pointing out that none of the objects of the senses can fulfil the mind's desire for happiness. He goes on to illustrate the point with the following story:

"There was once a merchant who was travelling along the road when he saw a blind man. His heart melted and he wanted to invite the man home with him for dinner. But he had another appointment to keep, so went up to the blind man, gave him his home address and said he would see him later.

Reaching home, the merchant asked his wife to prepare an extra meal because he had invited the blind man to eat with them. 'Fine', the wise woman replied, 'I shall prepare two extra meals'. 'Why two?' he asked, surprised. 'Well, if he is blind, he will not come alone. Another will have to come along with him to show him the way'.

"Like that, worldly happiness cannot come unaccompanied; sorrow is always waiting patiently as its shadow. Sooner or later, we all come to realise this through our own experience. Fortunately, there is a state of bliss that transcends the pairs of opposites; unlike normal happiness, it is not dependent on anything in the world, therefore it has no opposite and it meets no end. This bliss is our true nature and the whole world is nothing but a temporary and unbinding form of it".

Transcending ignorance

"How does ignorance operate, Master?"

"As long as ignorance remains, so long the soul appears to have the attributes of the body, the senses, the mind and so on. But the moment the individual soul realises its identity with the universal Self, which is pure Existence, ignorance comes to an end. This liberation is explained in the Vedic texts where it is signified by expressions such as 'You are That'.[272]

"However, whether it be active or inactive, ignorance has no fundamental effect on the soul. It is like a man who, in the half-light of dusk, mistakes a piece of rope lying on the ground for a snake. He runs away from it, calling out and shaking with fear. But then a bystander, who sees more clearly, reassures him: 'Don't be afraid, it's not a snake, it's only a length of rope'. The man then dismisses his fear and stops running.

"But all the while, neither his mistaken perception, nor its subsequent absence makes the slightest difference to the rope. It is always what it is, irrespective of anything that may be projected onto it. Exactly analogous is the case of the individual soul which, although in reality one with the highest Self, is made to appear different by what we call 'ignorance'".[273]

Unity and duality

The young man who arrives for the early morning *puja* at the ashram is from the hills. He is tall and good-looking, with a clear face, a bright intelligent expression and the independent bearing common among hill-folk. It is cold today and he is wrapped in a large woollen shawl typical of his home area, soft and warm and edged with lovely coloured embroidery. The winter sun hangs low above the horizon, a pale lemon orb, with little warmth in it. Weak though it is, the sunlight still causes innumerable pieces of mica to sparkle in the sand, while overhead flocks of birds are flying in long skeins, straggling out across the broad expanse of silvered sky.

"Honoured Maharaj-ji", begins the visitor respectfully in a strong Mewari accent, "I have been studying for some time with a teacher of Vedanta who bases his teaching on the *Ashtavakra Gita*. In that text it says that the world appears from ignorance of the Self and when knowledge of the Self is gained, it disappears. If this really is enlightenment, it seems to me to be too nihilistic a goal to bother pursuing".

"Indeed it would be!" laughs the Master. "You are quite correct in your reaction, but we must always remember that texts such as the one you are referring to are the confession of the illumined and as such can never be fully understood on the level of normal, waking consciousness. The words may be recognised, but their import will not be a living experience unless and until one shares that level of awareness, so one must be very careful how one interprets them. Nevertheless, they can serve as inspiration and encouragement, no doubt.

"Now, the verse you quote refers to two different levels: life before enlightenment, and life after it. In the former, it is indeed the case that, when the attention is focussed outwards on the world, there can be no awareness of the Self, because that awareness dawns only when the mind expands deep within and merges into the transcendental consciousness. And in that deeply introverted state, it is certainly the case that the world no longer exists. Not just the world but nothing whatsoever of an objective nature exists there – no space, no time, no boundary – because the whole mechanism that normally gives rise to the perception of the world – the senses, the mind, the individualised intellect and so on – all of that has subsided into the perfect quiescence of the Absolute.

"But the second level of the verse's meaning refers to the state of *sahaja samadhi*, permanent awareness of the Self that is never lost, no matter what the mind may be doing. When the mind is fixed in the Self, then whatever its mode of activity may be, whether it is asleep or dreaming or even fully active in the world – perceiving, thinking, doing – the Self is there. In this case it is certainly not true to say that with awareness of the Self the world just disappears for the sage – if that were so, he would bump into every tree and fall down into every ditch! Clearly, that would just be nonsense. No, what this verse refers to is the fact that for the enlightened being, the world ceases to exist *as an objective reality*, independent of the observer. In the state of freedom, the world in all its variety of different forms, very much continues to exist. How could it not? Only, now it is experienced in a radically different way. The relative world of duality is still there, with all its differences, all its comings and goings, but all that activity is perceived as being the fluctuations of one's own Self, which remains in the midst of all as inactive, tranquil and quite undivided. The world no longer exists as 'other' or separate from oneself, as one's own Self has become the Self of all beings – immaculate, untainted by action or its results. This non-attachment is the natural consequence of right knowledge, just as when a man realises that he has been trying to drink water from what is in fact a mirage, he no longer attempts to do so. [274] As there is no division in the seamless field of the Divine, so the sage sees that his very own Self is the uninvolved essence of everything, whether it be a brahmin *pandit* endowed with learning and tranquillity, a cow, an elephant, a dog or ..." he searches for an example to make the point "even one of those who eat the flesh of dogs.[275]

"Understand well: on the surface level of life, there is and always must be a difference between a man and all the objects in his field of vision. But that superficial difference does not, and cannot, blind the sage to the essential unity between himself and all these forms, whether they be *sattvic, rajasic* or *tamasic*.[276] It is a question of the difference between substance and essence. In the constant light of pure intelligence the divine harmony is primary and differences are a very secondary affair. So, let us hear the truth on this matter from the sage Ashtavakra himself!"

The Master motions to one of the *brahmacharis* who begins to recite some lines from the *Ashtavakra Gita:*

> *Oh, it is within me, the limitless ocean,*
> *that with the rising of the mind,*
> *diverse waves constituting various worlds are produced!*
> *How wonderful!*
> *It is within me, the shoreless ocean,*
> *that the waves of countless individual selves,*
> *each according to its nature,*
> *Arise, jostle against each other, play for a time,*
> *and eventually disappear.*
> *It is within me that all this world arises,*
> *inheres and falls away once more.*[277]

There is a long, rich silence.

"So, do you see now the relationship between unity and duality in the state of enlightenment?"

The young man nods, smiling. The Master closes his eyes and a great calm descends on the room. The visitors sit silently for many minutes enjoying the vibrant silence until, one by one, they rise, make their *pranaams,* and leave.

Unity and diversity

Question:

"If the Self is undivided and without parts as it says in scripture, how can it bring forth the unimaginable variety of the world?"

Answer:

"It's a perfectly natural phenomenon and, because it is, natural examples of the principle of variety emerging from unity are to be found all around us. Look at the minerals. They are all essentially modifications of the one material that we call earth, yet they take many forms. Some, such as lapis lazuli or diamonds, are valued as precious jewels, others, like crystals, are moderately valuable, and yet others are worthless like the common stones that are useful only for throwing at dogs or crows! Or consider the various types of seed: all are placed in the same earth, but some produce sandalwood, others give gourds and so on. And then all the various varieties that stem from these seeds have, in their turn, completely different leaves, blossoms, fruits, juice and scent from one another. Or yet again, take food: the one and same food gives rise to very varied effects in the body, producing blood here, hair there and so forth. Like that, the transcendental Self may very well be one, yet also appear as the individual soul, or personal God or whatever myriads of forms you may care to imagine. After all, there is no limit to what a single dreamer may dream up!".[278]

Use the gift of the mind

A naked *sadhu* has recently set up camp just outside the ashram gate. A wild, dishevelled character, he will sometimes dance and sing, sometimes sit quiet and motionless for hours on end, and at yet other times roundly abuse anyone who comes too near to him. The devotees are divided in their assessment: some think he is just an anti-social nuisance and should be chased off, while others praise him for having obviously transcended the limits of the mundane mind.

The Master is asked for his opinion.

"Let him be; whatever he is doing is his affair and he will not be there for ever. But as to transcending the mind, that in no way means we must act crazily! Far from it. The mind is our most valuable instrument. After all, it is only through using the mind, when it is suitably refined through the teachings of the scriptures, and purified by contact with the teacher, that one is eventually able to see the Self".[279]

After a few more days the *sadhu* leaves of his own accord and by then everyone is sorry to see him go.

Waking and dreaming

A student of metaphysics enquires as to what is the difference between the waking and the dreaming states.

"Their duration!" comes the unexpected reply.

The questioner does not understand.

"One lasts longer than the other, that is all. Essentially there is no difference, they are both just dualistic modes of the mind: impermanent, limited, egocentric. Our real state is beyond them: it is *turiya*,[280] the eternal, transcendental consciousness we call the Self. That is who we really are. All else is just a mirage, conjured up by the Self".

The questioner is shocked by the directness of the reply, adding that all this is too radical a vision for him fully to comprehend.

The Master nods.

"Indeed, we are getting to the very root of things here. Fine, let us imagine a flaming torch. You hold it aloft and there is just the unmoving flame. Then you start waving the torch around and you create fiery lines going here and there, some straight, others curved. Now", continues the Master, "where does this appearance of straight and curved lines come from? Do they emerge from anything external to the flame? No. And when the torch is held still and they don't appear, have they gone off somewhere else? No. Or, do they come out of the torch and go back into it in the same way you might leave your house and later re-enter it? Again, the answer must be 'no'. So, the actual status of these apparent fiery lines is mysterious and incomprehensible, is it not?"

The questioner agrees.

"Thus it is with all worldly experience when viewed aright. The absolute Consciousness is like the torch in that it is always stable and never changes. When that Consciousness appears to vibrate and create the waking and dreaming states, those vibrations do not emerge from it, nor do they come from, or return to, anywhere else. So these fluctuations in Consciousness are just like the fiery lines in our analogy: they exist, no doubt, but their existence is only apparent, notional. In reality, there is nothing but Consciousness, with various concepts superimposed upon it by ignorance".[281]

"Then in practical terms, Sir, what you are saying with your analogy is that although the former has a greatly superior status, unity and diversity somehow exist together?"

"Correct. The non-dual Absolute is mysteriously known in two complementary aspects: one appears to have limitations owing to the various attributes of the universe produced by myriad changing names and forms, while the other, in opposition to that, is stable, unchanging and forever devoid of qualities or qualification".[282]

Ways and means

The *pandit* is elderly, dressed in a worn but clean and freshly pressed yellow *lungi,* and walking very upright despite his years. A teacher, he has specialised all his life in the sacred science of grammar and mathematics, but is also interested in meditation and has studied the Upanishads. Though many years the senior, his attitude towards the Master is one of alert humility.

"I have long been confused by descriptions of the Self", he confesses. "Some texts speak positively about it, calling it the supreme intelligence, ultimate knowledge and love-bliss; but others use negative terms such as unknowable, unbounded and beyond all mental categories. And some sages even conclude that the only thing that can be said about the Self is 'Neither this, nor that!' To be honest, young Sir, I cannot reconcile these contradictory approaches".

The Master smiles at the older man with great tenderness.

"To stop thinking about the Self and actually *become* it, the seeker must transcend all words, all thoughts. The Self is like silence; the moment you open your mouth to describe it, you violate it. Being beyond definition, the Self is not knowable in the way that sense data are knowable, or quantifiable in the same way as are perceptible objects that have an origin and an end. Therefore, to bring the student to experience this most abstract level of his life, a teacher has to be highly pragmatic, resorting to any means necessary in order to achieve his aim. His attitude must be 'first let me set them on the right path, then in time I will gradually be able to bring them round to the final Truth'".[283]

Then:

"This is a principle you yourself know well. Think of how you instruct your pupils. First you take a stylus and scratch letters on a palm-leaf, then you fill them in with ink to make them legible, do you not?"

The *pandit* nods intently.

"And then you indicate a particular letter and give out the sound it signifies?"

"Yes, Sir".

"Now, your sole purpose in all this is to transmit the sound signified by each letter. It is certainly not to affirm that the stylus, the leaf, the incisions and the ink are themselves the sound?"

"Correct!"

"And similarly, when you are teaching mathematics, you draw lines and digits to signify numbers, first from one to ten and then on to a hundred and a thousand, and then with your more advanced pupils you can go on up to a hundred thousand billion! Yet in all cases, those lines are mere symbols; you would never suggest to your students that those signifiers actually *are* those numbers, would you?"

A shake of the head this time.

"Just like that", concludes the Master, "to teach the Absolute to ordinary minds the teacher may initially have to resort to many indirect means, such as ascribing it various qualities or powers, calling it the creator and maintainer of the world and so on. But all such attributes, positive or negative, are superimpositions on the Absolute, and none of them should be confused with it. Eventually, all provisional and particular notions about the nature of the ultimate must be transcended. Then, if one has to speak about it, all that can honestly be said is that it transcends all description, it is neither 'this', nor 'that'. With this, the silent power of the Self has a chance to shine forth spontaneously, in all its glory".[284]

The two sit for some time without speaking, while tears of release trickle down the *pandit's* cheeks. The gentle sound of a bell rings out rhythmically from a distant temple and a great feeling of peace engulfs the room.

What is renunciation?

The Master often mentions the sacred principles that uphold life. One of these is the fact that greater power resides in the subtler levels of creation. Here is one story he uses to illustrate this point, taking as an example the fact that it is primarily the mind, rather than our material surroundings, that determines the direction and quality of our life:

> There was once a *yogi* who was well practised in concentration but lacking in wisdom. He invited a powerful local king to join him in his peaceful forest retreat so that the man could gain enlightenment and be liberated from the onerous burden of having to be responsible for his kingdom. But despite his worldly persona, this king was actually a sage in disguise. He replied to the *yogi's* invitation with the following words:

'Honoured Sir, thank you for your kind invitation, but I fear you would be disappointed if I took it up. While it would be easy for me to get rid of my courtiers, palaces and retainers and enter your sylvan retreat, these are all just externals. By divesting myself of them, I would not have touched all my inner desires to create a kingdom and rule over it. These desires would not just remain latent but would soon start sprouting again and begin to attract circumstances and people conducive to their realisation. Before long your peaceful and isolated hermitage would suffer, becoming first an increasingly busy *ashram* and then the centre of a burgeoning new kingdom! This is the power of the mind, which is far greater than the power of any particular place'.

Why nothing matters

A serious young man approaches the Master, who today is in one of his irrepressibly playful moods.

"Mahatmaji, if you had to sum up your entire teaching in one sentence, how would you do it?"

"I would say that nothing matters!"

The questioner is shocked.

"But Sir, this is just nihilism!"

The Master laughs.

"The nothing I am talking about is the something that is everything. Only locate that no-thing and become That. Then all else will be experienced as it really is, a highly enjoyable passing show".

With five Buddhist monks

Some miles outside Kashi, surrounded by magnificent ancient trees, lies the beautiful Deer Park where Lord Buddha gave his first teachings. In this verdant and tranquil setting is a large monastic complex that houses monks of various Buddhist denominations and is served by a sizeable lay community that also resides there. The monastery is renowned as a place of great scholarship. Lively debate also flourishes there, both between the various Buddhist schools and the Hindu religious authorities entrenched a few miles to the south-west in the holy city on the banks of the sacred Mother Ganga.

News of the Master reached the Deer Park soon after his arrival in Kashi, but though he and his followers have seen monks from all over the Buddhist world – Thais, Burmese, Chinese, Central Asians – walking the dusty roads on their early morning alms round, he has not engaged in formal debate with any of them. Then, one morning around the May full moon,[285] five senior Buddhist monks come to the Shiva temple near Asi Ghat where the Master is currently staying. They are keen to question him on his teaching.

"Revered Sir", begins the first monk, going straight to the heart of the matter, "we have heard that you teach an eternal and unchanging self to be the supreme reality".

The Master smiles slightly. "I do", he replies softly.

"How can that be?" continues the monk. "The central teaching of our Master, the Enlightened One, is that there is no self whatsoever that is real, abiding or substantial and that all ideas of self are falsely imagined and conducive to endless suffering".

"Well, *bhikkus*",[286] replies the Master, "it all depends on what you mean by 'self,' so let us be very careful which words we are using here. If by 'self' you mean the limited and separate sense of 'I' that identifies with the body and is prone to sickness, old age and death,[287] the discrete individual that holds, 'I am the doer and the sufferer of the consequences of my actions', then I am in full agreement with your Master that there is no such thing as self, and that all ideas of self are falsely imagined and conducive to endless suffering".

"In that case, Sir", continues the second monk, clearly puzzled at this unexpected reply, "how can there be a self that you teach to be the supreme reality?"

"Let me ask you a question in turn, O, *bhikku*", counters the Master, smiling. "If a man were to see through, transcend and thoroughly repudiate the false idea of self, what would be left?"

"The state of freedom would be left, Sir".

"And what would this state of freedom be free from, O, *bhikku?*"

"This state of freedom would be free from the limitations of birth, decay and death, and the suffering incumbent upon the falsely imagined idea of self".

"And what would this state of freedom be called, O, *bhikku?*"

"It is called *nirvana*, Sir".

"And how would this *nirvana* be described?"

"It is described as being beyond description, beyond mind, beyond concepts, Sir", chimes in the third monk, taking up the debate.

"Well said, O, *bhikku!*" the Master laughs. "Yes, it is indeed indescribable because it is the unutterable delight of pure transcendence, for as you know the word *nirvana* comes from *nivriti*, which means 'delight'.[288] Does not your Master describe this indescribable *nirvana* as 'the incomparable security', 'the highest happiness', 'the unchanging stability', 'the extinction of craving' and 'the end of all suffering'?"

"Yes, Sir, he does describe it so".

"And in this context do not your scriptures quote his words that: 'There is, O, monks, an unborn, not become, not made, uncompounded, and were it not for this unborn, not become, not made, uncompounded, there would be no escape from what is born, has become, is made and is compounded?'"[289]

"Indeed he has, Sir", replies the fourth monk, astonished that this young teacher, notorious in the Deer Park community for his heretical views, should be quoting the Buddha's words to him as authoritatively and as naturally as if they were his own.

"And for your Master to taste and know and live and teach this unborn *nirvana*, must there not have been some awareness, some consciousness, some being present there to taste and know and live and teach it?"

The monk hesitates a long time before answering cautiously:

"He could not have known or taught the Truth without some vital awareness being present, Sir".

"Just so, in the way that I teach, that very awareness which lies beyond all limitation and is the end of all suffering and the witness of all, that one is known as the transcendental Self. That same *nirvana* is the eternal freedom in divine consciousness, the superlative joy of liberation known only to the enlightened; it is not a state caused by any external contact or circumstance, but the unborn absolute principle that is the goal of all seeking".

The monks are silent.

"And tell me, O, *bhikkus*," the Master continues gently after some moments, "was there not an occasion when your Master was asked to teach on the supreme reality and he remained silent, just holding up a flower?"

"Yes, venerable Sir, there was such an occasion" replies the fifth monk. They all wonder what is coming next.[290]

"Well, your Master was quite right, O, *bhikkus*, and his holding up of a flower was a teaching of immaculate purity and the utmost clarity. In our tradition of Advaita Vedanta there was a similar incident when the sage Bhahva was approached by the student Vaskall and asked to teach the nature of the Absolute. There was no answer; the request came a second, and then a third time. Finally, Bhava said, 'I am teaching It to you, Vaskall, but you do not understand. Its nature is silence'. Indeed, the Self is all silence; and in trying to understand this with the mind, people get stuck in words as an elephant gets stuck in the mud. The Truth is a realm beyond the senses, beyond words, beyond concepts, and beyond all distinctions. As our texts say, 'the eye does not reach it, nor speech, nor even the mind itself'"[291]

"Yet, be that as it may, as long as suffering and delusion exist in the world, it is necessary that there be teaching, and as long as there is teaching, so long will there be the teachers and the taught. Therefore, the great ones, out of compassion, go forth to teach for the welfare of all beings, and they teach at different levels according to the capacity of their hearers. Just as the doctor gives his medicine according to the nature of the disease, so is the teaching variously given; and a teaching is no teaching at all if it is not to the point. And mark well that what is taught by the great ones is not some conceptual fancy suitable only for the intellectuals and philosophers, it is the lived realm of realisation and open to all who earnestly desire it".[292]

To a man, the monks are amazed at the thoroughly Buddhist manner in which this young Vedantin has just expounded his teaching of the Self. As if reading their thoughts, he concludes:

"Whether they start from the north side, or the south side, or the east side, or the west side, all paths that climb a mountain eventually meet together at its summit. Just so, oh *bhikkus*, do the many ways meet in the realisation of that one Truth".

The monks prostrate low before him and return to the Deer Park, their minds clear and fresh and their hearts rejoicing that harmony now prevails where discord had previously been imagined.

Yoga and Veda

Question:
'What is the relationship of Yoga to the Veda?'
Answer:
"Close but not perfect! The Vedic literature mentions yoga as a means to the realisation of full illumination and many Upanishads also mention it in this connection. So, of course, do the yoga texts themselves. Then there is the Sankhya school of sage Kapila, which sets out the theoretical basis on which Yoga is to be understood. All these are accepted by good seekers after Truth; this is not in doubt.

"But what is very much in doubt is any claim that Yoga on its own, independently of the Veda, can bring about full realisation. Why so? The crucial point here is that both Yoga and Sankhya are dualistic, they do not teach unicity. Nevertheless, they contain much that is perfectly compatible with the Upanishads. Sankhya, for example, identifies the infinite character of the supra-individual Self, which it calls the *purusha*, while Yoga emphasises the necessity of radical detachment for those who follow the path it outlines. These approaches can lead one to Self-knowledge and as such are certainly conducive to liberation. But they stop short at the separation of the infinite Self and the finite world. Final liberation, which is the radical understanding of the Self's non-duality, can only come from the knowledge contained in the Upanishads, which are Vedic through and through".

"But the sage Kapila is revered as a perfected being, so how could his teaching be less than the final Truth?"

"A sage's perfection cannot override the Vedic scriptures. After all, there could be many different perfected beings each holding a different view and indeed, many of these divergent views are written up in texts that are held in high esteem. So if this variety of viewpoint is found amongst the perfected ones, what to say of the normal man? Even those of clear intellect have their own bias, and since the power of understanding differs from one to another, impartial comprehension can only come from recourse to the revealed authority of the Veda.

"As I have said, Kapila's shortcoming is that he stops at duality. When considering the individual he posits a plurality of souls and likewise, in his discussion of ultimate principles, he does not admit the unicity of the Self. This leaves him with a cosmic duality: on the one hand insentient matter, which he calls *prakriti*, and on the other, the sentient spirit which he calls *purusha*. These two are eternally distinct. Then, in order to explain the causal dynamism of nature, he is driven to posit an independent creative principle called *pradhana*, which operates as the original root of matter.

"Thus, although both Yoga and Sankhya are highly valued by the people and contain much true and worthwhile teaching, they fall short of the totality of Upanishadic wisdom. Our tradition is clear that the Self is forever one and undivided, and as such, it acts as God, the source of all. This *pradhana* of Kapila's is nowhere mentioned in our scriptures and anyway, if it is part of matter as he says, then according to his own theory, it must necessarily be insentient. How then could it create the world of sentient beings? No, such a power can only reside in the intelligent Self, which is Consciousness itself, all-creative and non-dual. So for all these reasons we cannot accept Kapila's system as complete. Any Yoga that is based upon it will certainly kindle the fire of knowledge, but can only take us half-way to the goal. What is then needed for full and complete realisation is the understanding of the great Upanishadic texts. That will yield the real yoga, which is union with *brahman*."[293]

Yogic wisdom will always endure

The darshan hall always has a wonderfully relaxed and open feeling to it. Today there has been a stream of visitors to the Master, who sits like some youthful grandfather surrounded by the ebb and flow of an extended family that stretches to all infinity. A young boy has been demonstrating his prowess at yoga *asanas,* which is considerable; then a woman came to give a very beautiful recital of some songs by a famous southern saint in praise of Lord Shiva. A local party of housewives came with gifts of sweetmeats, flowers and fruits. Lakshmi, the senior member of the ashram's herd of cows, has sat contentedly beside the Master's couch throughout the proceedings.

After some time, three *pandits* from the flat plains of the central land arrive. They are dark skinned well-built men, each wears a sarong of a pale coral colour fringed with gold thread and their long hair is piled up in a bun on the top of the head secured by brightly coloured threads. The three horizontal stripes of sacred ash on their foreheads and upper arms proclaim them to be devotees of Lord Shiva. They prostrate before the Master, introduce themselves as representatives of a famous temple, sit and then begin a recitation in mellifluous Sanskrit.

After a while, the Master holds up his hand to pause the chant:

'How beautiful these last verses are, beautiful! Bhagavad Gita, Chapter 4, verses one and two...'

Those who have spent any time with the Master have long since ceased to be amazed by his encyclopaedic knowledge of the scriptures. He translates to those present:

'The blessed Lord says to Arjuna: I proclaimed this imperishable Yoga to Vivasvat, Vivasvat declared it to Manu and Manu told it to Ikshvaku. Thus having received it one from another, the royal sages knew it. With the long lapse of time, O scorcher of enemies, this Yoga has been lost to the world.'

"Lord Krishna is explaining here the origin of our teaching. He says that 'this Yoga I gave to the Vivaswat' - who is Surya, the Sun - in the beginning. And the Sun gave it to Ikshvaku, and Ikshvaku gave to Manu, Manu gave it to the ruling dynasties, the warrior *Kshatriyas.* Now, why such a sequence? Because the sun is the origin, the source of all light, life and intelligence on this earth, endlessly generous, asking nothing from those who benefit from its attention. And then, on the human level, it is a ruler who is likewise looked upon by all his subjects for everything in life – material development from his policies, spiritual gain from his patronage – for any need that the subjects could possibly think of, they look upon the king. Manu was the first King and if the king is a man of integrated life, if the king is a man who could impart to his subjects, to every man in his kingdom, the wisdom of living, then what a tremendously joyful and graceful society he would be creating around him... and he will be the ruler of that great society. So, this wisdom was imparted to the most responsible people, the ruling class of *kshatriyas.*

"Today, things are different. People are paying less attention to what their rulers say and this will get worse, much worse. Not too far in the future, everyone will have to look to himself for every development of his physical or material wellbeing, because there will not be general trust those in authority, there will be no one to really look up to. In the coming days, freedom will be confused with license, and each person will have only their personal whims and aberrations to guide them through life. But nonetheless, our yoga will endure, and when needed it will be revived by great souls to overcome the evils that have crept into life. In this way it will always be available to bring balance and order and coherence back into human affairs. And why? Because this is the teaching of life itself, the knowledge of the oneness of all life and that state of unity is the undying Truth."

Totakacharya

After so many months of teaching and debating, and so much work reinvigorating the religious life of the spiritual hub of the Land of the Veda, it has become clear to the Master that what is needed next is a fresh body of commentary on the root texts of Advaita. So much misunderstanding shrouds these great works of spiritual authority that their true redeeming power has all but been lost. The time has come to restore them to their original glory. And so early one spring morning, along with a handful of his closest disciples, the young *sannyasi* leaves the Kashi ashram and sets off for the mighty Himalayas to take advantage of the purity and solitude of those vast uninhabited regions and focus uninterruptedly on this task.

Soon after they arrive in the mountains, after many weeks of travelling, an event occurs which has great significance as a teaching on the innocent power of devotion. It concerns a disciple who is to become one of the Master's closest companions. Giri is a simple man, totally unintellectual but blessed with an unshakeable devotion to his *guru*. His attachment comes from the heart rather than the mind and it is this simple empathy that binds his whole personality to his teacher. Realising his own limitations, Giri has humbly determined that the one thing he can do for his teacher is to save him the bother of having to worry about practical day-to-day necessities, so that his attention can be free to work on his commentaries and instructing those who come to him. So Giri busies himself day after day with sweeping, cleaning and organising various domestic duties around the ashram that has been established in a grove high above the river Alakananda. Realising he is no great intellect, he cares little for the abstract metaphysical debates so enjoyed by the other brilliant disciples, especially Padmapada and Vartikakara. Thanks to Giri's practical work, the other disciples too are freed from many tedious organisational duties, but they patronisingly regard him as a dullard – good-natured and hard-working no doubt, but of little importance in the greater scheme of things.

One day the disciples are sitting with the Master for a discourse, waiting to begin the customary Vedic recitations to start the session. They have all taken the ritual purifying bath in the river below, but Giri has stayed behind to wash his Master's clothes. Such a decision is nothing new, always preoccupied with his service, he is often late for such meetings, if he comes at all. The other disciples' impatience mounts as the minutes tick by. Whispers start going around. Why does the Master tolerate this simple fellow? To waste such precious time waiting for someone who can't even follow the discussion seems stupid. Eventually Padmapada suggests that as all the students are present the class can begin.

"Let Giri come also", is the Master's quiet reply.

Padmapada glances at the wall, muttering under his breath that it could just as well stand in for the absent Giri for all the benefit he would get from the class.

Just then, a beautiful sound is heard floating up the valley. As it gets nearer, the sound becomes recognisable as a lilting chant in a little-known and difficult Vedic metre called *totaka*. It is Giri's hymn of praise to his Master:

You have made the world happy with your brilliant insights into
the Self,
So help me to understand fully about God and the soul!
Let me take refuge in you O Shankara,
My Master, my giver of joy!
Oh my guru, the great ones wandering the world in various forms
Are hard to recognise, but amongst even them you shine supreme,
like the sun!
Let me take refuge in you, O Shankara,
My Master, my giver of peace![294]

Finally Giri enters the room, a radiant presence. Even the scholarly disciples can see his brilliance and recognise that through his simple devotion the man they dismissed as a dullard has achieved enlightenment ahead of all the intellectual giants. The Master immediately gives him the new name Totakacharya, after the metre of his poem, and in time he will become recognised as one of the greatest of the close disciples. Soon after this episode, again in front of the assembled students and to the astonishment of all his erstwhile critics, Totakacharya will spontaneously compose a lengthy and intellectually well-sustained discourse on the identity of the individual soul and the cosmic Self. It remains one of the classic treatises on Vedanta to this day.[295]

Vyasa's seal of approval

The Master and his party are visiting Kedarnath, a holy town high in the mountains of Kedar Khand, an area of great natural beauty where Lord Shiva is fond of spending time. While here, the Master decides to reinvigorate the main temple, which has fallen into disrepair due to lack of funds following the death of the local *raja* who was its chief patron. The place is revered as one of the *Char dhams* – the four great pilgrimage centres in the high Himalaya that were established by the ancient Pandava dynasty.

Immediately after he has performed the ceremonies and rituals that re-activate the sacred energy of the shrine, the Master is approached by an elderly man who requests a debate with him. The Master agrees. Although he appears very ordinary, the old gentleman soon shows he has prodigious and detailed knowledge of the Brahma Sutra, and he is able over several days to question and examine the Master on each verse fluently, with no recourse to written text or prompts. Everyone listening is amazed, and also delighted that at each turn, their beloved teacher seems able to counter his examiner's questions and satisfy his detailed demands for clarification on even the most minute and obscure points. The disciples come to realise that something special is taking place.

Later, it is said that the old man was none other than Vyasa, compiler of the four Vedas, author of the Mahabharata and one of the Seven Immortals. This divine being, so it is believed, had materialised to express his satisfaction that the brilliant young monk understood the profound import of the teachings and was the fit person to instigate a revival of sacred knowledge throughout the Land of the Veda for centuries to come.

PART FOUR:

THE MISSION

Long, long ago when the earth was still fresh and pure and humankind lived lives of righteousness, mighty Indra, the King of the Gods, inadvertently caused grave offense to the sage Durvasa by failing to show sufficient respect to Shri, the Goddess of Fortune. Deeply affronted on Mother's behalf, the holy man cursed the gods to forfeit their power, and so great was his thought-force that even those shining ones were unable to resist it. And so, as a result of his ire, they began to lose their everlasting battle with the demons. Before long, negativity gained control of life, and suffering became unbearable, so in desperation the gods repaired to Lord Vishnu, the Preserver of the Universe and sought his help. He advised diplomacy. The divine forces should pretend to form an alliance with their enemies and suggest that the two sides work together in churning the infinite Ocean of Milk, with a view to sharing between them all the wondrous treasures it yielded. As both groups knew well, the greatest of these treasures was the Nectar of Immortality, but Vishnu secretly promised the gods that this boon would fall to them alone.

The churning was swiftly organised. Mount Mandarachala was brought from the high Himalaya to be used as the churning rod, while Vishnu volunteered himself in the form of Kurma the giant turtle, on whose back the rod would be balanced. Vasuki, King of the Serpents, kindly offered his body as the rope, and so the stage was set. The demons took the serpent's head and the gods his tail, and as the two armies pulled in tandem the mountain began to rotate and the churning began. The first thing that happened was that a terrible poison gushed out of the depths, threatening to envelope the universe. Seeing the impending disaster, Lord Shiva compassionately intervened and swallowed the venom, which was so putrid it stained his neck indelibly. Ever since he has been known as Neelakantha 'the Blue-Throated One'. Then, one after the other, fabulous life-enhancing treasures began to rise up from the frothing milk. These included Mother Lakshmi, Goddess of Abundance, Kalpavriksha the Wish-Fulfilling tree and Kamadhenu, the divine Cow of Plenty, who is the mother of all earthly cows. But when Dhanvantari, the heavenly physician and father of

Ayurveda, finally emerged from the deep, bearing a pot containing the prized Nectar of Immortality, the co-operation of the two armies ended abruptly and fierce fighting broke out between them, for both gods and demons coveted this ultimate prize above all.

To protect the precious ambrosia from falling into the wrong hands Vishnu was true to his word and sent his vehicle Garuda, King of the Birds, to snatch the pot and carry it safely away from the battle-scene. As Garuda soared high over the globe lustrous drops of the divine nectar fell to Earth at four spots across the Land of the Veda. These places became charged with an extraordinary spiritual power and to this day a great religious fair, the Kumbha Mela or 'Festival of the Pot', is regularly held at each of them to commemorate this unique and precious descent of the divine energy upon earth.[296]

The commentaries on the great scriptures are finally finished. For over two years the Master has been staying in the remote Himalayan vastness, writing what is destined to become the authoritative canon of Advaita Vedanta: his explanations of the wisdom of the Brahma Sutra, the major Upanishads and the Bhagavad Gita. Each of these three mighty pillars of knowledge has now been recast in the light of an all-encompassing understanding that relates and reconciles each of the various extant schools of interpretation, whilst transcending them all in the experience of Divine unity. The ancient teaching has been restored in its fullness and the pure light of Truth established once more, to shine for all generations to come. What else is there left to do? With no thoughts of what may lie ahead, the Master decides to return to Kashi with his disciples and see what Mother Nature has in store. Ever contented, he is free of all the compulsion that might well accompany such a prodigious output in a normal man; it is as if the bounty of life flows effortlessly and with inexhaustible freshness from him, already fulfilled at every stage of its manifestation.

Winding its way back south along the mighty Ganges, the party of saffron-robed monks makes a stop at the sacred city of Prayag Raj.[297] This holy place is revered as the navel of the world, for it is here that Brahma, the Lord of Creation, performed the sacred fire offering that inaugurated the present age. All the gods were born anew from that holy pit and throughout the succeeding centuries untold numbers of holy beings, both human and discarnate, have come to join them at this hallowed spot. And it is to cool the awesome strength of that primal fire that the three mightiest river-goddesses – Mother Ganga, Mother Jamuna and Mother Saraswati – chose to meet together here. The pellucid green of Ganga, icy from her long journey down from the serene Himalayan heights, has gathered speed as she flows down through Rishikesh and Haridwar, hermitages sanctified by the meditations of yogis and saints since the beginning of time. And now she lies becalmed, mingling with her sister Jamuna, who, fresh from her dalliance in the heart-land of Braj where the Dark Lord of Love dances to fill the world with celestial happiness, is still flushed with his ethereal blueness.[298] And deep in the earth, watching over these two, runs their silent elder sister, Saraswati, the embodiment of the intelligence that governs all life, who retreated underground when the folly of humankind became too gross for her to countenance. She lies there patiently waiting for the time when the earth will be pure enough to receive her blessings again and she can join her sisters and flow freely up on land once more.

The Master's heart is thrilled to be at such a place. The whole area seems to be scintillating with subtle magnetism and the world is an even more brilliant play of divine bliss than usual. And what is more, as the configuration of the planets - sun, moon and Jupiter - is auspicious, the Kumbha Mela festival is in full swing. The dried-up river beds have become a vast field of saffron, an encampment set up to house an army of spiritual warriors. As far as the eye can see, stretch tents, *pandals*[299] and huts made of earth, leaves and bamboo. Above them flutter banners and flags and streamers of all sizes, colours and designs; each standard proclaiming the sectarian affiliation of those who gather beneath it, for every type of actor on the limitless stage of the sacred is represented here.

The assembled company divides into two main groups. Most eye-catching are the various followers of one or other of the many forms of Shiva, the Lord of Transformation, who dances the universe in a delicately controlled ecstasy only to retire to the burning ground from where, wearing nothing but ash from the pyres, and accompanied by innumerable spirits, he orchestrates universal impermanence. These *sadhus* are the spiritual anarchists, temperamentally unable to conform to the restrictions of any institution or ordinance. Among them are the Vratyas 'those who have taken the vow', nomadic brotherhoods outside the Vedic orthodoxy who have roamed the Land of the Veda since the beginning of time. Identifiable by their red or black bordered loin cloths, red turbans and lavish silver ornaments, they travel by horse-drawn carts and practise arcane rituals. Some Vratyas generate spiritual energy through sexual continence, while others consort freely with the communal women that travel with them. Then there are the Keshavins, 'the long-haired ones', trance-shamans from the highland plateaus of the far north, who are hung with animal skins, feathers and necklaces of amulets made of teeth and bones, and carry spears and ritual drums. They whirl and dance, and leave their bodies to get messages from the spirit realms.[300] The Pashupatas are there, worshippers of Shiva in his form of Pashupati 'the Lord of all Beasts', each bearing his *nagpani* trumpet shaped like a coiled cobra to communicate at great distances when on the roam, and there are the Kapalikas 'the Bearers of Skulls' whose only possession is a human skull used as a drinking bowl. These spectral souls practise their shadowy rituals with human bones amidst the embers of the cremation grounds, and are rumoured to offer not only wine and blood to the dark elementals they worship, but pieces of their own body too. There are the Aghoris, 'the Fearless Ones', who inhabit their own liminal universe that is closed to all outsiders. These *sadhus* are experts in incantation and witchcraft and controllers of ghosts and *djinns,* and they scorn all social norms: drinking alcohol, eating meat and offal, and casting spells for a fee. And alongside them are the Kanphatas, the 'Ear-pierced' brotherhood, easily distinguished by the huge earrings of wood, ivory or gold that designate their place in the group's hierarchy. And then are the Naga *babas,* naked *sadhus* who sport long tresses matted with cow-dung, their lean bodies protected from the sun of the desert or the cold of mountain heights by being smeared with ashes from the funeral pyre. Organised into regiments whose leaders often possess considerable scholastic learning, the Nagas are ascetic body-building warriors armed with swords, cutlasses, daggers and spears, as they move around the land, a mobile army of the righteous perpetually alert in their defence of *Sanatana Dharma.*[301]

Less unconventional are the worshippers of Lord Vishnu, the divine protector of hearth and home and the householder life. His forms as the ever-charming Rama, the ideal ruler, or Krishna, the beautiful blue-skinned Lord of Love, are especially popular among the devotees here. These Vaishnava *sadhus* are generally treading a less rigorous path than the followers of the Lord of the Cremation ground;

they seek their bliss in plumbing the depths of the world rather than rejecting it as insubstantial folly. They play and sing and dance with wild abandon in devotion to their Lord; others cook and offer food to gain admission to the court of the Divine. Some even dress as women, mimicking the cowgirl *gopis* who fell so hopelessly in love with the amorous Lord Krishna and, lured by the sound of his flute, abandoned all their duties to follow him. But even amongst these various Vaishnavas there are austere renunciate cadres, especially from the low-lying lands bordering the great Eastern Sea, where they are particularly numerous. As part of their penance, some of these never walk but move everywhere at a relentless trot; others have abandoned human company altogether to live in remote caves and forests, alone with their god.

Here and there amidst the swirling flow of bodies, the great *gurus* and abbots of the settled acetic orders stand out. Regally bedecked in flowers and brightly coloured cloths, they sit in magnificence atop painted and decorated elephants and camels or astride the white horse that is the traditional symbol of renunciation and the mount of Lord Kalki, whose fierce sword of judgement will bring the current age of ignorance to an end. Bands playing music and groups singing *bhajans* and chanting scriptures attend them, for these are the crowned Monarchs of *Maya*, the Sovereigns of the Spirit, and the whole of the widespread *mela* ground is their royal court.

Then there are also devotees of Mother Divine, She who takes countless forms in order to watch over every particle of the universe. Sometimes when She is feeling gentle, Mother deigns to materialise as the gentle maternal Ambika, giver of love and protection or as the ever-bountiful Annapurna, from whom even Lord Shiva, in his guise as a fasting mendicant, accepts food. But at other times Her fierceness knows no bounds and then she becomes embodied as Durga, riding astride a lion and brandishing all the weapons of her fellow deities at once, or as her terrifying sister Kali, garlanded with skulls and hot blood dripping from her long, lolling tongue.

The second main group is composed of various orthodox orders of monks and it presents a very different aspect. Vedic *sannyasis* are clearly visible robed in various hues of orange; they live and travel singly or in small groups and only meet together during the annual four-month monsoon retreats or at religious fairs such as this *mela*. There are Viraktas, who move around the country in small orderly groups while keeping silence and there are many serious *brahmacharis*, white-robed apprentices to various spiritual teachers, serving their mentors as they tread the long path of scholarship and devotion. The followers of Gautama, the Great Renouncer from the foothills, are easily distinguished. Their hair shorn, their school announced by the colour of the robe – red, maroon, ochre, yellow, brown, black – these monks and nuns have travelled here, not only from all over the Land of the Veda, but from places far beyond the high Himalaya and across the great Eastern Sea. And then there are the two orders of Jains, rigorous ascetics who follow the teachings of Mahavir, last in the ancient lineage of twenty-four *tirthankaras*, 'those who have crossed to the other shore'. On joining the life of the religious, these novitiates have every hair plucked from their body and as they walk the length and breadth of the land they wear cotton masks and brush the path in front of them with brooms made of softest cotton, lest they inadvertently destroy some tiny creature. One of these Jain orders wears spotless white; the other is as naked as the sky.

There have been many days of *yajna* and *puja*, meditation and worship of deities, devotional singing, mass feeding of holy men and women and the poor, numerous religious assemblies where doctrines were debated and disputed, and recitations of scripture and epic tales of the gods. Also, for the common pilgrims, there have been wrestling competitions and gymnastic displays featuring practitioners of *hatha* yoga, as well as acrobats, magicians, jugglers and popular storytellers, and huge communal kitchens that work all hours of the day and night, dispensing food in a never-ending stream. The climax of the *mela* is now to come, and, as always it is the ritual immersion at the Triveni Sangam, the confluence of the three sacred river goddesses. Tradition decrees that the most ascetic orders have the right to go first into the water to take the *shahi snanam* 'the Royal Bath' at the astrologically auspicious moment. Throughout the crowds the atmosphere is electric in anticipation of this communal immersion that has the power to wash away the debt of accumulated *karmas* and ensure liberation from the cycle of birth and death.

But this time something goes terribly wrong. The emotional tension is always high as the moment of immersion approaches, and around midnight, a disagreement arises amongst the Naga *babas* about which of their various orders is entitled to be the first to enter the water. Suddenly, as if from nowhere, a pitched battle breaks out between different groups and spreads with the rapidity of a forest fire. Hundreds die in the fighting and countless bystanders are crushed to death in the chaos that ensues.

The next day a darkly sombre atmosphere hangs heavily over the *mela* ground and the air is thick with the sweet stench of death. The Master has taken his followers far downriver, away from the wailing crowds, the bodies in the water and the scrawny vultures that hop and flap and peck around them, bloody strips of flesh swinging from their beaks. The orange-robed group sits quietly together on the river bank as the wintry sun climbs slowly higher in the grey sky. Since hearing the terrible news, the Master has been in deep meditation, and now he emerges to speak in a tone his companions have not heard before.

"The spiritual life of our holy land is in chaos", he begins. "Wherever you look there are so many disparate groups, each one turned in on itself, each claiming to have the truth, each wrapped up in its own subjective visions and fantasies, and limited by its conditioned perspective to the exclusion of the others around it. The only well-organised seekers are the Buddhists and the Jains – but they have rejected the Veda and its authority because their founders lived at a time when our tradition was in decline and no longer served the needs of the people. Our own monks are quite numerous, but disunited and scattered with no real sense of community, they wander like wild swans here and there as individual itinerants or in small cadres, rejecting organisation, without cohesion or purpose. And because of this, they cannot exert a powerful influence on the people at large, and their ability to guide and transform the ways of society and bring true understanding and righteous living to the people is very limited. What is the hope of ending suffering if even the so-called spiritual fight amongst themselves to gain some petty advantage? It is a ludicrous situation".

He gestures disgustedly upriver towards the *mela* ground. "No, no, no! What is needed is a totally new structure, an organisation through which the truth can be efficiently disseminated and can begin to exert its rightful and necessary influence on the lives of the suffering and ignorant". The disciples have never seen their Master in such a mood, and it awes and thrills them.

"Now!", continues the young *sannyasi,* his eyes blazing. "Let us consider the Land of the Veda as a sacred *yantra*". Taking his bamboo staff, the symbol of renunciation, he draws a square on the sand and marks on it the cardinal points: north, south, east and west. "What we must do is to draw this *yantra* together into a coherently functioning whole. So, we must activate and re-energise it by establishing vibrant *chakras* at its unifying centre and at each of the points radiating out from there. These five *chakras* will be great monasteries, places of learning, refuge and enlightenment, and their enlivening influence will allow the country to breathe freely again: its in-breath will draw the people to the monasteries for instruction and inspiration and its out-breath will send them back outwards, refreshed and renewed in their understanding of life's great purpose. These centres will circulate spiritual energy and spread the celestial light throughout the body of the Land of the Veda, their role will be to restore its health and reinvigorate its noble heritage of Vedic wisdom. To this end, each institution will be the custodian of a particular Veda, have responsibility for its specific teachings, and act as its material form.

"You have seen this pattern before", he continues with mounting enthusiasm, as the plan unfolds as if spontaneously. "In our temples, the central holy of holies houses the main deity, and the four subsidiary shrines contain affiliated deities that radiate the central energy out to the four directions. The temple complex gains its power not only from the deity that lives there, but because the physical structure of the place reflects eternal principles. These are laid down in our texts on sacred architecture and have served their purpose for millennia, but the time has now come to apply these principles on a larger scale and thereby extend their influence throughout the land for the good of all.

"Now, how shall we ensure that the sacred influence generated in each of these five great monasteries is at its purest and most powerful? Each must serve as a continuing home for Lord Shiva and his Shakti, so in each place the most potent *lingam* will be installed and the appropriate image of Mother Divine will be enthroned there also. This will balance the masculine and feminine energies and will also provide a focus of worship for householder rituals, for these sites must act as spiritual nourishment for the people at large, and not just feed themselves and the religious who are housed there".

The Master pauses here, deep in thought. Then he continues:

"And then, once these places have been established, how will we ensure that their sacred influence radiates most effectively in a way that is kept lively and dynamic? Now, look again! Superimposed over this *yantra* we add a *mandala*", so saying he draws a circle over the square and deftly marks off ten points equally spaced around its circumference. "We shall establish a highly disciplined and intellectually capable order of monks divided into ten groups corresponding to each of the ten directions, and they will be known as the *Dashanami sannyasis* 'the Renunciates of the Ten Names'. Each of these groups will have its own family name, its own responsibility and its own character. Once again, this ten-fold organisation is nothing new, but marks a revival of a principle of universality we are already familiar with. The source of all our wisdom, the collected primordial sounds of the Rig Veda, is divided into the ten-fold *mandalas,* and this structure is then replicated at a grosser level of materiality in the physical form of the ten directions of space embodied and acknowledged in our temple compounds.[302] So, each of the ten orders of *sannyasis* will be affiliated to its particular monastery, owing allegiance to the institution and its unbroken lineage of teachers. Their lives will be of an exemplary simplicity; moving from place to place, they will spread the Teaching, and for the most part living singly, for if ascetics gather too much into groups, a gradual deterioration of purpose will set in. But, if appropriate, they shall return to their parent monastery for the four-month rainy season each year; this arrangement will serve to keep the orders unified and coherent. It is a system that Gautama ordained in his time and it has worked well for the Buddhists, so we can learn from this. If the Vedic teaching is organised in this way, it will stand firm with its continuance assured; it will be the everlasting Wish-Fulfilling Tree that nourishes and protects the Land of the Veda! This is the vision of possibilities that has been born today, my inseparable companions, and it will transform human life!"

The disciples are quiet, stunned by the boldness of the plan and the speed at which it has unfolded. After some moments Sureshvara speaks up: "I can see how this will reform the life of the religious, Master, but the householders...?" The Master smiles fondly at the man, recalling his previous affiliation as the champion of the householder way of life and the momentous debate they once had when he was known as Mandana Mishra. "Ah yes, our friends the householders. Well, no problem there!" He laughs and quickly draws a second quadrant next to the first. "Now, we just follow the *Vastuvidya* temple pattern again. All the gods are but forms of the one Absolute and, as such, all are interrelated. But as we know, a person generally feels an affinity with one or other of these forms, so no one single representation can serve all devotees equally. Therefore, we install the chosen deity in the centre of our *yantra*, and to that deity worship is directed, but the other deities are present too, stationed at the cardinal points, witnessing and partaking in the whole process indirectly, as it were. They are not the guest of honour at the feast but honoured guests none the less, in a subsidiary role. So, let us say a man is temperamentally drawn to Lord Ganesha as The Remover of Obstacles. The appropriate image will be duly installed in the central position, while Shiva, Devi, Surya and Vishnu occupy the outer positions. Or, if Lord Vishnu takes the centre stage, then Ganesh and the others stand on the periphery. Actually, it makes no difference in the end. In this scheme, all the expressions of the Absolute are enlivened, each brings its blessings to the worshipper in a way that satisfies his partiality and, eventually he will be drawn to transcend them all and reside in their source, the Absolute that is his own Self.

"See, it is a beautiful way to manage the progression from the outer to the inner. This five-fold structure, with the hidden sixth as the backdrop of the unmanifest Absolute, is already a principle that governs life at different levels: remember the five elements, the five senses, the five *koshas*. All we are doing is consciously recognising its operation in the celestial realms of the deities also. Yes, yes! This will be the way to bring some coherence into the daily worship of the people ..."[303]

After a moment he adds thoughtfully "We are establishing a new dawn here, the dawn of the new Age of Enlightenment!"

Then, after another pause "So, as this is the new dawn, we shall follow the course of the sun and begin with the east. No time is to be wasted; we shall start tomorrow! "

The next day as the sun rises over the horizon, the Master and his party set off for Puri, a sacred city on the east coast that is a great pilgrimage centre due to the special form of Lord Vishnu as the Ruler

306

of the World who resides in the great temple there. Thousands of pilgrims regularly come to the city to get *darshan* of the deity, and it is not long before the Master is able to secure the patronage of local well-wishers and establish the Govardhana Math, set back from the mighty ocean that stretches as far as the eye can see eastwards. This will act as a spiritual powerhouse, teaching the Veda, training *pundits*, looking after the health and welfare of the local people and tending to the needs of visiting pilgrims. Padmacharya is appointed as the first abbot of the monastery.[304] The Master's influence ensures that many local people are initiated into *sannyasa* and three orders of *sannyasis* are founded in affiliation with the *math*: the brotherhoods of *Vanam* 'forest', *Aranya* 'jungle' and *Sagara* 'sea'. The monastery is appointed as the custodian of the Rig Veda, the summation of all Vedic wisdom, and a teaching institution called the 'Hall of Freedom' is also founded and left in charge of a group of scholars whose special responsibility is to preserve the purity of Vedic recitation and textual analysis. So delighted is the local raja that he insists on giving the Master the extraordinary privilege of being able to enter the temple wearing his wooden sandals, with a parasol to use and a mattress to sit on once inside. The practice is still followed by Shankaracharyas today. Before leaving the city, the Master also installs as the presiding deity an image of Shiva in his form as *Ardhanarishvara*, 'the Lord who is half-woman', to symbolise the conjunction of matter and spirit and the mutual embrace of the masculine and feminine principles. And so the founding stone of the revival has been laid.

Filled with energy and enthusiasm, the Master decides to continue his mission by heading south. His reputation spreads rapidly before him and whenever the party reaches a new town, they will stay for some time as crowds assemble to take *darshan* of this young man who is known to be the living embodiment of Vedic wisdom. As well as religious and philosophical authorities, many ordinary people come to see the Master to get his blessings, for they know that a saint is a force-field of spiritual energy who can transform lives by only a glance.

Sometimes he sits in radiant silence as an open door to the infinite, while the descended energy purifies all those present, cleansing minds and opening hearts; sometimes there is recitation of the sacred Veda or singing of popular *bhajans* praising the many faces of God; sometimes the Teaching emerges through parable, debate or textual analysis, according to the needs and capacity of those present. This results in an extraordinary flow of knowledge, given out as naturally and effortlessly as a flower gives out its scent. And wherever he goes, his presence is a consistent invitation, offering those who come before him a glimpse into their own divine nature through the medium of an imagined other.

A farmer asks the Master about the Teaching and he replies:
"You are an expert in growing things. And what is the secret of growing? As you know very well, the way to nourish a wilting plant is not by attending to each individual leaf but by watering the root. Just so, the way to nourish our life is to purify the mind, for our mind is the root of our life and our thoughts of today build our life of tomorrow. Take the mind to the reservoir of inner silence and this will refresh all aspects of your life in a natural and balanced way, making it strong and healthy so that all your legitimate desires will mature and yield their fruit in due time. And once you have learned to water your own root, you will naturally grow yourself in the plants, grow yourself in the crops, grow yourself in the goats and the cattle and grow yourself in the hearts of others also".

A young bride asks the Master about the Teaching and he replies:
"You women stand at the pinnacle of creation, for you incarnate the great goddess Shakti, who governs the entire material creation. It is because of this that women are more in touch with the material side of life than are men and they act to organise daily life behind the scenes and at the subtler levels. But with this blessing comes a great responsibility. Always remember that the material world is only half of life and do not forget that materialism on its own will soon degenerate into mere worldliness and vulgarity. Born with a more refined nervous system than a man, you women naturally entertain those

finer feelings which are the gateway to the Divine. Because of this you are the guardians of the purity of tradition. You bear and nurture life; what you eat, think and feel affects even the children you are carrying in the womb. You feed, teach and shape the family and by this you stabilise and civilise the whole of society. So the safety of tradition lies in your hands. And, as it is said in our scriptures[305] once the age-old traditions are lost, unrighteousness overtakes the entire family, the women of the family become corrupt and the whole social order suffers as a result. And remember that marriage is a path of devotion, and devotion entails sacrifice – each for the other, mutually. Husband and wife are one soul in two bodies. They should treat each other as gods and in this way one can help the other, and both can reach the Divine together. This is the spiritual purpose of the marriage you are entering into".

A cloth maker asks the Master about the Teaching and he answers:
"Just as when you are dyeing a white cloth, you must first dip it in a vat of colour and then expose it to the heat of the sun to dry, so must you dip your mind in the inner peace and expose it to the demands of the everyday world. The colour will fade in the sun, but a layer has been laid down fast. And just as you have to dip and dry a cloth many, many times before it becomes saturated with a colour that remains indelible, so the mind has to be dipped in the inner peace many, many times before that tranquillity will stand fast under each and every circumstance that life may throw at you".

A weaver of silk brocades asks the Master about the Teaching and he replies:
"Each life is a tapestry of unique design and hue, and it is woven of the threads of our thoughts and the actions that follow on those thoughts. You always have the choice of which threads to use and combine, and which to discard and whether to weave them too tight, too slack or just right. So see that the tapestry you weave is true to your best nature: strong, even and beautiful both inside and out, and not

just some showy, glamorous affair that has no inner strength and ends up smothering your true Self".

A woman who makes and sells flower garlands outside the temple asks about the Teaching and he answers:

"May the gods smile on your life for the work you are doing. Take one of those flowers and split open the stalk. Inside you will see the colourless sap that has taken form as the flat dark green leaf, the stiff straight stalk, the soft red petals with their beautiful scent. All these are just the manifestations of the colourless sap; that sap is present everywhere in the flower, the unseen cause and nourishment of all its different aspects. Like that, everywhere within this endlessly varied universe there is the underlying causal energy, hidden and silent. This unifying intelligence is the Absolute, it is the source and goal of all life, and that is your real nature. And now see how your flowers are strung one by one on the thread, one after the other, in succession, ready to be offered to the image of the deity. Like that, your different lives will continue, strung on the thread of *brahman*, one after the other, until you realise your real nature, your real Self".

A wealthy merchant asks him about the Teaching and he responds:

"Each creature naturally seeks for more and more until it is satisfied, for this is life's longing for itself. Just so it is your nature to seek for more. In fact, everything that you may need has been sent into the world well before your arrival here but, until you realise this, your seeking may focus on anything – money, possessions, family, fame and all the rest. There is nothing wrong with making money, but you must remember that the purpose of doing business is not just to make money, it is to provide what is really useful and nourishing to the people and thereby to make some money into the bargain. And when you have made your money, take care to use it wisely, otherwise you will end up being used by it. Be generous to those less fortunate than yourself and always keep your income purified by donating regularly to religious and spiritual causes. Sooner or later you will come to see that the real wealth, the treasure all people are seeking, is the inner abundance that no money can buy. At that time you will realise that the wealthiest of all are those who possess nothing, but own everything. For if you could only see it, you would realise that there is no lack anywhere whatsoever; all you really lack is the infinite plenitude of your own being".

A rajah asks the Master about the Teaching and he answers:

"Just as you can only govern the hearts of your people if you treat them with respect and kindness rather than harsh discipline and punishments, so you should treat yourself on the path to self-mastery. Self-mastery is a state of being that is more regal than anything you could imagine, but it has nothing to do with outer power and magnificent trappings, and it cannot exist where there is domination or fear of being dominated. Truly you are the lord of all you survey, but to realise this you must use the inner eye of wisdom. When this eye is opened, then your commands will be carried out quite naturally by the hidden forces of nature. The gods and goddesses will spontaneously do your bidding, because your wishes will be for the good of all. Then you will be like God, who is the greatest of all Maharajahs – witnessing everything but doing nothing!"

A *brahmin* devoted to the spiritual path asks him about the Teaching and he replies:

"Life is precious, fragile and short; not one of us knows what the future holds. It is extraordinarily fortunate to have achieved a human form among the eighty-four thousand possibilities of embodiment. Even the angels envy mankind, because they are trapped in their heavens by the blissful atmosphere there, and lack the incentive to develop any further. We humans, on the other hand, have been born into a realm which, sooner or later, will prove to be inherently unsatisfying, and this dissatisfaction turns out to be the greatest blessing, because it will push us on through the insufficiencies of the world to seek for the ultimate. So devote as much time as you can to spiritual development, for if Yama snatches you from this little body before you have achieved enlightenment, then you will have sold a diamond for the price of spinach".

How can the One become many?

As the guest of a local landowner, the Master is seated in a pleasantly airy room overlooking large well-tended gardens, surrounded by a group comprised of both disciplined, critical thinkers and some more emotionally committed disciples. He is equally and effortlessly at home with all of them, his bright gaze genial and penetrating by turns.

A student of metaphysics asks:

"Master, it is said in the scriptures that the One becomes the many. I don't understand how this can be unless the Absolute enters into something which is different from itself?"

The answer is accompanied by a serene smile.

"Very good! The text you are referring to has the Absolute say: 'Let me become many, let me be born!', and so on?"[306]

The questioner nods.

The Master continues:

"Now, the multiplication referred to here does not imply becoming something extraneous to oneself, as you might do by having a child, for example. So what then does this text really mean? It means that the way the Absolute creates is by manifesting the many worlds of name and form that lie latent within itself.[307] Once these get manifested they evolve in time and space, while still remaining inseparable from the Absolute as their intrinsic nature, just as time and space themselves are also intrinsically inseparable from the Absolute. And it is just this evolution of myriad names and forms that is called the appearance of the One as the many. As the Absolute is an infinite, unified mass of Consciousness without parts, there is no other way it could become finite and multiple.

"So we can see that there is nothing whatsoever, whether in the past, present or future, here, there or anywhere, which is disconnected from the Absolute, nothing that is remote from it or separated out from it by time or space. On the contrary, it is only because of the Absolute that the manifested worlds – the visible and the invisible, the formed and the formless – exist in the first place, and they are all dependent on their source , always and completely. But the Absolute *brahman* itself is utterly and perfectly independent; it stands free of its creations and does not consist of any of them, singly or taken together".[308]

"If this is so, Maharaj-ji, how is it taught that the world is unreal?"

"Because the world has no reality when it is considered apart from its essence, which is the Absolute".

The Self is omnipresent

At another time when in the land of the Andhra tribes, near the great temple of Tirupati where Lord Venkateshvara resides in all his splendour, someone approaches the Master and asks:

"Swamigal, will you not come to our village to give *darshan*?"

"I am already there!" he laughs.

In Kanchipuram

The party continues southwards, with the Master giving audience at temples, ashrams, pilgrim rest-houses and the residences of well-wishers. Eventually they reach the country of the Tamils, many of whom are devoted followers of Shiva. They have their own scriptures that derived from Sanskrit originals many centuries previously. The young *sannyasi* is clearly happy to be back this far south after such a long absence, enjoying once more the language, customs and food of the people amongst whom he grew up.[309] Although he is spending much of his time engaging in metaphysical debate with philosophers and pundits of various religious schools, he himself at this time seems to be filled with an unusual devotional fervour. Some attribute it to the personal contact he has been having with many of the great Goddesses who live in the temples and shrines that lie scattered through this part of the country. He appears to enjoy a particular affinity with these forms of the universal Mother.

Swept up in the mood of revival, people have joined him at each place he stops. With what is now a large group of both monks and lay people he travels on down to the ancient city of Kanchipuram, one of the seven sacred 'Cities of Liberation' celebrated in the holy texts. The great poet Kalidasa celebrated Kanchi as 'the best among cities' and the city has long been known as the Kashi of the south. As befits the capital of the mighty Pallava dynasty, Kanchi is indeed a splendid place with wide, well-laid out streets full of fine buildings and water courses. It is also a thriving centre of devotion and learning. Many orthodox temples and institutions flourish here, while orders of various heretical schools, such as the Jains and the Buddhists, are also patronised and supported. With such a culture of open-minded enquiry and sincere seeking, the Master is confident that here is somewhere that will be receptive to the great spiritual transition that is taking place, an evolutionary movement seemingly conducted by Mother Nature herself.

However, on their arrival, the Master and his followers are met with unexpected news. Kamakshi Ma, the presiding deity of the city, is mightily out of sorts; offended by laxity in the performance of rituals, she has angrily recoiled within herself and withdrawn her blessings from the people. As a result, the rains have not come this year, crops are withered in the fields and wells dried up, illness is rife amongst both humans and animals. A heavy sense of gloom hangs everywhere, and the senior temple authorities, well aware that the blame for this unfortunate situation lies on their well-oiled shoulders, turn to the young visitor, whose reputation has long preceded him, in near desperation.

His response is authoritative and immediate. What is needed is the revival of an ancient branch of wisdom that has long fallen out of use: *Shri Vidya* 'the most auspicious knowledge', a spiritual methodology that worships the Goddess as the three-fold personification of the supreme Consciousness. In this understanding, the Goddess is to be approached as that personal intelligence which unites all levels of manifestation. The gross, subtle and causal worlds, the three *gunas* that structure the material universe and the three states of waking, dream and deep sleep – all are aspects of Her, every being, every situation and every occurrence is Her playful form alone.

Central to the *Shri Vidya* ritual is the *Shri yantra*, a lotus *mandala* of nine intersecting triangles that symbolise the interplay of the male and female principles and the interpenetration of consciousness and matter in varying degrees of density. Focussing on this microcosm with appropriate purifying mantras and meditations aligns the practitioner's awareness with the deity and establishes a connection with Her that brings extraordinary powers and eventual liberation. A skilled adept, who has achieved the inner illumination that enables him to perceive the depths of reality, can practice these techniques on behalf of the community. This the Master duly does and, gratified, the Goddess responds favourably. Harmony is restored to the Kanchipuram community and to perpetuate a living connection with Her, a monastery and teaching centre is duly established near her temple in the heart of the walled city. It is known as the Kamakoti Pitham; to this day it continues as a great spiritual influence throughout the Land of the Tamils and far beyond.

In celebration of this event, the Master composes a great poem of praise to the Goddess[310] which emphasises that the supreme Reality is always non-dual, whilst generously including, yet simultaneously transcending, all dualities. The poem is also a practical textbook of ritual, containing many *pujas* and *mantras,* and detailing *yantras* with instructions for their correct worship and the benign results that will follow. With great focus and an unrelenting energy, the Master also teaches the techniques of *Shri Vidya* to some *brahmins* who are suitably qualified, instigating a tradition of ritual expertise that continues today.

Among the Buddhists

During his lengthy stay in Kanchipuram, the Master comes into contact with many followers of the various Buddhist schools that have long been firmly established here. Very often they are highly intellectual people, who in their search for truth seem to have lost touch with the natural warmth and spontaneity of everyday life. Each school claims it had the original message of the Buddha and often highly charged debates ensue. Generally, the Master takes a very common-sense approach with such people, sometimes showing them short shrift.

It is early afternoon on a hot spring day and the Master is lying on his simple couch at one end of the *darshan* hall enjoying a rest. Yet his body is also emitting a powerful energy, so much so that it seems inconceivable he is asleep. Various people are sitting in the airy room; some are lost in contemplation while others converse in whispers. A feeling of safety and intimacy pervades the room as soft light dapples the floor while birds fly in and out of the open windows. Suddenly, the figure on the couch sits upright with an easy and natural movement, without the slightest strain, as flexible as a child. The sage turns to face the hall with a gaze that is clear and shining; it is evident that he is stationed somewhere inherently beyond what we call waking and sleeping. His complete openness invites immediate engagement.

Near the couch sits a group of local Buddhist monks. One of them, a proponent of a celebrated idealist school[311], is the first to speak up.

"I have studied your teachings closely, Sir, and I think we are in complete agreement. We both teach that everything takes place within the mind, that thought is the only reality. We define a perception as a solely internal process, made up of the process of knowing, the object of knowledge and the result of that knowledge. Do you agree?"

"Well, I do not teach solipsism", replies the Master briskly. "Of course there is an outward reality – pillars, walls, pots, cloths, whatever – that corresponds to each act of perception. There can be no serious debate with a view that denies the existence of such outward things and events. Holding such a view is like eating a meal and enjoying the food, but at the same time denying you are doing so!"

"I do not hold that I do not perceive anything", replies the other carefully, "but only that I do not perceive anything apart from the perception itself".

The Master gestures around the hall.

"The very nature of daily living argues that the outward world exists apart from the individual perceiving consciousness. Anyone who perceives a pillar or a wall is aware not only of their subjective perception, but also that all others present are perceiving the same pillar and the same wall as well. Indeed, the very fact that you attempt so hard to distinguish the inner world of perception from the outer world of objects shows that, at bottom, you accept the outer world does in fact exist!"[312]

The idealist falls silent and after a moment another member of the group, who allies himself with the dialectic school that teaches 'universal momentariness'[313] now takes up the debate:

"Honoured *sannyasi*, I just cannot accept that there is any permanent self and I do not understand why you are misleading the common people by promulgating this erroneous notion. Our teaching is clear that nothing in the world is permanent, everything without exception is only momentary. Therefore it follows that reality is just an uninterrupted series of momentary phenomena, devoid of any lasting substratum. These discreet phenomena may well create the appearance of an abiding entity, but that is only because of their similarity moment to moment – just as a flame appears to be one and the same but is in fact a rapid succession of different jets of flame. So for us, the goal of life is to transcend this conditioned series of phenomena and achieve liberation, *nirvana*".

The Master's eyes, clear and wide open, show he is communing deeply not only with what is being said, but with what lies behind it.

"Certainly", he replies, "nothing in the world is permanent. Quite correct. But the Self is not in the world! We are talking here about the pure awareness that is the transcendental root of both the perceiver and the perceived. Now, you maintain that all things are momentary, including the perceiver himself. How then is it that any of these momentary perceptions are maintained in the memory? The memory belongs to the perceiver, does it not? It is an impression retained by the subject. No one is in confusion as to whether it is he himself or another person who has a particular memory; nobody thinks: 'It is I who am remembering this event, but it was someone else who had the original perception of it'. So then, what is it that grasps the similarity and the continuity of these successive moments of perception? It must be the perceiving subject and, to do so, that subject cannot itself be momentary, it must be permanent. This is borne out by our everyday experience. It is really just common sense, is it not?

"Moreover," – the Master is warming to his theme now – "your teaching undermines the practicality of the very path to relieve suffering that you claim to follow. Since, according to your view, every flash of consciousness is but momentary, it must naturally subside by itself, without any effort on the part of the perceiver. This being so, of what use then are traditional Buddhist spiritual practices such as the meditation on momentariness? Nothing has to be done to bring anything to an end, because being momentary, everything comes to an end automatically!"

"But what if the suffering individual is in fact just a series of these momentary flashes of consciousness?", comes the reply.

"In that case, a further factor would then be needed to terminate them! And because, according to your theory, this factor is also momentary itself, it could have no lasting connection with that on which it acted. The logic of this line of argument is that if everything were only momentary, nothing would depend causally on anything else, and conversely, anything could then be the cause of anything else! This is patently absurd. Only when two things exist simultaneously can they act on each other, and from this fact comes the sequence of cause and effect that your teacher the Buddha designated 'the law of dependent origination'".

Unable to counter this reasoning, the man then asks how the Master's teaching of Vedanta would resolve the problem.

"Very neatly!", comes the reply. "What I teach is that when a false superimposition is destroyed, the destruction is confined to that superimposition alone, not to its substratum. This is the situation that pertains: on the one hand there is the erroneous assumption of a limited selfhood run by ever-changing desires, and, on the other hand, the eternally abiding Self. You people who deny any such abiding Self, yet argue that liberation is the total destruction of everything conditioned, must answer this question: who or what is it that remains to gain anything from this cherished liberation?"

The Master lets the question hang in the still air a moment, then continues:

"No, all clear thinkers must eventually agree that something ultimate exists, whether they call it pure awareness, the Self, the Void or whatever they may care to. But as the witness of being and non-being, it cannot itself be non-existent, as you are effectively arguing. If no-one or nothing exists to experience a gain, then that gain must surely be worthless, even if it is the incomparable gain of enlightenment! So we see clearly here: that which is aware of non-existence must itself exist and it must be real. If not, people would not be able to determine the existence or non-existence of anything whatsoever and such an absurd situation just cannot be accepted".[314]

The group is quiet now and a timeless silence blossoms in the room. The Master sits regally immobile, like a lion. At times like this he seems balanced on the very cusp of finite existence. After a while, the men make their salutations and leave the hall. Following their departure the Master gives his own followers some advice:

"My friends, whenever learned philosophers refuse to admit something that is perfectly obvious from everyday experience, be very careful! Clever minds may play with words to advance their own opinion and demolish contrary views, but by doing so, in the end they cannot really convince either themselves or others. Even these Buddhists will manage to attract seekers of truth because a thirsty man will always be drawn by the promise of water. But as we have just seen, whatever their Master may originally have taught, their systems are in fact without foundation. And so, rest assured, sooner or later they will give way, like the walls of a well dug in sandy soil".[315]

Householder or recluse?

A well-respected headman from a large village to the south of the city comes to see the Master. He is an elderly man of great dignity and carries a quiet serenity about him. The Master receives him with great courtesy.

"I have listened to your discourses on several occasions over the last few weeks, Swamigal", the visitor begins, "and I have to say that I am astonished at the intellectual brilliance of what you have to say. You exhibit a conviction and clarity all too rare in someone twice your age, let alone a young man of your tender years. And there is no doubt to me that you speak so eloquently about ultimate reality from the depths of your own personal experience. But there is one thing that I find disturbing about your teaching as I have understood it, and that is that you tend to disparage the life of the married householder in comparison to the life of a recluse. How can such a bias be helpful to the vast majority of people, who may well not be saints in the making but simply wish to live properly in society, raising a family and doing their best to lead a virtuous and religious life?"

"My dear Sir", replies the Master, his gaze saturated with compassion, "I do not mean to disparage the married state or the life of the householder. How could I? I myself owe the precious gift of this human body to the union of two beings who were united in the state of marriage, and all my work here", he indicates with a sweep of his hand the ashram courtyard where they are sitting "is made possible only by the generosity of those householders who are giving alms and offering service. So I have no intention of denigrating the life of the married householder; indeed, I consider it to be the foundation of both the secular and the religious life".

"But do you not extol the virtues of the renunciate life over and above those of the householder?"

"Actually, as I see it, the outward form of any particular life is not what matters, it is the inner disposition that is important. You may be a recluse in a remote mountain cave, lusting after women and gold or you may be a householder embroiled in the busy market place, living a life of rectitude, equanimity and dispassion".

The headman nods slowly, somewhat reassured.

"My point on this matter" continues the Master, "is simply that for any human being, time and energy are very limited. Not one of us knows when Lord Yama[316] will come, but come he must. So each of us must choose very carefully how we spend our energy and attention in the few years allotted us, and this is especially so if we want to make any progress on the spiritual path. The scriptures tell us there are 84,000 types of birth to be endured before the gift of a human form, so is it not incumbent upon us to make the very best use of this rare blessing? Look at the animals: they spend all of their time getting food, securing territory or reproducing. As human beings, should we not aspire to more than this endless search for survival and continuance? All the holy texts and teachings tell us there is a human possibility greater than the limitations of mere individuality, so should we not aim to realise that great destiny and seek the Truth?

"Considering all this, one thing that can be said about the householder life is that it places very great demands on a person's time and energy. There is the need to earn a living, to provide for children and relatives, to maintain a house in good order and all the rest of it. There is always something to be done, for such is the nature of the world, and to satisfy the weight of family demands and social obligation, the attention must continuously be employed outwards, in the realm of the senses. All this activity in the outer world is a great source of joy and satisfaction no doubt, but it generally leaves no time to investigate who or what we really are, to discover what is the inner nature of this person who is always so busily occupied. And it is also undeniable, is it not, that the end of so many of our worldly endeavours is sadness, disappointment or pain? The fact of the matter is that the world and its insufficiencies wear us all out sooner or later, and it is all too easy to miss the opportunity to explore the possibility of a radically new way of being in the world, one which will spread joy and light all around".

The Master pauses to let the weight of this analysis sink in. Then, he takes his argument a stage further:

"Also, it must be admitted that there is impurity inherent in the householder way of life. Constant engagement in the world involves desire, and through desire and accumulation, one is constantly accruing more *karmas*: bounced this way and that between friends and enemies, attachment and aversion, kindness and aggression. This makes it very difficult to avoid lying, causing harm to others, wasting life-energy through excessive attachment, and so on. So we can see that a life-long celibate who lives the renunciate life can be considered to be in a better position to avoid these entanglements of desire and the resulting emotional reactivity. He lives a life that deliberately circumscribes the advancement of the personal ego, and thereby the reduction of *karmas* and the cultivation of non-attachment come more easily to him. This is the advantage of lessening engagement in the whirlpool of the world".

"But adopting the recluse way of life is no guarantee of enlightenment, surely?"

"Indeed not. But the effects of a man's life, the type of mind that has been created during his sojourn in this present body, will surely affect the direction he takes after death and determine which subtle realm he goes to, and what experiences he encounters there.[317]

"So it is for all these reasons that the life of the contemplative recluse has always been extolled for those who are really serious about breaking out of the general mould and making significant progress on the spiritual path. It is simply a matter of using one's time to the best advantage, that's all. Otherwise, when Lord Yama does come, there could be only be tears and regret".

The two sit in silence for some time; the younger man serene, the older deep in thought. Above them, the huge evening sky glows rose and deep mauve, and the dark, massing clouds promise overnight rain. As the last rays of the sun gild the contours of the venerable trees whose branches loom over the courtyard, the bell from a nearby temple announces the evening *puja*. The visitor rises, bows low and deeply to the young teacher, and leaves to make offerings to his god.

Desire

A wealthy landowner complains of his dissatisfaction.
  "I wish I had more land".
  "But why?" asks the Master. "Don't you have enough already?"
  "If I had more, I could raise more cows".
  "And what would you do with them?"
  "Sell them and make money".
  "For what?"
  "To buy more land and raise more cows ..."

Among the Jains

Kanchipuram is also a thriving centre of Jainism. Many of its inhabitants are dedicated to the teachings of Mahavir, the twenty-fourth and last in the lineage of Jain saints, who is said to have travelled with Prince Gautama, the future Buddha, during his search for enlightenment. The Jain parts of the old town are spacious and well laid-out with gardens, many temples, monasteries and large renunciate communities that are all generously supported by a pious and hardworking lay population. Several of the renunciate orders go about naked to demonstrate their total disregard for the things of the world; they are known as 'the sky-clad'. Forbidden by their religion from causing harm, Jain householders reject such livelihoods as farming or agriculture, in order to avoid any unwitting destruction of life. As a result, they tend instead to be bankers, jewellers, merchants and the like, and it is their generous donations that have ensured the healthy continuance of the monastic way of life.

A group of such Jain householders comes to seek the Master's *darshan*. All are wealthy merchants; they appear pure, humble and respectful. After a few polite formalities, one of the party, a dealer in grains, initiates the *satsang*:

"Revered sage, we Jains have long been taught that the process of *karma* and its fruition in an appropriate rebirth is an inviolable law of life. Yet recently we have heard other teachers say that this is just a clever device to motivate the ignorant to act in a law-abiding way and deter them from indulging in harmful behaviour. Can you shed any light on this dichotomy? Personally, I have become very confused by it".

The Master smiles graciously, evidently pleased by the sincerity of his visitors.

"I know of your religion, and it is the beautiful legacy of a long and hallowed tradition of realised souls".

After a pause:

"Now, as regards your question, the first thing to realise is that all the great spiritual teachings that have stood the test of time – the Veda, the teachings of Lord Buddha and your own lineage of *gurus* such as Adinath, Parshvarnath and Mahavir – all these great systems teach the law of *karma* and rebirth. So, if this idea really is a fiction, then all the holy texts and respected teachings have been deluded and, wittingly or otherwise, the sages have perpetrated deception all these years. In truth, however, this is just not possible, because these teachings embody the sacred law of life, and it is a law that that has been corroborated and exemplified by the lives of countless great beings throughout the ages. The principle is clear: as long as one is identified with the body and bound to the individual sense of agency consequent on this identification, there must be rebirth. There is no doubt about it; rebirth is a necessary consequence of the usual way of being and acting in the world".

The Master pauses to let the weight of his words sink in, and it is as if one of the great teachers from the time of the Upanishads – a Yajnavalkya or an Uddalaka Aruni – is seated here before us, such is the power of the historical continuity of living truth.

"On the other hand", he continues, "what we call enlightenment is precisely the undoing of the knot of egoistic attachment that binds one to the usual shrunken sense of being. Once this knot has been undone, the individual finds himself not only unattached to his own body, but to anything whatsoever! He has become one with the universal Self, the real and essential Being that persists unchanged within and beyond all physical boundaries. This unicity sees clearly that not only are all states of matter an illusion because temporary and unbinding, but that the individual soul is one with the universal Consciousness. This realisation – 'I am the Eternal' – is the very nature of purified intelligence, and it is the spontaneous confession of the enlightened, verified by innumerable sacred texts.[318] Now, for such a one, how could there be rebirth? Who, or what would reincarnate?

Where would he go? If he has become the all, the Totality, where is there he could move to that he is not already present? So we see from this that only the isolated part could think in terms of reincarnation, of moving from here to there through time and space. To the unbroken wholeness, such a concept is like the son of a barren woman, self-contradictory and without meaning".

"So, in the end, the teachers who declare there is no reincarnation are right?"

"Yes and no! What we always have to bear in mind when discussing these ultimate matters is that experience is different in different states of consciousness. Now, for one who lives the enlightened state categorically to declare, 'There is no such thing as reincarnation' would not be right, because what is manifestly true in his own case is not the truth for the generality of men. His is the truth of enlightenment, while theirs is the life of ignorance. Now, it may be that in the ecstasy of enlightenment, overwhelmed by joy and freedom, he makes some such declaration, but a mature consideration of the case would not allow him to say such a thing unequivocally, because his own freedom from reincarnation does not mean that others are also likewise living that liberated state. How could it? It is like a man who, on becoming rich, declares that there is no such thing as poverty. This non-existence of poverty is true in his own case, certainly, but to claim that it is true for all those who continue to be poor, is manifestly absurd.

"So for a realised soul to deny reincarnation would only spread confusion. Moreover, to do so would contravene the scriptural injunction that it is the responsibility of the wise not to confuse the ignorant. [319] Make no mistake here, the wise and the ignorant live in two entirely different realities, as distinct from one another as are waking and dreaming for the normal man".

"Is it the ability to honour these different levels of reality that distinguishes the great teacher?", came the question.

The Master smiles and nods but remains silent, his countenance luminous.

After some time another of the men, a wealthy jewel merchant, speaks up.

"Swamigal, you teach that the Self is eternal Consciousness. If this is so, then it must always be present. Why, then, are we not aware of it in dream or sleep?"

The Master:

"In the normal man, both dream and sleep are untrustworthy mental states that habitually obscure the Truth. Dream is simply a false and confused cognition, whereas sleep is a dullness that fails to perceive anything, let alone one's real essence. This essence lies beyond these two mental states, and it shines forth only when their errors are removed. And once the essence is realised, the whole phenomenal world is seen to be nothing but That, which is one's own Self. Any other ideas of separation and duality simply vanish, just as the erroneous perception of a rope being a snake vanishes as soon as a light is brought to banish the darkness".[320]

"I can understand why the activity of dreaming would obscure the real essence, but how can the non-activity of sleep do the same? It seems a contradiction in terms somehow ..."

"In fact, in dreamless sleep the sleeper experiences a blank, not because of the absence of Consciousness itself, but because his mind has ceased to function, and therefore there are no longer any objects to reflect consciousness. See, it is like light. We do not perceive the light pervading the empty space between two solid objects, not because it is not there, but because there is nothing for it to reflect off, nothing for it to illuminate. But when the mind is clear, its inherent ability to reflect is always retained, and therefore even in the absence of specific objects to cognise, awareness of just being conscious, as the omnipresent Self, is always there. It is there whether the mind is sojourning in its dreaming mode or its sleeping mode, whether it is entertaining objects or is free of them".

"Fair enough, honoured Sir. Let us then leave the illusory states of dream and sleep and return to where we are now. You say that the Self illumines this, our present world, yet we are not even aware of it in our everyday waking state, here and now. How is that possible?"

The Master, delighted with his visitor's persistence, begins to be a little playful:

"Well, you have seen in the bazaar how the jewel merchant tests the quality of an emerald?"

Intrigued, the merchant smiles: "I have, indeed".

"He puts it into a container of milk to see if it adds that peculiar greenish lustre to the milk, does he not?"

The merchant nods, wondering to himself how this extraordinary young monk could be so equally at home with both the highest abstract philosophy and the everyday details of commercial life.

"Just like that, the Self, which is the very nature of light, imparts its own lustre to the entire material world. This brilliance manifests in a hierarchy of successive stages from subtle to gross, each stage denser and more solidly material than its predecessor. First the Self illuminates the intellect, the subtlest and most transparent aspect of the individual, then it illuminates the various levels of the mind, then the senses and finally the body and the outside world.

"As a result, all our experience of everything, everywhere, depends on the light of the Self. But living beings typically suffer under the delusion of limited selfhood and so are unaware of this fact. The Self remains hidden, so to speak, because as we were saying a moment ago, just as one cannot separate light from the objects it illuminates, and hold it up in its true nature as light, so one cannot separate the Self from matter and hold it up as one could exhibit any other object. Therefore, people constantly superimpose all sorts of activity onto the ever-inactive Self, as if they were mistaking light itself for the objects that are reflected in it. They say the Self 'thinks', or the Self 'moves', whereas in fact the Self does nothing whatsoever but illumine everything that is less than itself. And because the Self cannot be objectified in the normal way as some sort of a temporary, active agent, there are all sorts of doubts and confusions about it, and people wander around quite unaware of who they really are, and what the nature of life really is. It is all very curious, is it not?"[321]

So saying, the Master erupts into carefree laughter, his face suffused with the innocence of a child. Everyone else sits in silence for some time, their verbalising minds suspended for a long moment. The visitors have never heard such a fluent and perfect exposition of the Self, delivered in a way that leaves no doubt the teacher is speaking from his depths of his own experience. Eventually, feeling deeply satisfied, they respectfully take their leave and depart.

The effects of this meeting are to prove lasting. Each of the men will feel his life has somehow been subtly transformed and from that day onwards they all become staunch followers of Vedanta. For the rest of their lives they will do much to help the material upkeep of the Kanchipuram ashram and the work of the Master's order in the city.

That evening, one of his close followers asks the Master about the value of the Jain doctrines.

"These Jains are very pious people", he replies, "and that is all very well, but it must be said that they do not have a clear understanding about the nature of the Self. Their monastic teachers have developed a very complicated system of analysis and argumentation that points out, quite rightly, the relativity of all philosophical positions framed within the waking state. But in fact, this relativism undercuts their own stance, because if there is only shifting relativity, nothing can be definitely determined by anyone. Thus they attempt to promulgate an authoritative system which is detailed in all sorts of lists and categories yet is at the same time based on the idea that nothing definitive can be said about the means of knowledge, nor the object of knowledge, nor the knower, nor the knowledge itself! How can a system of knowledge claim authority while teaching that something is true or perhaps not true, real or perhaps unreal? This just ends up in absurdity and presents a teaching that is no more acceptable than the ramblings of a drunkard.

"Moreover, because they are confused about the Self, they are also confused about its reflection as the individual soul. They teach that the soul is eternal and yet it transmigrates; but we know that if it transmigrates it must be finite and transient, not infinite and eternal. What is more, they avow that the soul is the same size as the body it inhabits. Does this then mean a person's soul is the same size when he is a strong young man as when he is aged and shrunken? What happens to the size of a human soul if, due to bad *karma*, it takes birth in an elephant or an ant? Does it shrink or expand to fit the new body? And again, if all this is indeed the case, such a soul cannot claim to be eternal, because it shows itself to be highly mutable and, if it is mutable, it is by the same token limited, transient and partial.

"No, there are far too many logical inconsistencies here for us to accept. As Vedantins schooled in the wisdom of the Upanishads, we know the individual soul to be a faithful reflection of the universal and unchanging Self. Whatever it may once have been, the teaching of these Jains is now surely less than supreme knowledge".[322]

Death of the mother

A few days after this discussion, whilst in deep meditation the Master has a vision of his mother lying on a bed, in some distress and approaching her end. It is an experience of what is known as 'the infallible knowledge' gained when the introverted mind is so silent, empty and expanded it is able accurately to cognise events that are far distant in time or space.[323] Mindful of his promise to her that he would attend her deathbed, no matter what, he immediately quits Kanchipuram alone, and heads westwards over the spice hills towards his native village. Before he leaves he arranges to meet his disciples later and also promises the local people that he will return to the city and inaugurate the monastery when its construction is finished. Some say he fulfilled this promise and took up residence there in the years leading up to his own death.

Arriving in Kaladi, the young *sannyasi* enters the ancestral house to see his mother lying on the bed, just as he had envisioned. A few neighbours are sitting around the edges of the room. Even though her features are startlingly familiar – almost his own – she now looks very distant, a stranger, shrunk into a private and impenetrable world from which she will not return. There is nothing more that needs saying and nothing more that has to be done; her time has come and the unstoppable process has begun.

The Master sits beside her bed, every so often gently lifting a bowl of warm *tulasi*[324] water to her lips. In mid-afternoon one of the neighbours prepares a meal; the Master encourages the others to eat, but he himself does not. Some of those present are softly invoking the name of Ram. For his part, the Master remains silent, focussing his attention on the supine figure with great tenderness and intensity. The old woman lies there for another two hours, with her chest heaving and her breath coming in loud, uneven gasps. Different expressions of joy and sorrow pass in rapid succession over her gentle, lined face; she seems to see some things she recognises, and others which startle her. The Master sits serenely at her side all the while, resting his right hand on her chest and his left on the crown of her head. He sits like this for a long time; feeling whether her soul has subsided into the heart, he seeks to guide it to leave through the highest subtle centre, the crown *chakra*. Towards the end, a bright lustre suffuses her features. Then, finally, her breath croaks and splutters for the last time, and she is gone.

The Master stands up with a serene expression and announces to those present that his mother has made an easy transition and she should be cremated without more ado. At this, there is an instinctive wave of resistance from the assembled villagers, who are already suspicious about this young man who has renounced the world, deserted his mother and ancestral place, and then suddenly turned up again out of nowhere. Now he is proposing to perform a rite that the scriptures clearly state is forbidden to a *sannyasi* such as he, and can only be performed by a householder relative, ideally the eldest son. As high-caste Namboodiri *brahmins*, their desire to abide by the scriptures is matched by their reluctance to incur the ritual pollution of being near a corpse, let alone handling it. Nevertheless, one of the men brings a machete and a pot of *ghee* and points wordlessly to the grove of trees behind the house. The group files out, leaving the Master alone in the room with the body that once bore him. Single-handed, he begins to hack down guava branches to build up a funeral pyre in the yard behind the house. Almost as an afterthought, he adds some banana stems to the pile. Then with great tenderness he carries the frail cloth bundle outside and lays it on the pyre. He pours the *ghee* over the wood, and rubbing sticks together to get a spark, lights the pile, and sits down beside it in meditation. He stays there all night without moving, until only a smouldering heap of ashes is left. Then, as the rising sun shreds the morning mist into long thin wisps, he wraps bones and ashes in banana leaves, takes them to the riverbank and casts them far out into the sparkling golden water.

It is said that since that time there has been a curse on the *brahmins* of Kaladi. When one of their kind passes away, the body has to be cremated in the backyard of their own houses, for there is no separate cremation ground set aside for them. When you go to that part of the country, you will find their houses facing the street, but the backyard is always an open space and anyone who enters it will have to take a purifying bath. And, to this day, unlike other parts of the Land of the Veda, banana stems must always form part of the funeral pyre.[325]

A meeting with Mookambika Devi

After many days' travel, the Master rejoins his followers in the peaceful forests of the Kodajadri hills. Always the first to be blessed by the monsoon rains, this whole coastal strip is now lush, verdant and fertile and these woodlands have an especially enchanted atmosphere.

It is said that while sojourning here, the young *sannyasi* has a vision of the Great Goddess, this time in her form as Mookambika, Mother of the Universe, who appears before him and offers to grant him a boon. The Master replies that his only wish is she should consent to dwell in the area to act as a source of inspiration and blessing for the local people. Full of divine grace, the Goddess agrees, but lays down a condition: while the Master is looking for a suitable place to build a temple and install her image for worship, she will follow behind him, but he must not look back at her until he finds it. The Master agrees and with his monks following at some distance, begins to descend from the hill through the spice-scented woods that overlook the brilliant paddy fields below, stretching to the far distance. As he walks, the Goddess is so close behind him that he can hear her ankle bells delicately tinkling. But, after a while, being in playful mood, she decides on a whim to test him. Suddenly, she pauses. No longer hearing the bells and fearing for her welfare, the Master instinctively turns around to see what had happened. Too late he realises he has broken his side of the bargain, and so he is caught like a fish in her silken net. The Goddess stops short, and refuses to move further. Feigning petulance she demands her image be installed on that very spot. No other will do. There is no option but to concur with her cosmic play.

And so the Mookambika Devi Temple is duly founded on the banks of the broad river Sauparnika.[326] As if by magic, funds flow in, buildings spring up and the Master installs a particularly fine image of the Goddess in a youthful and beneficent form, seated on a *shri chakra*. He also institutes the rite that on the last day of the annual festival of the Nine Nights, which celebrate Mother Divine, small children should come to the temple to be initiated into the alphabet of their mother tongue. This custom has persisted to this day, and the place continues to be a centre of traditional instruction in music and dance, as well as being a potent spiritual site attracting millions of pilgrims each year.

The founding of Shringeri Math

After prolonged *pujas* and celebrations, punctuated with Vedic recitation, devotional hymns and performances of classical music and dance, the Master and his followers leave Mookambika to travel inland in an easterly direction. Before long it becomes evident that some supernatural energy is infusing this part of the Master's mission, as a number of inspired events take place in a short space of time.

Firstly, they reach a place near the source of the holy river Tungabhadra where a local warrior chief named Veerasena receives them with great enthusiasm and piety. He immediately provides the funds to build a temple, which the Master dedicates again to Mother Divine, but this time in her form as Shri Sharadamba, the ever-pure patron deity of learning. Many scholars and pundits attend the opening festivities, and the master Vedantin is evidently thrilled by the waves of devotion and happiness that tangibly pervade the atmosphere, casting a warm glow of sweetness and feminine lustre over the whole proceedings.

Adjacent to the temple, on the high bank overlooking the river below, a monastery is founded and the brilliant Sureshvaracharya installed as its first pontiff. Three orders of 'The Renunciants of Ten Names' are assigned the place as their base: the Saraswati 'well-learned', the Puri 'town-dwellers' and the Bharati 'unbounded'. The Master determines that the knowledge and preservation of the Yajur Veda shall be the special responsibility of this seat of learning and that it shall henceforth be known as the Shringeri Math. Its *dharma* is to act as the stabilising central point of the sacred *mandala* that is the Land of the Veda.

Hastamalaka

The next significant event occurs while the party is travelling further north along the coast. Before long, they reach a *brahmin* village called Shri Bali, located not far from a place known as Gokarna that long ago was inhabited by *rishis*, and ever since those days has been a thriving centre of Vedic learning where many *brahmacharis* come to study with their tutors. The Master gives *darshan*, as is customary whenever he reaches a new place, and among those who attend and are captivated by his presence is an affluent landowner called Prabhakara. Apart from his wealth, this man is well-known in the area for the devoted way he looks after his son, a deaf-mute who has not spoken a single word in his thirteen years of life.

The man has been in the habit of taking the boy to all the holy men he can, in the hope that one day his affliction could be cured by the proximity of spiritual greatness. After the discourse is over, he approaches the Master and bows down respectfully to him, pulling his son to the ground beside him as he does so. But the boy remains lolling there, as if senseless. As the compassionate sage lifts the lad up, his father, greatly embarrassed, apologises profusely, explaining his son is simple-minded, and has long been habitually listless, showing no interest in education, and even being indifferent to food. What could be the *karma* that is causing such a state?

Taking the boy's face tenderly in his hands, the Master looks directly into his eyes and asks:

"My boy, why are you behaving in this way? Who are you really?"

At this, it is said that the lad's eyes filled with light, and in a loud, clear voice he began to recite:

'I am the Self, the universal Consciousness dwelling in the inmost heart of all! Giving life to the mind, the senses and the world, its plenitude is forever untouched by the limitations it assumes. The Self remains alone, unmoving and untainted like the pure, boundless sky!'[327]

Eleven more verses praising the glory of the Self pour out, to the utter astonishment of everyone present. Prabhakara himself is speechless as the Master smilingly informs him that his son is no idiot, but a great being, to whom the truth of life shines forth as clearly as 'an *amalaka* fruit sitting in the palm of his hand'.[328]

Greatly perplexed, the man returns home with his son, but once there the boy immediately relapses into his idiot-like state. Early the next morning, the two arrive at the house where the Master is staying. As soon as they enter the compound, the boy begins to act more normally; intelligence returns to his face and his eyes shine with clarity. Prabhakara salutes the Master humbly: "Maharaj-ji, please adopt my boy as your disciple. He obviously belongs more to your family than to mine". It is clear that Prabhakara is certain about his decision; there is nothing more to be said.

And so the brilliant lad joins the Master, who immediately initiates him into *sannyasa*, and gives him the name Hastamalaka – which means 'the *amalaka* fruit in the hand'– by which he will be known ever after. In time, he is to become one of the foremost disciples and most revered *gurus* of the holy lineage of Vedanta.

Travelling on further north, the party reaches the legendary city of Dwarawati.[329] This place has a renowned history: it was built by Vishvakarma, architect of the gods, on the banks of the holy Gomati River, by order of Lord Krishna when he renounced war and wished to relocate his capital here on a peaceful spur of land on the western fringe of the Land of the Veda. Since Krishna's time much of the area has been engulfed by the sea, but the city still has the aspect of a royal capital, being spacious, well-planned and full of fine buildings, elegant waterways and many prestigious and well-supported temples. Naturally, the main religious affiliation of the people here is with Lord Vishnu, in his incarnation as the enchanting blue God of Love, but the Master soon proves so popular and his teachings on the role of devotion in the spiritual life are so well-received that he decides on the spot that this would be the ideal place to establish the western limit of the sacred *mandala*.

Accordingly, a monastery and centre of learning is founded on land given by the local *raja*. It is to be known as Sharada Math, and dedicated to that aspect of the Goddess who presides over sacred knowledge and the refined intellect. Building begins immediately. The institution will be given responsibility for the Sama Veda, and two more of the ten *sannyasin* orders – the Tirtha 'pilgrimage spot' and the Ashrama 'hermitage' – are created to serve it. To the surprise of many, the newly-joined disciple Hastamalaka is installed as its first abbot.

In just a few short months, the Master's mission has progressed rapidly. Four of the five principal monasteries he envisaged at the Prayag Kumbha Mela have now materialised, while many shrines and temples along the way have been restored and re-energised, and numerous groups of initiated disciples, both *sannyasi* and lay people, established. All in all, it is clear that Mother Divine herself is directing everything from behind the scenes.

Devotion

A local follower of Krishna is keen to understand the relationship of devotion to non-dualism.

Q: "What is devotion, guruji?"

A: "There are different stages. At one level, devotion is the singing of *bhajans*; at another, it is carrying out the dictates of the Lord implicitly."

Q: "But is not love of God involved?"

A: "Of course, this is just what we are talking about! Now, the love you are speaking of implies a duality does it not? On one side there is the lover and on the other, the beloved. But this separation is only provisional. On the path of devotion, the devotee passes from an experience of 'I belong to the Lord' to that of 'The Lord belongs to me'. Finally, the process culminates in the experience: 'The Lord is truly my Self'. So on the path to non-duality we see action, devotion and true knowledge, but in fact all are just aspects of the one process, stations on a single, glorious journey".

Everything is as it should be

The Master is laughing in a carefree, childlike manner. Those around him find themselves laughing too, for no reason other than their teacher's own overflowing happiness. In such innocent enjoyment, the chronic knots of selfhood are easily loosened.

A devotee asks: "Master, how does the world look from the highest state of consciousness?"

"You see that everything is exactly as it should be", comes the reply.

The devotee hesitates before asking a little diffidently: "But why then, Maharaj, are you always working so hard to improve the situation in the world?"

The Master's eyes twinkle with gracious humour.

"Because that is exactly as it should be."

Maya

There have been many months without rain. In recent weeks, heavy dark clouds have gathered, but day after day passes slowly in an eerie, sunless half-light, waiting. The land itself seems squashed by the stifling pressure of the clouds, the dry air sticks in the throat, and there is a sense of stultifying and unfulfilled expectation, a brooding silence that presages something enormous, unnamed. Even the animals are finding it hard to summon the energy to go on as usual. Before much longer the warning wind will come and those sullen clouds will unleash their burden; the weeks of waiting will finally be broken and the skies will open. The rain will cascade down with a breathtaking ferocity, drumming on the roofs so hard that one can hardly hear oneself think, and turning the parched earth into a sodden quagmire within seconds. Overnight, bright green shoots will sprout, and in a single day the earth that has been lying dead will be sprinkled with tiny multi-coloured flowers, fresh and brilliant. Frogs will fill the air with their croaking and their little leaps will draw the birds to swoop down hungrily. Once again, life will return from its state of suspension, and everything will be able to breathe freely once more. But for the moment, there is no relief. One can only suffer and wait.

The Master and his party are staying in an old Shiva temple by the sea just outside the city. The air is a little fresher here, and away from the lethargic crowds, there is a lighter atmosphere. A local official, a man without religion who has been involved in the transfer of land for the Sharada Math, has come for *darshan*. It is only mid-morning, but already hot and tired from his journey, he is in a belligerent mood.

"I am a practical man, young Sir, and I value commonsense. I just cannot accept your teaching that everything is an illusion!"

"I do not teach that everything is an illusion", comes the measured reply. Then, laughing: "How could I? If I did, this teacher himself would be an illusion – and then what to say of his teaching?" [330]

The devotees present are thrilled by the master Advaitin's keen intelligence which, as always, cuts straight to the heart of the matter.

The official is not to be put off.

"Well, I have heard many reports that you teach the world is an illusion and only the Absolute is real. What sort of a philosophy is that? You will just drive ordinary well-intentioned people to lethargy and despair, and let us not forget it is the generosity of these good people that supports you and your monks".

"It is very good that you have had the intelligence to come to hear the teaching directly, rather than pick it up second-hand in the bazaar", comes the even reply. "Actually, the tradition does not teach that the Absolute is real, and the world is an illusion. What it actually says is that the Absolute is real, the world is an illusion, and the Absolute is the world.[331] There is an infinite difference between these two statements!"

The official frowns. "And what does this mean, exactly?" he asks, somewhat defensive now, as he is aware that he is in the presence of a mature intellect, and not just some youthful polemicist.

"It means that although the universe is commonly conceived to exist as somehow apart from the Divine, that perception is erroneous, it is an illusion. The universe, which is multiple, contingent and limited, is nevertheless the unfailing manifestation of the non-dual, self-sufficient and limitless Reality".

"Where does *maya* fit in with all this, then?"

"Look to the word itself. *Maya* means 'that (*ya*) which is not (*ma*)'. So *maya* is understanding that the world has no reality in, and of, itself. On its own, it *is not*; it has no substance apart from the underlying Reality of which it is a temporary appearance. So, the world is real when cognised as an appearance of the Self, but unreal if it is understood to be self-sufficient, and in some way apart from the Self. In truth, there is only the one Self, omnipresent and non-dual".

"But how can one thing be real and unreal at the same time?"

The Master laughs, clearly enjoying the turn the exchange is taking.

"Indeed! It is all a question of perspective. Now, imagine you are walking along the path at twilight, and you see a snake lying there. Your heart starts pounding and your mind races. Panic! Then someone brings a light, and you see there is no snake, but only a length of rope – the snake and everything associated with it was an illusion. Like that, everyone is running here and there, fearful, preoccupied and self-absorbed, because they are labouring under an illusion they call 'the world', which is perceived as being external to another illusion they call 'myself'. Yet, when seen in the light of true understanding, that same world and that same limited self both stand revealed to be nothing but the one Self: ever radiant, blissful and serenely unperturbed".

"And in your analogy you are the bringer of the light?" There is a hint of a sneer in the official's tone.

The Master pauses, then murmurs softly "The tradition, the tradition ..."

The official sits silently for some time, considering what he has heard. He begins to realise the inappropriateness of his previous aggression. In a more conciliatory tone, he continues:

"Well, young Sir, I think I see what you are saying here. But according to your analogy, once knowledge of the Self dawns, the world just vanishes".

"Oh no! Not at all", the Master is laughing again, playful now. "But you are correct insofar as the first analogy explains essence rather than substance; the first picture must be completed by a second. So, now imagine you are taking another walk, this time along a path on a hot day like today, and you see a puddle of water ahead of you. You are thirsty and go to drink. As you draw closer you see there is in fact no water; it is just a mirage. Yet even when seen for what it really is, the mirage is still there, it continues to exist, giving the appearance of water. It does not vanish, but you are no longer deceived by it, this is the crucial thing. Like that, even after its true nature is revealed, the world certainly continues to appear, but it is now transformed, as it its appreciated as the Self, and not as something independent or devoid of the Self".

After more thought, the official softens further.

"Well, this analogy is a neat one as far as it goes, but again, young Sir, it seems to me there is a flaw in your argument. The phenomenon of the water in the mirage is purely illusory because that water is useless, you cannot drink it. But the phenomenon of the world is quite different: it is purposeful, and it has its practical usefulness, no doubt about it. How do you account for this difference?"

"Indeed, but just because a phenomenon serves some apparent purpose does not mean it is ultimately real", counters the Master. "Consider your dreams. They are full of creations that are purposeful, things that are useful in the dream world and occupy their own logical place in it. The dream water slakes the dream thirst. But as soon as you wake up, the unreality of the dream and all that happened in it becomes self-evident. Whatever happened in the dream state is contradicted by the waking state – indeed, not only by the waking state, but by the sleep state also! In this you are ascribing reality to something that does not last, whereas Vedanta teaches that to be real, a thing must enjoy continuity – something cannot be real one moment and unreal the next. So, if discontinuity is its salient characteristic, then that thing is actually like a conjuror's trick, a sleight of hand[332] that has all the superficial appearance of being real, only as long as one does not know the secret of it".

"I must admit you have disposed of the world very neatly! What then is this Self you speak of?"

"To those who see clearly, the sensible universe and all the hidden subtle realms are revealed to be nothing but the Self, which is the single, limitless Consciousness. After the dawning of this supreme knowledge, the entire cosmic drama continues to unfold with perfect legitimacy, but it is realised to be nothing but the display of Being, Consciousness and Bliss".

"And the suffering of the world?"

"Rest assured, the display of Being, Consciousness and Bliss contains all that may not appear to be Being, Consciousness and Bliss".

The discussion has reached its natural conclusion and the official sits for some minutes in silence. Then he rises and respectfully takes his leave. After he has gone, the Master appears pleased by the meeting and comments to the monks around him:

"Excellent! This discussion will bear fruit in time; no doubt about it. It will have its effect".

Everything is silence

Devotee:

"Maharaj-ji, why did you leave the silence of the Himalaya and come out into the mud of the world?"

Answer:

"I have never left the silence of the Himalaya".

A thought is just a thought

An elderly householder has come to meet the Master. He has studied with many teachers over the years. The saints he has seen have told him that everything is a form of God; the yogis he has met instructed him that all is *brahman*. In an attempt to follow their teaching, he has tried to create this realisation for himself by holding in his mind the idea of an omnipresent Unity. He has also applied himself to practising the intellectual discipline of discriminating between the ever-changing relative world and the unchanging reality of the Absolute. These continued attempts have not brought him realisation. Now disillusioned, he carries with him an air of disappointment.

The Master listens to the man's story for some time and then gently asks:

"And are you enjoying your life?"

"Well, Sir, I can't say that enjoying is the right word, because wherever I look I am reminded of life's insufficiency".

"Yes, taken on its own, life will certainly not provide undying satisfaction. But that resolute happiness you seek is not gained by spinning words about the Absolute or by trying to understand it through thinking. It is good to hear about the Absolute again and again, no doubt, because it is inscrutable and unlike anything else, but what is needed is direct experience of it. The mind must go beyond the movement of thought in order to touch that which is unchanging and without parts, uncaused and therefore undecaying".[333]

"Go beyond thinking, because ...?"

"Because the thought is not the thing itself. The thought of *brahman* is just a thought, it is not the experience of *brahman*. Even the thought of thoughtlessness is just another thought and all these concepts will continue endlessly in the extraverted mind just as a flame will continue until the oil that fuels it is completely used up. So merely to superimpose the idea of *brahman* on an object or a situation, as a worshipper might superimpose the idea of Vishnu on an image of the deity, is a conceptual act that can never by itself lead to liberation. To say it could, is to say that one could achieve liberation without having to transcend the tedious and circular thought-habits of the normal waking state. At the least, this is a contradiction in terms, is it not?"[334]

"What then is the answer, Master?"

"The mind, which is the maker of all concepts, gives rise to the idea of a limited selfhood constricted to a limited body. So, the mind and all its mischief must be transcended".

"How is this done?"

"By pursuing spiritual practice. Only then will That which lies behind the mind be revealed".

"And what is that?"

"Have you not heard descriptions enough by now?"

Consciousness is eternal

She is a handsome middle-aged woman, fair-skinned, with an aristocratic bearing, and clearly very intelligent. Her family, wealthy and cultured, had for generations been followers of the prophet Zoroaster, worshipping the Eternal Fire and living by the codes of behaviour laid down in the sacred Avesta scriptures that emphasise fairness, equality and honesty. Then, some years before, she and her relatives were driven out of their homeland by the invasion of nomadic tribes from the west, warlike followers of a new prophet from the empty deserts, who claimed his teaching to be the final and perfect revelation of God. All who resisted were destroyed; many ancient institutions were laid waste. Fleeing eastwards, the woman's family reached the sea and set sail for the Land of the Veda as they had heard it was a country of great religious plurality and tolerance. Safely arrived, they bought land from a local raja and settled near the coast. They are now already established as a powerful merchant group dealing in foodstuffs, so materially her life is again very comfortable. But spiritually the woman feels bereft. While destroying her ancestral temple, the invaders had extinguished the Eternal Fire that was its heart, scorning an idol that they said attempted to usurp the one true God of whom there is no image. On arriving in her new homeland, deprived of her usual religious focus, the woman had immediately felt a spiritual affinity with the Vedic fire rituals she saw, but being a foreigner had been excluded from participating in them by the *brahmin* priests. This rebuff turned her towards seeking the company of wandering holy men, who seemed to live pretty much apart from the strict routines and prohibitions of the orthodox. On hearing that the Master is temporarily encamped at an ancient Shiva temple, she has come for *darshan.*

The Master puts his attention on the woman, welcoming her kindly to the assembled group and having her sit right at the front. As all present are aware, such a focus from a great being can by itself have a transforming influence on the recipient. Having listened to her story, he begins his response by quoting some verses from the Gita that refer to yoga as 'the fire of Knowledge' which burns up worldly desires by destroying the seeds of egotistic action.[335] He goes on to describe the 'Eternal Fire' as an outward symbol of the inner consciousness of the soul which, lying beyond all change, is the ultimate goal of the religious life.

"Whilst I recognise your words, honoured Sir, I cannot see any consciousness as being 'eternal'. In my experience consciousness comes and goes: it is not there when I am asleep or if I fall into a faint or even if I get distracted in the midst of doing things. And then there are people who have had their consciousness taken over by spirits and so on. When they eventually return to themselves, they say they were not conscious during the possession. So to me the soul's consciousness is intermittent and therefore a random happening, adventitious even".

"Yes, you are quite right," comes the warm response, "This is indeed the common experience and it will continue as such unless and until the little self comes to realise its identity with its source, the universal Self which is the unchanging Consciousness".

Here he quotes some more verses on this theme, this time from the Upanishads.[336]

"Now, as to not being aware when you sleep, this appearance of not being aware is not due to the absence of consciousness itself, but due to the absence of any objects to be conscious of. See, it is like light. In itself, light is imperceptible, yet it spreads through endless space. When all objects are removed, that light is not perceived anymore because all the objects that reflected it and made it visible have gone. But that does not mean that light itself, in its own pure nature, has vanished.[337] So it is with consciousness. What is therefore needed is to train the mind to remain conscious in the absence of any object; that is, to be consciously aware without thought, feeling or perception. This is meditation, and it is time for you to start the practice".

The Master initiates her into meditation later that same day.

The following afternoon, a party of learned priests from the Land of the Dogras[338] visits. This lushly wooded stretch of the mighty Himalaya is famed as a great centre of learning. Recently a Buddhist pilgrim from China called Hsuan-Tsang has written of his travels there; now monks from the east and other travelers and merchants from the west are coming to the Land of the Veda inspired by his account. The valley kingdom is considered the Crown of the Land of the Veda, and boasts many varied and highly accomplished schools of thought, especially in the field of *tantra*.

The visiting party is composed of high-born *brahmin* priests who are all devoted servants of the deity Sharada, and they attend to her in her preferred place, generally considered the most prestigious temple in the land. Now they are on a pilgrimage to holy sites in the south, and having heard of the master Advaitin are naturally keen to have his *darshan*. Delighted to find he has been busily engaged in setting up a local abode for their beloved Mother Divine, they cordially invite him to visit their homeland, assuring him that all the appropriate arrangements will be made. Somewhat to their surprise, he accepts the offer without further ado.

The Throne of Knowledge

The last few weeks have been quite extraordinary. After arriving in the Dogra country, the Master and his party were escorted with great courtesy and pomp to the Sharada temple at Shardi on the banks of the sacred river Kishanganga, courteously attended by the same pundits who had invited them to visit. A formal welcoming ceremony took place, followed by celebrations of Vedic *yajnas*, *pujas* to the Goddess and much high-quality recitation of the Veda.

The ancient stone structure, long renowned as a high seat of learning, has four entrances aligned to the cardinal points, each guarded by a magnificent door made of dark wood intricately carved in the fashion that is the speciality of this heavily forested area. At the centre of the shrine sits a high throne, known as The Throne of Omniscience, reserved for those deemed by consent amongst the learned to possess infallible knowledge. Scholars, pundits and saints from various parts of the Land of the Veda have in the past won the right to occupy the throne, but not one teacher from the south, and so the southern gate has remained closed. Because of the Master's extraordinary reputation, rumours soon begin to circulate that at last the southern gate will be opened in honour of a great sage from the far distant land of the Tamils.

A large group has assembled awaiting the visiting party. A programme of debate lasting several days has been organized, and as the whole area is steeped in veneration and scholarship, there is no shortage of the learned eager to debate with this precocious young teacher. The dualistic Samkhyas are there, as are the ritual specialist Mimamsakas, alongside Buddhists of different affiliations, as well as representatives of both the White, Robed and the Sky, Clad sects of Jainism. Shaktas, those who worship the Mother Goddess with complex rituals, sacrifice and symbolism, are also present, as are leaders of many Tantric schools who practice *kundalini yoga* and follow Lord Shiva as the exemplary ascetic yogi. There are also assorted atheists, rationalists and secular philosophers of all shades of opinion, for it is the tradition among these Dogra people that everyone is allowed their say in the search for supreme knowledge and no-one can predict from which quarter the truth may emerge.

One by one, each expert comes forward to present his argument, and time and again the master Vedantin steers the discussion back to the ultimate authority of the scriptures. He is well aware that this adherence to orthodox texts may cause problems to many who hear him, as not only are they unfamiliar with such priestly complexity but often find the Veda downright confusing. He will counter such arguments by pointing out that, because the scriptures deal with realities that are hidden from normal sight, they must employ a twilight language that only reveals its import gradually. This use of implied meaning silently opens the door to greater and more universal truths that lie behind and beyond the literal word. When his opponents criticise this as a circuitous and lengthy route to understanding, the Master replies that such an approach is the only one suited to unfolding truths which, being by their nature subtle and recondite, will always elude the conventional mind and its rigid concepts.[339]

Each scholar thoroughly interrogates the young *sannyasi*. One by one, they are made to retreat by the force of his pellucid logic. His replies are delivered in a sweet and unruffled manner, underlined with a self-assured dignity and decorum. Finally, recalling the liveliness of the public debates he had when establishing his reputation on the *ghats* of Kashi, the Master calls on anyone else in the audience to speak up if they wish. Some of the religious experts look surprised at the invitation, no doubt considering the opinions of the common people irrelevant, but they say nothing.

Two men in early middle age step up to the podium together. The elder explains they are brothers, born into an orthodox *brahmin* family who for many years practised their inherited craft of priestly ritual. But then, confused by the difficulties of the texts and disillusioned by the corruption of many of their fellow priests, they gradually lost their faith and have now abandoned the priesthood. Like many disappointed idealists, they have become highly cynical, choosing to guide their lives by a mundane rationality that accepts nothing it cannot easily explain. But they have not lost the love of dispute native to their caste, and are renowned in the community as formidable and plain-speaking opponents in any theological debate. So now even the haughtiest of the scholars present sits up and takes notice, knowing something of interest is about to ensue.

The elder man begins bluntly.

"The trouble with the Veda is that the canon contains so many blatant contradictions. The mantras just don't hang together as a coherent body of teaching. To take but one example among hundreds, there is a *mantra* in the Yajurveda that says: '*There is only one Rudra, and not a second*'.[340] Then, at another place further on, this statement is flatly contradicted when the very same text says: '*There are thousands and thousands of Rudras on this earth.*'[341] How can these two *mantras*, completely contradictory, both be said to be equally authoritative? It is as if someone tells you: 'I have been dumb since birth'. If he has never spoken in his life, how can he suddenly do so now? What is more, he is telling you he has always been unable to speak! Such mutual contradictions are nonsensical and, by the same token, so are many passages of the Veda".

A stir runs around the assembled company. The Master nods slowly, then begins in a calm voice:

"In fact, the *mantras* you quote contain no contradiction; their purpose is to show that there is but one undivided God who nevertheless assumes many various forms. This apparent paradox of unity creating diversity without sacrificing its unicity is often alluded to in texts, and in describing the process they themselves necessarily appear paradoxical. You know the Upanishadic passage when the sage Yajnavalkya is quizzed on the number of deities there are?"

Both brothers nod; it is a celebrated text.

Having subtly won a measure of agreement, the Master proceeds: "Then you will remember that when Yajnavalkya is asked by an intelligent and motivated student how many gods there are, he initially replies: 'Three hundred and three'. Then, when pressed further, he says 'Thirty-three', then 'Six', then 'Three', and then he comes down to 'Two'. And then, when the student keeps on pressing him, he comes down to 'One and a half', and then finally crowns it all with 'Just one!'".

There are smiles in the crowd; for many the passage is an old familiar friend.

"It is a marvellous teaching, in which a string of contradictions is employed to show that the multitude of deities can, indeed, be successively reduced to one and one alone, and that the non-dual singularity that is the supreme intelligence contains, nonetheless, limitless limited aspects".[342]

After a moment's reflection he adds: "And actually, we don't even have to talk of divinity here. It is mentioned in our scriptures that a yogi who has acquired supernatural powers can divide himself into thousands of forms and indulge in assorted different actions at the same time, and can then collect back all these forms into himself, just as the sun draws back all its rays within itself.[343] If this sort of thing is possible for a mortal creature like a yogi, then what to say of great immortals like Rudra?"[344]

The questioner remains silent; his younger brother now speaks up.

"My principal objection, Sir, is not so much scripture's inconsistency as its absurdity."

Again, a shock passes through the audience at the strength of the language.

"If we take the Yajurveda again as an example, we see there are *mantras* when the priest solemnly intones: 'O. grass, protect him' or 'O. razor, do not hurt him' or even 'O. stone which presses the Soma plant, listen to me'.[345] Now, how can a tuft of grass, which is incapable of protecting even its own self, possibly protect anybody else? How can a sane person address a plant, or ask a piece of inert stone to hear what he is saying? Does a stone have ears? It is absurd to confuse insentient objects with sentient ones and to anthropomorphise nature in this way".

The Master replies:

"Yes, there are certainly many passages in the Veda in which inert elements appear to be treated as sentient, on some occasions they even appear to indulge in action. We are told, for example, 'the clay spoke' or 'the water saw'.[346] But you have to realise that wherever such passages occur, they allude to the fact that each object in this world, including the elements and the human organs, has a sentient deity identified with it, a subtle impulse of intelligence that governs it and of which it is the gross material expression. So it is not that the objects in question are themselves assumed to be sentient; what is being referred to is the presiding deity which inheres in that particular object".[347]

He continues:

"Scriptural language also exemplifies the important principle that the unfamiliar is most easily approached through the familiar. For example: there is a passage in Yajurveda that refers to the patron of the Soma *yajna* having his head shaved before the ritual begins. The *mantra* recited at this time is: '*May the waters wet you*'. Now, from a literal point of view it might be argued that this merely repeats what is already obvious – that hair is wetted before being cut – and there-fore the passage cannot claim any special spiritual authority. But ac-tually we have heard only part of the *mantra*; the full line goes: '*May the waters wet you, giving you long life and fame*'.[348]

"Now what is being conveyed here is not just the well-known fact of wetting the hair before cutting it off, but something else that we did not know, which is that during the *yajna*, when the patron has his hair wetted, the presiding deity of water graces him with long life and fame. In this way, the text uses a known situation to acquaint us with a subtle reality of which we were previously ignorant. Like that, the Veda is always educating us in the hidden realities of life. And these texts are actually the only authority for disseminating this kind of knowledge; it cannot be known by any other means".

"I see, Sir. Are you saying then, that understanding the Vedic texts is all that is needed?"

"Scriptures serve their purpose by revealing their import in a gradual manner. Initially, they create a fertile doubt in the mind of a seeker, which makes him think more deeply and then question the commonplace view of reality. Searching for answers, and finding none, he then takes shelter at the feet of holy men who are not only well-versed in the traditions of scriptural interpretation, but who are also living embodiments of the wisdom those texts contain. These wise ones guide him on the path and are able to reconcile apparent textual anomalies while not discarding even a single *mantra* as useless. In this way, saved from falling into the pit dug by his own tired patterns of thought, the seeker is eventually brought to full realisation".

When each and every query has been dealt with, the Head Priest of the temple orders that its southern gate be opened. The normal procedure of a formal committee decision is dispensed with, as the decision is clearly unanimous. Each of his opponents presents the master Advaitin with a garland of orange marigolds, and then, accompanied by the blowing of conches and the waving of banners, he crosses the sacred threshold and ascends the Throne of Knowledge. It is said that such a profusion of flowers was showered on him that day that even Shachi, the wife of Indra the King of Gods, had to go without blossoms for her hair.

The next day the sage visited the Chakreshvari Goddess temple on Hari Parbat hill overlooking the great lake that lies at the heart of the valley. Here he installed a Shri Chakra in stone, and instructed local pundits in its correct worship. Some say that shortly after this he composed the *Soundarya Lahari* or 'Wave of Beauty', a collection of hymns and associated *yantras*, that remains a prime textbook on tantric ritual to this day.

Two wings to fly

The ancient temple perches on the summit of a densely wooded hill overlooking the lake far below. It is a scene of great natural beauty; the unbroken stretch of water sparkling in the sun is speckled by birds of many sorts that live around the lake. Here and there a small boat can be seen, drawing long lines across the water's calm surface and all along its banks are trees, flowers and gardens growing food. So profuse is the vegetation that the dwellings can hardly be seen; only the smoke drifting up from a thousand cooking fires showed where humans are living out their little lives. A drowsy drone of bees mingles with the distant chanting of scriptures, birdsong and the occasional ringing of temple bells. The whole area lies becalmed and the warm, deep silence is immense, its enfolding embrace in no way disturbed by the many different sounds it contains.

After his triumph at the Shadi shrine, the Master and his entourage have moved here to the hilltop temple of Gopadari where they are spending some time enjoying the serene atmosphere, beautiful climate and spectacular surroundings. Each day, he likes to walk around the hill, moving with an easeful gait and stopping every so often to commune with the wild deer that live there. But there is also a steady stream of people, both individuals and groups, climbing up the winding path to the summit in search of *darshan*. As is his custom, the young *sannyasi* deals tirelessly with the demands made upon him, receiving everyone and attending appropriately to their needs with grace, humour and compassion.

One day a householder asks about the relative roles of meditation and activity in spiritual development.

"Both are very important," is the prompt reply. "Just as a bird needs two wings to fly, so we need to both rest and be active. Each will complement the other; both are very necessary".

"But isn't practising yoga alone enough to reach the goal?"

"A seeker on the path of enlightenment must certainly perfect and purify himself by yoga, but yoga has two aspects: *karma* which is activity in the world, and *samadhi* which is silence in meditation. Regular and sustained practice of these two aspects of yoga, will in time surely bring the seeker to discover spiritual wisdom in himself".[349]

Non-attachment

"Maharaj-ji, what role does non-attachment play in enlightenment?"

Answer:

"An absolutely central one! The enlightened being has no sense of agency whatsoever. Whatever action he may be engaging in, he has no feeling of being the doer, such as: 'I am doing this, I am doing that'. For him, everything is just happening by itself, spontaneously, and he is just the witness of it. There is no attachment to action, whether his own or anyone else's".

"But how can this be?"

"Such non-attachment is a state of effortless being. It is quite natural to the wise man, because he has realised his identity with the absolute Self which lies beyond the realm of action. Even those actions which he appears to others to be performing are experienced by himself as being carried on only by the body, senses and mind. They do not actually touch him, because he is the Self, which is forever inactive".[350]

"But what about those actions such a person performed before he became liberated? What happens to those *karmas*?"

"Exactly the same; they are washed away, nothing to do with him. The one who is liberated has the unshakeable realisation that just as he is now nothing to do with action – he does not undertake it and it has no effect on him – just so, he realises that even before he was liberated, he never really had anything to do with the action that he then undertook. It was merely his ignorance that lulled him into thinking he was the doer, and that he suffered the consequences of his actions and all the rest of it. But once he has consciously recognised his identity with the Absolute, the enlightened sage sees very clearly that nothing in the past, present or future has, can, or ever will bind him, because the Absolute is not bound by anything whatsoever. It exists quite free of all time, space and causation, and he is It. Indeed, if it were not so, how could we talk of liberation? If the infinite flow of actions and their results just continued on their habitual course, raining down joys and sorrows on his head to bind and limit him, how could such a man ever be called liberated?"

After a pause:

"And what is more, just as liberation is total freedom from space, time and causation, so it can never be brought about by any particular combination of these factors. For if it could be so caused, liberation would have a beginning, and if it had a beginning, it would necessarily have an end, and thus it would be rendered impermanent, like everything else in the world. Therefore, and mark this well, liberation is of quite a different order. Being the conscious identity with the non-dual Absolute, this freedom is eternal and forever beyond anything in the relative realm of particulars".[351]

Humans and animals

A Jain *sadhu* dedicated to complete non-violence comes up to the temple early one morning. He is wearing a white cotton cloth over his mouth to avoid breathing in insects, and uses a soft white cotton brush to clear the ground in front of him when he walks, or wherever he is about to sit, for fear of inadvertently crushing some tiny creature.

He has sat silently for several hours and then in the evening *satsang* addresses the Master in a very sweet tone:

"The animals seem to follow their *dharma* and conform to the natural laws, in spite of changes to the environment and circumstances. Man on the other hand flouts social and religious laws and does not seem bound by any definite system. In fact, he appears to be degenerating, whereas animals hold steady as they are. Is it not so, Maharaj-ji? "

After a long pause, the Master nods slowly:

"The Upanishads and other scriptures say that human beings are only animals unless and until they are Self-realised. This liberation is the unique potential of a human birth. In other cases, humans can certainly behave worse than animals, yes".

Do the enlightened reincarnate?

A renowned local saint has recently died. He was a great devotee of Vishnu and often counselled his followers that once identity with the Supreme Lord had been realised, sojourning in heaven or taking re-birth on earth was no longer necessary. But soon after his death, the man he appointed to be his successor announces to the mourning followers that their guru has been welcomed into heaven by all the celestial beings and is now enjoying eternal happiness. This causes considerable confusion among them, as it infers that their master was not fully enlightened, for if he had been, according to his own teaching, he would have been unattached to even the heavenly realms of bliss, having, as it were, already passed beyond them during his lifetime.

A group of the saint's devotees come seeking guidance from the Master. He receives them courteously, paying compliments to their departed *guru-ji*.

The group's spokesman begins:

"Honoured Sir, we are confused over this business of reincarnation and whether it applies in the case of the saints. Some say they choose to return to the earth plane to do more spiritual work, while others claim that they remain securely stationed in heavenly bliss, united with the deity to whom they have been devoted. Others have different theories. Some even claim the enlightened have passed beyond any limit we normal mortals can conceive of. We are feeling confused by all this; can you help us at all? What is your perspective?"

The answer goes straight to the nub by explaining the subtle mechanics of the mind:

"To understand reincarnation in the case of the saints, let us look first at reincarnation for the ordinary person. Why does such a one come back to earth, life after life? What could impel such a cycle, time after time?"

A pause.

"He comes back because deep in his subtle body, at the deepest stratum of his mind, there lie seeds of desire that are awaiting the opportunity to sprout into action. These seeds were planted by the mind's reacting to various experiences during life, and because these seeds were planted by earthly experience they need the conditions pertaining on the earth plane to sprout, manifest and flower. Such seeds embody a particular quality of desire and so they need the same quality of environment in order for that desire to be expressed. It's like the mango seed that needs the same soil as produced the mango tree, the guava seed the same soil as gave birth to the guava tree and so on. This is observable all through life, the law of affinity. In fact, there are other qualities of desire along with their corresponding realms, but here we are talking just about human life and earthly desire.

"Now, along with their personal desires, the orthodox also have the duty to perform various obligatory rites that can only be performed while in this earthly body – such as the rituals that speed the further evolution of the soul of a departed ancestor. So this is another reason that brings the individual back to this earth – the karmic duty to perform the necessary Vedic rites. Is this clear?"

Nods all round.

"Now" – the master Vedantin is warming to his theme with that particular blend of enjoyment and enthusiasm that his followers know so well – "what is happening with all this in the case of the enlightened? Well, how do we define such a being?"

He lets the question hang in the air a moment, rhetorically; no one wishes to interrupt or deflect the flow by offering some speculative answer.

"An enlightened being is one who has passed beyond the grip of desire. He is united with the source and goal of all desiring, the absolute Self as unbounded awareness. This unity is so fulfilling that all earthly desires just fade away in its light. Such a one is ever contented, he feels no lack, no need, as he himself is all plenitude. Being relieved of the irritation of desire and released from its binding influence, his mind is freed from subjection to past impressions and he is thereby exonerated from the compulsion to repeat. Desires do not spring up in his mind owing to the destruction of their causes".[352]

"If this is so, good Sir," interrupts one of the group, unable to stay silent any longer, "then what is his motivation to act?"

"His action is a spontaneous response to the needs of the environment. He acts for the good of others, to kindle insight and alleviate suffering. Such action has no personal motivation. The sage is doing the work of the Self in the realm of the Self. It is all and always the Self for him: the actor, the action, the acted upon. There is no personal motivation here. In fact, his experience is that he does not act at all; it is Nature who does the acting and he is just the spectator of the whole thing, enjoying the passing show".[353]

"Now," continues the Master, "along with this freedom from personal action, he also free of the need to perform rites. Rites are performed to enlist the support of the celestial beings, to help us humans either here on earth or in the afterlife. But one who has become the Self is already stationed beyond those celestial realms, beyond even the gods. He is one with the Absolute that underlies and interpenetrates all levels of existence, even the most glorified. This being so, he has passed beyond all forms of action, whether mundane or ritual".

"If this is so, where does the enlightened go at death, then?"

"Nowhere! Where could he go? He is already one with the omnipresent Self. And as the Self is omnipresent, what place could he go to that he is not already inhabiting? This is what 'omnipresent' means; it means being everywhere – up, down, inside, outside, here, there and everywhere. And being already everywhere, it cannot leave one place and go to another. Omnipresence is not just a poetic metaphor, but the living experience of the enlightened: he exists everywhere, all at once, now. So there can be no question of his coming and going – where would the omnipresent come from and where would he go to?"

"Then what happens to the enlightened at the time of death?" The questioner is having trouble grasping the implications of the answers he is hearing.

"As I have just said, nothing happens to him! He is one with that pure consciousness that is absolute, beyond any movement, time or space. Nothing happens to him, just as nothing ever happens to the Self, because he and that Self are one and the same".

"I'm sorry sir, I can't follow this". The man is unable to grasp the idea of a consciousness that transcends personality.

The Master smiles at him with great compassion.

"No. Your problem is that you identify the sage with his limited physical body and his apparent self. But these are not what the enlightened being *is*. He is the Self, immortal, unbound and everywhere present. So all that happens at the time of what we call his 'death' is that this apparently limiting physical shell drops off. This is what we call death – the dropping of the physical shell, the vehicle that has sustained individualised life up to that point. In fact, the true sage has long since discarded any identification with this shell. That is precisely what we call enlightenment, transcending the illusion 'I am the body'".

"So there is no individuality, just a nothingness ...?"

"He remains what he always was. His individuality has long since become the cosmic; this is his enlightened status. At death, the functioning individuality just drops off with the body, leaving the cosmic status of the Self remaining undisturbed. Nothing can happen to it because the Self is absolute, non-relative. That is why in the case of the enlightened sage we cannot really speak in terms of death. We can only talk about his body ceasing to function. In the eyes of those around, he ceases to be located, because they see only the body and mistakenly take him to be that body. When that medium of experience goes, then all its operations cease, because the means for their continued functioning no longer exist. But, in such an event, the Being that lies beyond individual functioning and dwells prior to it, simply remains as it always was. It is undisturbed by any changes in the limited world of form, even the collapse of the body. What does all that matter to the Self? The enlightened sage has already become cosmic by virtue of his enlightenment, so none of this business touches him".

After a pause to let all this sink in:

"So, to return to our starting point: if the realised sage doesn't go anywhere, then there is certainly no question of his coming back!"[354]

Individual soul and universal Self

A teacher called Ashmarathya arrives, keen to promote his teaching. Highly intellectual, he is well-known to oppose the Master's teaching of Advaita Vedanta, preferring a doctrine technically known as 'difference in non-difference'. Many local devotees of Lord Krishna adopt his metaphysical position, believing that in the highest state, the soul unites with the Divine, yet somehow retains its separateness as well. [355]

He begins to put his case:

"In our understanding, the relationship between the individual soul and the Self is like the sparks and the fire they arise from. The sparks are not absolutely different from the fire, because they are made of fire, yet, on the other hand, they cannot be said to be absolutely non-different from the fire, because if they were, they could not be distinguished from it nor, indeed, from each other. In the same way, individual souls, which are a reflection of the Self, are neither absolutely different from the Self – for that would mean that they are not made of pure intelligence – nor can they be said to be absolutely non-different from the Self, because in that case they could not be distinguished from each other and they would all be omniscient like the Self. And if that were the case, it would be useless to give them any instruction! Therefore, to be accurate, we have to say that individual souls are somehow different from the Self, yet somehow non-different".

The master Vedantin usually loves to engage in intricate debate, but today he is in no mood to humour this particular visitor. Shaking his head vigorously he replies:

"According to Vedanta, which is the highest point of view, the individual soul and the supreme Self differ in name only. The perfect oneness of the two is attested by both the experience of the enlightened and countless textual authorities. [356] It is senseless to insist on a plurality of selves, as some teachers do, or to claim that the individual soul and the highest Self are different from one another. Certainly, the Self is called by many different names, but it is always and only singular, non-dual. Those who insist there is a distinction between the individual soul and the supreme Self act as obstructions to the perfect knowledge vouchsafed by the Upanishads, thereby blocking the tried and tested doorway to supreme beatitude". [357]

Ashmarathya makes no reply, but, shocked by the forcefulness of the reply, sits quietly for the rest of the *darshan*.

Life is the play of the Lord

The subject of the real Self is never far away. Abstract though such a topic is for most seekers, many of whom are preoccupied with what they think are more relevant personal concerns on which they are hoping for guidance, it generally ends up exerting a great fascination on them. Yet they are often surprised when such weighty discussions melt into laughter under the force of the Master's brilliance.

A master logician who runs a local academy is in the mood for a keen debate:

"Honoured Sir, you teach that the transcendental Self, in its capacity as the supreme Lord, is the intelligent cause of the world. But surely any act of creation presupposes a motive? We know from ordinary experience that a man, who is an intelligent being, begins to act only after due thought. He does not engage even in an unimportant undertaking unless it serves some purpose for him and this is particularly so if the activity is an important one. Now, the creation of this world, with all its unfathomable variety, is certainly a mighty business. So as all action serves some purpose, then the Lord must have had a purpose when he undertook such a huge task as this creation. However, if he did have such a purpose, this fact necessarily undermines the self-sufficiency which sacred scriptures are always emphasising is part of his nature. If, on the other hand, the Lord is without motive, as you orthodox Vedantins claim, then it follows that he cannot really act at all because devoid of intention, and this being so, he cannot have created the universe".

It is a powerful opening salvo; pleased with the neatness of his argument, the man continues:

"On the other hand, even if we allow that the Lord really *did* create this world without any motive, then his action must be similar to an otherwise intelligent person's falling into a mindless frenzy and acting without sense, randomly. But then if this were so, it follows that the Lord cannot be omniscient as the scriptures claim him to be.

"No, all in all, there are just too many contradictions here for me. The only logical conclusion is that the doctrine of the creation proceeding from a supremely intelligent Self is untenable".

The Master smiles contentedly; evidently pleased by the intricacy of the man's arguments he murmurs:

"Well said, Sir, well said!"

It seems as if that is all there is going to be by way of a reply, but then, after a pause, he begins:

"This may be well said, but actually, it is not so. For example, look at those princes in their pleasure palaces down in the old city – they do nothing but enjoy themselves. The same is true even for men of high position who have achieved everything they want in life and have no unfulfilled desires left. They too act without any extraneous purpose, but just for the fun of it. Still, act they do, and life for them is just unending pleasure, a play".

Then, sensing the objection that grandees or royalty constitute special cases, the Master continues:

"Or, on a less elevated level, consider how your own body breathes. The process of inhalation and exhalation goes on continuously without reference to any extraneous purpose. The body is merely following the law of its own nature. Like that, the activity of the Lord is natural and effortless and without any purpose beyond itself. As such, his activity can be considered mere sport. His power being infinite and his desires all fulfilled, there can be no extraneous motive attributed to his action, such as might be the case with others. To him, even such a huge endeavour as creating the universe is a mere pastime, a play. So our reasoning does not find fault with scripture here – we can find no purpose in the activity of the Lord. Similarly, it cannot be said that he does not act or if he does, it is like some senseless person as you have said, for again, scripture affirms the fact of the creation on the one hand and the omniscience of the Lord on the other".

After another silence, the Master adds with a smile:

"And anyway, let us not forget that all these scriptural teachings on creation do not accurately describe the highest reality. They only discuss the impermanent world of appearances, which is characterised by innumerable names and forms and is everywhere hedged in by all the trappings of ignorance. The true aim of the scriptures, on the other hand, is always and only to propound the fact that the real Self of everything without exception is the non-dual Totality we call *brahman*".[358]

Body and soul

Q: "What is the relationship between the body and the soul?"
A: "Sheath and sword, carriage and driver!"

The benefit of debate

The Master always emphasises that Self-realisation is not a matter of mere intellectualising, but requires sustained and self-transcending practice. Nonetheless, because of his scholarly brilliance, large numbers come to debate their various understandings with him. Some of these are *pandits* learned in Vedic ritual, others metaphysicians of various orthodox and unorthodox schools, and yet others who hold their own idiosyncratic opinions. From his side, he seems always happy to engage in such discussions as long as the seeker is sincere and there is a chance of real insight. However, not infrequently his visitors are emotionally attached to their particular viewpoint and some are unwilling to change it, even when the Master's pellucid reasoning exposes the fallacy of their position.

After a particularly argumentative scholar has left the *darshan* hall, a senior *brahmachari* laments the fact that such people waste the Master's precious time in fruitless discussion by doggedly continuing to advance their own opinions, while not really paying attention to the answers he gives.

The Master's reply surprises him.

"Oh no, argumentation is quite alright. You see, any understanding that is based only on the surface levels of life must appear to contradict the Transcendent. This apparent dichotomy is quite natural, even though whatever is on the surface is in fact only an expression of the hidden depths. It's like the ocean and its waves. The waves could be very varied: some huge tidal swells and others tiny rippling wavelets, but they are all equally water, all equally expressions of the one ocean which, irrespective of all the different waves, is forever silent at its depths. Like that, the silent ocean of the Absolute contains everything, and so nothing can be in ultimate contradiction with it! And because that Oneness is all-encompassing, there could be innumerable expressions of it, many of which may well appear to be mutually incompatible. So in the search for truth, every viewpoint has its function in expressing one of the possible forms of the Absolute. Even error, which is certainly opposed to truth, can inadvertently serve to point towards it".

One of the monks seeks to add a comment, but the Master is in full flow now, buoyed up by a happiness clear for all to see.

"And, and, and ..." he continues, lightly striking the table in front of him with a flower he is holding, "what is more, how do you get to the depths of the ocean anyway? By penetrating the surface. You have to start on the surface, with the waves. Like that, to get to the Transcendent you have to pass through all the more superficial levels of opinion, discussion, argumentation, challenges and so on, and keep on diving deeper. Deeper and deeper: that's how one gets to the core of things. You remember the text: *'Through discussion and yet more discussion is born the awakening of That'*?[359] It is as if every possible doubt, angle and viewpoint may have to be exhausted before the questing intellect can finally acknowledge 'Aha! So *that's* how it is!'

"So, there is nothing wrong with argumentation. Whatever arises, the wise see that the Absolute is present there, just as the water is present in each and every wave, no matter how various or contradictory they may appear. In fact, the greater the challenge, the more the Truth is brought out. In fact, the teacher actually feels indebted to the student who really challenges him. We love such students!"

There is general laughter. Then:

"Just as the experiences of the *sadhaka*[360] proceed in the direction of enlightenment, so does his intellectual understanding advance towards the same goal. One limited opinion is replaced by another more evolved one, one partial perspective gives way to another more comprehensive one. Like that, it's a natural evolution".

The *brahmachari* who originally asked the question:

"Thank you, Master. I can see how those whose minds are flexible enough will benefit from discussion and evolve, but those who cling to erroneous opinions presumably remain stuck and their evolution is stalled until they can move on at some later time?"

"Not so", comes the reply. "Evolution always continues, no matter what. Everything that lives is evolving, by the very nature of things. Look at the common man. First he is a child, then he grows up and his views mature and he gets a profession, then he marries, has children of his own, assumes parental responsibility as a stable member of the community and so on. Then by the end, he has become an elder and his knowledge and life-experience win him the respect of his juniors. So there is always evolution going on, even if one does nothing more than survive and live one's life in the ordinary way".

"How, then, is it different for the spiritual seeker?"

"The speed, the speed. The normal sort of evolution, just surviving, breeding and continuing, is very, very slow; the whole thing can be a woefully lengthy business. What differs in the case of the genuine aspirant is the speed of his evolution, the rate of his growth. If a man consciously participates in his own spiritual development, then the pace of his evolution is enormously quickened".

After a few moments of silence, he repeats in an abstracted, almost dreamy tone: "Enormously, enormously".

Sleep

Someone has asked about sleep.

"Sleep? There is a dialogue in the scriptures where the teacher Ajatashatru teaches his pupil Balaki about this. Out walking together one day, they come across a man sleeping by the road. Ajatashatru wakes him up, then turns to his pupil and asks: 'Balaki, tell me, where was this person when he slept? Where has he just come back from?'

"Now, it is taught in Vedanta that at the time of deep sleep the soul becomes one with the highest Self, the absolute consciousness from which the whole world proceeds. As we know from our own experience, deep sleep is characterised by an absence of individual awareness and utter tranquillity; nothing happens there and it is delightful! In other words, sleep is a state devoid of all those specific cognitions which, being produced by the body and mind throughout the waking and dreaming states, continuously superimpose limits on the soul and cause it all sorts of mischief thereby. Likewise, it is from the universal Self that the soul returns when sleep is broken. This is why we enjoy sleep so much and miss it once we have returned to the waking state once again".[361]

Death as evolution

A man whose wife has recently died in childbirth comes for *satsang*. Deeply saddened, he is seeking some answers.

"Sir, does the soul reincarnate?"

The Master nods gently. "It must", he replies, "yes, it must."

"Why is that?"

"It is the unavoidable process of evolution".

"How so?"

"Well, what happens at the time of death? What we call death is when the vital force leaves the body. Deprived of vitality, the material form gradually disintegrates and returns to its own constituent elements, which eventually return to their causal level. At the same time the life force departs, all the inner intelligences – the senses, mind, intellect – follow it, and as they go, they take with them the impressions of the past experiences undergone by that person. Once this departing self, the *jiva*, withdraws from the gross realm of material existence, it passes into the subtle strata of creation and then, after some time spent there, this discarnate entity takes a fresh form, a new body".

"Is this process automatic or can it be interrupted?"

"It is automatic. All the intelligences follow the vital force like a prime minister who follows the king without question. And by using the word 'follow' here, I am not implying a sequential movement but simply that they move in conformity to their respective leaders, they all go together".

That the physical presence of his late wife is still very much with the man is evident from his next question.

"That new body, sir, how is it made? Is it that the self, so to speak, crushes up the elements of the old one and somehow refashions them or does it employ new materials every time?"

"No, no", replies the Master gently. "It is just like a goldsmith who breaks off a little quantity of gold from an old piece in order to fashion a new and better form. Like that, the intelligent *jiva* uses the five elements [362] to fashion a new form, so as to enjoy the appropriate rewards of its past actions that are to be experienced in whatever realm the new birth may be. But it is always a new and better form than the previous one. Therefore, however painful a death may be for those who are left behind, from a wider perspective and for the one who has departed, it is always a step forward".

"And what, Sir, is the cause of taking these new births?"

"The driving force of desire. Action holds the foremost place in this world and all action is driven by the desire to achieve something. There is normally no end to this, because anything experienced as separate from oneself could become the object of desire. Therefore, only those who have realised their true Self are freed from the grip of desire. How so? Because there is nothing that is not the omnipresent Self, nothing is separated out from it, and so once that satisfaction is attained, all partial desires are already effectively attained. Thus the Self-realised have nothing left to desire, no sense of want remains for them, and so they are no longer caught in the process of rebirth".[363]

The mind is not self-luminous

One topic that often causes confusion is the difference between the mind and the Self. Many people entertain concepts about the Self – as a guide, a protector, an inner authority or conscience – that more properly apply to different levels of the mind. What follows is an example of such confusion and the Master's response.

Disciple:

"Maharaj, the other day at *darshan*, I think I heard you say that the mind is not conscious. With all due respect, Sir, this is quite incomprehensible to me. Surely the mind is the source of what we call consciousness or awareness? Can you explain what you meant please?"

Master:

"Be careful! What I said was that the mind is not self-luminous, by which I meant the mind does not shine by its own light, it is not the source of its own awareness. The thing is: the Self is Consciousness alone. It is just simple awareness, unlocalised, omnipresent and perfectly unobstructed intelligence. This intelligence we call the Self is all-seeing and it alone is truly conscious. Everything else is insentient and only enjoys sentience by virtue of its association with the Self as consciousness. As it is all-seeing, the Self is also a witness of everything that is other than its own pure nature, unsullied by any object. So the mind, along with its perceptions, ideas and objects, are all external to the Self and by the same token, external to consciousness. Hence, the mind is not self-luminous".

"Hold on a moment, Sir! Can you explain why the mind or the world are not of the same nature as the Self?"

"Because they are made up of various combinations of the three *gunas*, whereas the Self is pure awareness alone, quite separate from the *gunas* and absolutely unattached to them. It is the unchanging power-of-seeing in itself, the one Seer that is itself unseen, and as such it does not pass over into whatever it sees. Nevertheless, it *appears* to have passed over into the mind, and thence into the changing objects that the mind perceives. But in fact, it only witnesses the mind and its contents, which are quite separate from it".

"Yet we still perceive, think, remember and enjoy all the other functions of consciousness?"

"As I say, the power of seeing appears to have passed over from the real seer - the Self - to what it sees, the mind. So the mind seems to be the source of its own consciousness, but that consciousness actually belongs to the Self and the Self only. In fact, the mind borrows awareness, so to speak, from the Self. It is a reflector of the consciousness of the Self, like a face in a mirror, and as such has no ultimate reality. We can see this from the fact that the mind is always changing from moment to moment. If it were unchanging, the same object would always be present in it but, as we know, the mind contains a cow one minute, a clay jar the next and so on. With the Self, however, the reverse is true: its object – the mind – is always known to it. If it were not, how would we be aware of the continuous changeability of the mind? So the Self is unchangeable and real, because it always knows its object, which is not the ever-changing content of the mind but the mind itself, in all its varying modes".

Seeing the abstract nature of the discussion is eluding his listeners, the Master introduces a simpler analogy.

"Look, imagine a piece of black iron that is placed in close proximity to a roaring fire. Before long the iron begins to glow with heat and we say that it is on fire, but its appearance of being on fire is due solely to its proximity to the real source of heat and light, which is the fire. The relationship of the mind and the Self is like that".[364]

"If what you are saying is the case, how is it that we are completely unaware of what is really going on?"

"We are blinded to the reality by the long habit of erroneously identifying with a limited mind housed in a limited body. Because of this erroneous identification, we fail to experience awareness as it is: unlocalised but reflecting off various localised media, such as intellect, mind and so on. This failure to discern correctly is what our teaching of Vedanta calls 'ignorance' and it is this ignorance that is the sole cause of all our manifold suffering".

Even those who did not follow the argument intuited that what was being presented was an essential and radical truth about life and one that deserved careful consideration.

The power of silence

Although the Master spends much of his time teaching and instructing, there are also many occasions when he gives silent *darshan*, saying nothing but just radiating the ineffable peace and happiness he always carries with him. All who encounter this atmosphere feel its effect; for many it is a life-changing experience.

One day a question arises about a great saint who lives on the other side of the lake. He has a powerful reputation and many healing miracles have been attributed to him, yet he never leaves his small hut and rarely even speaks to those who make the effort to come to see him. The questioner, a woman who devotes her life to helping the poor, is critical of the inactivity of this man; she feels he should at least make the effort to go about and preach the truth to the people at large. The Master will have none of it, however, animatedly interrupting her criticisms with:

"How do you know he is not doing so? Does preaching consist in mounting a platform and haranguing everyone in earshot? Preaching is simply the communication of knowledge, and that can be done in many different ways. And as it happens, silence is the most effective of them".

The questioner looks bemused.

"Look, imagine two men. One listens to a sermon for an hour and then goes off without having been affected in such a way as to change his life, while the other sits in a holy presence with no words exchanged, yet goes away with his outlook on life totally changed. Which is the better?

"From the point of view of the teacher, sitting silently and sending out the inner force can well be the most effective method of teaching. If the word can produce an effect, judge for yourself how much more powerful must be the silence from which all words spring. Words are limited. After all, how does speech arise? First there is the abstract consciousness, that silence out of which the ego, the limited sense of 'I' arises. This 'I' in turn gives rise to thought, and from thought is born the spoken word. So we can say the word is the great-grandson of the original silent source. Therefore, to repeat: if the word can produce an effect, how much more powerful must the teaching through silence be?

"Mark well, the realised soul has no need to go out among the public; anyway, if necessary, he can always use others as instruments. The sage naturally emits potent waves of spiritual influence which can draw many people towards him. He may sit all his life in a cave and maintain perfect *mauna*[365] yet just coming into contact with such a soul will certainly have its effect, even if he says nothing. His silence is the ultimate Reality. Contact is what is important; if the eyes of such a being meet the eyes of the disciple, words have no more significance".

Immortality

The foothills of the mighty Himalaya, with their pure soil and heavy rainfall, are carpeted with healing plants and herbs, and their verdant valleys have since earliest times been known as an important source of Ayurvedic medicine.

One afternoon a renowned local *vaidya* [366] calls on the Master. He is desirous of achieving immortality and over the years has apparently subjected himself to many experiments to that end. One, which involved the use of mercury, very nearly cost him his life.

When he has heard the *vaidya's* story, the Master asks:

"Why are you so interested in achieving immortality when you are already immortal?"

"I don't understand, Sir".

"The one immortal Being gives birth to innumerable mortal beings. You are that One. It would be better to forget all your medicines and remember who you really are".

The value of Yoga

A *hatha yogi* comes for *darshan*. He is famed for his extraordinary flexibility and looks healthy and vibrant. He is probably much older than he appears.

"What is your opinion of Yoga, Maharaj-ji?"

"You mean Hatha Yoga? A cart with one wheel! But it is useful for those who are still under the thrall of worldly desires".

"And the Yoga taught by Maharshi Patanjali?"

"Its value lies in kindling the fire of knowledge".[367]

"So is there no real value in doing *asanas* themselves then?"

"Oh, there is. Doing a few *asanas* helps purify the body and steady the awareness but all this is a preparation only. True Yoga consists in making everything that one has learnt about the theory of spirituality a direct and immediate perception. So we can say that of all the *asanas* by far the best one is *nididhyasana!*"[368]

"And is the practice of meditation an aid to this perception?"

"Indeed, it is indispensable. There are many attributes that cultivate ripeness for supreme realisation: fearlessness, persistence, charity, modesty, settledness of mind, and so on. All of these will be enhanced by correct meditation, but even the best meditation is also just a means. In the end, one's awareness must be fully absorbed in the metaphysical experience of the one Pure Intelligence that is Reality. So note well - the meditator's attention cannot just be directed to the tip of his nose or that is all he will be left with!" [369]

The process of reincarnation

A group is gathered by the riverbank, in a clearing amidst grasses that are lush after the recent rains. The headman of the nearby village has just been cremated, and the conversation, as it so often does amongst the older devotees, turns to death and reincarnation.

Master:

"It is clear that, as a consequence of its past actions, each self has fashioned a particular type of consciousness throughout life. It is the quality of this consciousness which will determine the direction he takes after the death of the body. This is why our Master Vyasa[370] says that a man attains whatever he thinks of at the moment of death, because it is that last thought which indicates the predominating quality of his mind; it is the summation of his mental tendencies so to speak".

Disciple:

"So we should think good thoughts at the time of death then?"

Master:

"Of course! Ideally the mind is fixed on an aspect of the Divine".[371]

A pause. Then:

"But I'm afraid it is not that easy. This process is not under the conscious control of the person who is dying, it is an automatic response, a spontaneous consequence of what has gone before. In order to have some say in the whole business, one should practice Yoga and purify the mind during life, for nothing can be done at the last minute, when death comes knocking at the door. At that time we are quite powerless. This is one reason all the sacred books teach that we should do good in life, rather than evil, because whatever we have done in the past will determine the quality of our heart and mind, which in turn will determine what happens after the body falls off. This is why study of our Upanishads is so valuable: it nurtures the type of mind needed to make the best not only of life, but also of death"

Disciple:

"What is the mechanism involved here, Maharaj?"

Master:

"Well, imagine you are setting off on a journey with a creaky old cart loaded up with provisions to sustain you on the road. Like that, when the self leaves the body at death, it carries along with it the knowledge, actions and experiences garnered during life. We take the impressions of our past actions along with us when we leave, compressed, as it were, into the heart centre of the subtle body. These impressions are like seeds waiting to sprout and, as such, they will have their effects. They influence the direction the departing life-thread takes as it leaves its gross shell, and they determine which of the bodily openings will be its gate of departure. Later on, they will initiate further actions in the next life, and these will in turn be the means for bringing past acts to fruition there".

A sceptic asks:

"This all sounds coherent enough, good Sir, but is there any proof?"

Master:

"Well, we see the results every day. Have you not frequently observed that some people are from birth naturally clever in all sorts of activities – such as painting, for example – without needing any practice? Now, organs and faculties are not normally skilled without practice, but if they carry over skills from before, then that practice is not needed. They enjoy a natural ability by virtue of the force of their past impressions working themselves out. By the same token, we commonly see others who are unskilful even in relatively easy tasks; they have no such latent impressions. Similarly, there are all sorts of variations observable amongst people – some are bright, some are dull – and all of this is due to the revival or non-revival of their past experience. In this way, it is the knowledge, actions and experiences we take with us that determine the body we have for our next life, the circumstances of its birth and family, our talents and so on. Mark well, cultivating only what is good in life benefits us, not only for now, but also for the future".

A Jain monk speaks up:

"We are taught that when the self leaves the old body, it travels to a new one like a bird going from one tree to another".

A follower of the Devatavadin school, a sect that believes in angel guides adds:

"As I understand it, Swami-ji, another body – a subtle being – carries the dead soul to the place it is to be reborn".

The Master answers:

"These are nice images, but actually, it is more like the light in a lamp. Imagine: as long as the jar which encloses the light remains intact, so long that light remains localised. But when the jar breaks, the light becomes all-pervading. Then, when a new jar is made, it contracts again once more. Like that, the organs which are by nature infinite, contract and expand according to whether or not there is a localised container for them. This is how the mechanics of individuality operate, and it the same process whether for an ant, a mosquito, an elephant – right up to the entire universe".

The disciple who asked the original question comes back into the discussion:

"I still don't understand how the self can move from one body to another, Maharaj?"

"Well, you are already familiar with something similar each time your awareness moves into the dream body and roams around there under the force of its previous impressions. What happens after death is not so dissimilar to that. Now ..."

He looks around, then reaches down and plucks a handful of grass from the ground bedside him.

"Look here! You see this little black leech at the end of this piece of grass? Observe it closely. You see how it gets to the end of one stalk, then stretches itself out to grasp the tip of another stalk close by, then draws its body behind it into a ball and leaves its former perch?"

Not for the first time, the group is spellbound by the Master's ability effortlessly to draw out profound knowledge from his everyday surroundings.

"Like that, the transmigrating self we are talking about leaves its old body senseless, and projects its accumulated impressions to take hold of another body that is being formed. Then it pulls itself into the new body, like this leech grasping its new stalk. When the physical organs have been arranged in the new body appropriately to the brought-over past impressions, and in such a way as to manifest the effects of those *karmas* in the new life, then the presiding intelligences that are to animate that new body come and settle in. So, you see how a new body gets formed from the old? It's an old, old story ..."[372]

The ocean refuses no river

A man arrives at the temple one day; still in his thirties, he is known locally as having been addicted to opium for many years. Recently he has managed to stop the habit, but is a sorry spectacle: thin, unhealthy looking and nervous. Nevertheless, something in him still burns bright with the hope of improving his lot. He tells his story briefly, ending plaintively with the words:

"I suppose, Swami-ji, there is no hope left for someone who has wasted their life as I have?"

The Master's reply is brisk:

"Of course there is hope. Whatever happened in the past is the past, gone. All that matters is the present and the future. So do not bog yourself down with thinking about the past and what could have been or might have been or should not have been. That's gone. Just focus on improving your situation in the present, that's all. If you do that wholeheartedly, things will get better, no doubt".

Then, with a sudden tenderness:

"And remember, the ocean refuses no river, even the muddiest".

The renounced life

After many enjoyable weeks in the Land of the Dogras, the Master and his followers are now travelling eastwards to revisit the area where he spent such a productive time working on the textual commentaries. It is clear he always feels particularly at home in the serene atmosphere of the mountains, and greatly enjoys the powerful purity of their energy.

As the party travels up and down the high river valleys, the Master is approached by many who are living there in isolation, people who have abandoned social commitments in order fully to dedicate themselves to the life of the spirit. Some of these he initiates formally into *sannyasa*, and they join one of the monastic orders he has already established. At the same time, villagers committed to their hard life of surviving in the world also come for *darshan*, some seeking help and advice with their problems and concerns, others just wishing to get a glimpse of a famous saint. Often these simple householders bring with them the feeling that somehow their way of life is inferior as regards the attainment of spiritual progress. So preoccupied are they with the mundane tasks of earning a living and raising a family that, apart from regular visits to the temple, and attending to the needs of their family or village deities, there is little they can do in the way of the journey to ultimate liberation. Not a few express the desire to renounce all their family commitments and adopt the reclusive way of life as a means to speed up their spiritual progress. The Master, however, will generally reassure such people that their born way of life is appropriate to their *karma*, reassuring them that if they are sincere in their efforts, meagre though they may appear, progress on the spiritual path is in no way barred to them.

What follows is a typical exchange on the matter.

Seeker:

"Revered sage, I have been seriously contemplating renunciation. I have a family and a job, but feel that these commitments do not allow me sufficient time to focus on my spiritual advancement. Should I not enter a monastery or take to the road as a *sadhu* and just abandon myself to God's will?"

Master:

"For you, it is better not to know the recluse way of life. It is a very difficult path to follow, suited only to a few. All kinds of difficulties are there. Once you have left the home and the support of your family, there will be no solid basis to provide the essential standards of living. It is as if you are lost, adrift, and for most people, this is a very great hardship. The life of a recluse is a very hard life. The householder's life is one of relative comfort – he has regular routines, practical and emotional support from family, good food, a comfortable bed. In the recluse life there is none of this: no bed, no food, no home, no shelter, nothing. Really nothing".

Seeker:

"Well, I don't believe it can be so bad because you chose that path and you made that decision. There must be something good about the recluse way of life?"

The response provokes laughter in the group and the Master chuckles.

Then:

'Yes, you are right! There is one good thing in the recluse life and that is the Teacher. The Teacher is the sole resort of the recluse life, its centre and its circumference. Just a good Teacher and that's it. And why? Because the life of a recluse is not his own life. He lives for the Absolute, the Divine, and the absolute Divine is, for him, located in his Teacher. So he lives for his Teacher. Because of this focus, he doesn't mind where he sleeps – on the thorns or on the rocks or on the earth or in the fields, a damp cave, wherever. He doesn't mind what he eats. He has no material certainty whatsoever, all he knows is that his whole being is centred in the Teacher. He breathes with the breath of the Teacher, he lives with the life of the Teacher. All his mental and emotional energies are rooted in the heart and mind of the Teacher. He just lives for him and that's it. So this is a life of complete dedication.

"But this should be something very natural. If it is in any way fabricated, then there will be all sorts of inconveniences, the thing will not work and the whole purpose of the recluse life will be damaged. This centring on the Teacher must be a natural thing, a one-way flow, like a river flowing on to the ocean. The ocean doesn't flow to the river, only the river flows to the ocean. So it is only the one-way relationship between the disciple and the Master. It is the responsibility of the disciple to flow on to the Teacher and live with him a life of complete surrender, complete dedication. One-way flow. His whole life moves around the Master – thinking, feeling, everything, all for him. And yes, you are right, I have been fortunate to live that life; therefore I know all the mechanics of it. Otherwise, the life of a recluse could be very, very torturous. Because there is nothing of physical comfort. Actually, basic physical needs are barely met, so what to say of comforts? In the householder`s life there are comforts of all different sorts; but in the recluse life there is only this one-pointedness".

Seeker:

"And those who live in monasteries?"

Master:

"I am talking here of recluses, those who live far from other human habitation, in the wilds of nature, in the forests, jungles and all that. These people live under the trees or in the damp cave or some such thing. Now, life in the monastery is a different life. Monasteries are a little bit more protected; there is more structure: physical protection and the support of a community. The recluse life is something different. It enacts the extreme edge of human existence, right up close to the Divine that transcends the material world".

For a moment he seems as if lost in some far distant realm, before continuing:

"And then, over and above that, there are the tests that a student has to go through, set up by the Master to see the genuineness of dedication. These tests can be terrible, and if there is any lack of dedication, then one fails in the test and does not come up to the mark. But, again, if the dedication is natural, one doesn`t feel as if one is being tested. It is just a natural thing, part of the natural flow of events, nothing to bother about specially. There is discomfort, for sure, but it is a very fortunate discomfort".

The Master laughs softly, as if to himself, and there is a subtle relaxation of tension in the group, all of whom are electrified by such an unusually personal disclosure from their *guru*.

Then a high-born woman with a young son speaks up:

"How does the institution of *brahmacharya* fit into this pattern, Sir? Those young *brahmin* boys spend twelve or fifteen years of their lives as a recluse and, after having established the devotion to their Master, they then come back into society and become a householder?"

Master:

"Yes, but their training is different again. This is the beauty of our Vedic system, you see: all the different areas of society are catered for. Different people have different roles to play and this accords with their born *dharma*, their individual *karmas* and their overall evolution. It is all set out in the Veda; all we need to do is follow the sacred traditions correctly.

"Those *brahmin* boys are suited by their birth to become students of sacred knowledge and, as there is quite a good level of enlightenment along with that training also, they become grounded in the spiritual realities, the deep hidden principles that guide and conduct everything on the surface of life. Then, when they have to enter into the householder life at the age of twenty or so, fine, they are properly prepared for it. At that point they assume their appropriate role and carry on the duties of the world according to their specific training. They are not trained into the recluse way of life, they are the qualified students of the Veda. And, as experts in that knowledge, they are then able to guide the daily lives of the people".

Someone else asks:

"Is this dedication you speak of, the dedication of the recluse to his Master, anything like the devotion to God?"

Master:

"Indeed, it is just like that. Exactly like that. When celestial vision dawns for the seeker, his whole being is transformed, he becomes naturally one-pointed in the light of God, everywhere, even unconsciously. He has no choice in the matter at all. Like that, the surrender to the Master has the same status. His life just moves with the thought of the Master, the intentions of the Master".

Another question alters the flow of discussion:

"Sir, you always teach that life when lived aright is all joy. How do you reconcile this with what you have just said about the hardships involved in the reclusive way of life?"

Master:

"Ha! Even those deprivations are a joy! Because, as I said, if that dedication is complete then the discomforts experienced in that way of life have no weight, no force. In such a self-transcending state, everything is a joy, no matter what. Such a dedication means that the will of the Master, the feelings of the Master become my will, my feelings. If he wants me to go this way, fine, this is my way. If he wants me to turn that way, fine, that is my way. So the burden of agency is taken off one's shoulders and that itself is a massive relief, a real joy! This way the whole of life takes a shape, takes a flow, spontaneously. With no effort. And that movement is deeply grounded in love and one-pointedness of purpose, that's all".

The questioner is not convinced.

"Yes, Sir, but what is the purpose of the hardship in the recluse way of life? If the devotion is really there as you say, why must the hardship be there? If they have no force, then surely they are unnecessary?"

The Master chuckles:

"Well, hardship is the usual condition of living, so there is nothing additional to provide!"

"Couldn't one be just as devoted while living under a roof'?"

"If the Master is found under the roof, fine!"

"Does this sometimes happen?"

"It could sometimes happen, yes".

"Why then is it that a Master tends to be found out of doors?"

There is general laughter. The tone of the discussion has suddenly lightened, but those who are alert enough sense that a precious sweetness, a rare level of intimacy, has taken flight too.

Master:

"It depends upon the liking of the Master. There are reclusive Masters and Masters who stay in monasteries – with rooms, cots, blankets and all the rest of it – and that way of life is set. But, if the Master is not the owner of a monastery, if he is like a wild swan, then homelessness will the life of his disciple also".

"But the knowledge gained can be just as great, whatever the circumstances?"

As if relieved, the Master brings things to a conclusion:

"This is the real point here. The way of living has little to do with the storehouse of knowledge. The storehouse of knowledge may be sitting here or there, or anywhere. All we have to do from our side is to bring ourself in tune with him, wherever he may be, and then the knowledge will flow."

He gestures outside the room.

"It's just like the water tank in the yard out there. It is sitting there quietly, full of water. Now, the water doesn't have a spontaneous tendency to flow out, because it is contained, in one place, but on the other hand, it will certainly not resist flowing out freely if a pipeline is brought to it. So, the pipe must always come to the tank, not the other way around.[373] If we want to have the benefit of the water in our fields, we just raise the pipeline to the right level, and the water will flow naturally. Like that, the disciple has just to bring himself – his feelings, his mind, his life – to the level of the mind and feeling of the Master, and then the wisdom will flow. But the effort must be made; if we can't be bothered to take the trouble to raise the pipeline to the correct level, how and where can the water flow ?"

An empty house

The path criss-crossing the mountain side is broad enough, but steep and rocky. Overhead, long tendrils of liana snake down from the twisted, moss-coated trees that line the path, sticking out at fantastic angles as they stretch upwards for light and life. Three thousand feet below, the river rushes full and clear, leaping over outcrops and swirling frothily around the small islands in its centre. The silence of the mighty peaks is present everywhere, magnified rather than obliterated by the constant sounds of nature. Against such a vast background, the human beings who wend their patient way up and down the path are frail specks. But they are as purposeful and determined as a line of ants, for the difficult path leads to the shrine where Shiva in his benign form as Pashupatinath, 'The Lord of all Creatures' likes to come and spend time. Surely, any amount of hardship can be endured if there is a hope of having a taste of his sweet grace.

That rich and poor are as one to the Lord is attested by the fact that although the shrine is a wealthy royal establishment, long patronised by the Licchavi kings who rule over this valley and its capital of Kathmandu 'The Place of the Wooden Temple', the dense woods that surround it are home to hundreds of *sadhus* of various sects. They camp out here, living on alms and, barely clothed, they wander freely in and around the temple as if they own it and all its riches. Many of these wild men are *aghori tantrikas* who congregate around the cremation *ghats* on the bank of the holy Bagmati river that flows past the shrine. They are feared for their skill in dealing with spirits and casting spells, and it is because of this that the Master has been drawn to visit the area with a view to re-establishing the purity of worship here. A massive programme of education follows his arrival. Some of the *jadu babas*, resenting any interference in their way of life, clear off but many foreswear magic, and are initiated into the *sannyasi* orders.

The grateful monarch pledges his royal patronage for monasteries and institutions of Vedic learning. The Master also instructs some of the southern *brahmins* who are travelling with him to stay on as priestly experts to care for the great four-headed Shiva *lingam* that presides over the holy of holies. Their duty will be to perform the correct rites, as well as ministering to the local people and the many thousands of pilgrims who descend on the shrine for the great festivals, especially the annual spring festival of Shivaratri. The descendants of those southern families continue to run the Pashupatinath temple to this day.

Satisfied that the true teaching has been re-established after many years, the Master is now returning with his party to the valley far below. Two wooden carts crammed with orange-robed figures sway and lurch from side to side, bouncing along as the mules that draw them pick their way fastidiously across the uneven surface. Suddenly, one of the mules skitters and slips on a large flat stone. Sparks fly from its flailing hooves as it goes over on its side, thrashing wildly and dragging its fellow beast down with it. The cart lurches, bucks and clatters over, tipping its occupants out. The Master is thrown onto the road and one of the *brahmacharis* falls heavily on top of him. Everyone is worried that their beloved *guru* may have been hurt, but he himself is quite unconcerned. Springing to his feet, he dusts himself down, chuckling:

"Don't concern yourselves! The tenant of this particular house was evicted long ago. After all, when the landlord chooses to show his face, who can resist his command?"

Siddhis

Some days after this, a teaching takes place which will linger long in the memories of those fortunate enough to be present. What is so remarkable about the event is not only the depth and purity of the teaching – qualities which his followers have come to expect from all the Master's discourses – but the extraordinary atmosphere of loving

compassion that suffuses the gathering. The Master is like some solic-
itous and beloved elder at an intimate family gathering, even though
most of those present are older than he is, and some considerably so.
Moreover, in this meeting he speaks of his personal experience, which
is a very rare happening, and an added delight for his followers.

The discussion began with recalling the time spent at the Pashupatinath temple and then naturally turns to the subject of *siddhis* –
the so-called 'supernormal powers' documented in several yoga texts.

"Yes," begins the Master, "these days the majority of people is searching for *siddhis*, that's what they seem to want out of their efforts".

"How are such powers accomplished, Guru-ji?"

"Well, the texts tell us that there are various ways.[374] In some
cases, it is a matter of *karma*. Because a person has done good
spiritual work in the previous life, they are born with that merit in
this one, but along with the merit, there are some worldly desires
still remaining. So their *prarabdha*[375] works itself out in that way
and draws them into the experience of *siddhis*. The texts are full of
such examples from the Golden Age, when life was much purer and
human consciousness much higher, but even today some *mahatma*
can be born a natural *siddha*.

"In other cases, for less advanced beings, *siddhis* can come from
special herbs, the so-called *aushhadhi*. When I was spending time in
seclusion in the jungles, there were *sadhus* who used various concoc-
tions; the *kantakari* was an especially popular ingredient.[376] Herbs
like this can give you the strength to live for a very long time, they
inhibit the decay of the body, so a person can live for huge spans of
time, because disease just cannot get a hold on them. Such herbs can
have other remarkable effects. I remember there was one *baba* living in a cave on the banks of the Narmada, who had infused *siddhi*
into his sandals. When he needed *ghee*, he would cross the river by
walking on the water, collect *ghee* from the bazaar on the other side
and return the same way. Then there was another *sadhu* who was
quite famous because he had developed the *gutaka siddhi* which is
gained by placing a magic ball made of herbs in the mouth. It grants
invisibility. So these herbs can grant many *siddhis* and fulfil all sorts
of desires".

The Master chuckles at the memories.

"And then, *siddhis* can also come from *mantras*. If the *devata* associated with the mantra becomes pleased with your repetitions of it
then, whatever power that being has, it will grant you the same. And

here too there is a huge range of possible effects. After all, it is said in the texts that there are numerous *devatas*[377] each with their preferences, powers and appropriate rituals. Living in the jungle there were a good many practitioners of *shabara mantra*s – those sounds gain subtle support for a specific occasion. With this *siddhi*, a man can get help in achieving success in some particular undertaking or other.

"Now, *siddhis* may also come from *samadhi. Samadhi* may seem a great mystery for the ordinary person; to them the life of the *yogi* is something perplexing. But in truth, *samadhi* is just the abandoning of the senses, and the untying of their grip on objects. Until this happens, worldly desires cannot be left behind, and one remains like a king living in exile in the forest of illusions. But once the mind is pure, then this mental restraint is maintained naturally, and one can live the regal life of an unattached *yogi* even while surrounded by wife, family, work commitments, and all the rest of it.

"The important thing here is to let *samadhi* purify the mind. Rid the mind of *tamas* and *rajas* and allow it to become *sattvic*.[378] Then spiritual work will yield its real benefits and the *kleshas* will be destroyed.[379] Only then is a man pure enough to be a person of Knowledge, and liberation comes from Knowledge, nothing else. And what is Knowledge? It is the apparent 'attainment' of what one always and already is – the limitless, omnipresent consciousness that is your own real Self. And those beings who enjoy this realisation have all their desires already fulfilled by the happiness that Self-realisation brings. Nonetheless, though they desire nothing more for themselves, they naturally merit the unceasing and direct support of that which is their own deepest Self, the Divine consciousness, which is almighty.

"The main point to be understood here is that all these specific powers are limited; they cannot grant the great happiness, which is intimate experience of the Self. This supreme state of pure Being, on the other hand, has limitless power, so by having recourse to that transcendent level, everything can be done. Those who claim the scriptures teach otherwise, and who insist on the performance of rites, are like those who claim to trace the footprints of birds in the sky or to catch the clouds with their clenched hands. But something else is operating here as well, because what really pleases this Divine consciousness is the fact that from our side, we have gone beyond desire. Our little entreaties don't touch that level, so the trick is to be truly disinterested, without personal desire. Then you will have a natural connection with the Divine, and because you also have no egocentric desires, the Divine will bless you in return. So the lesson here is: don't trouble the Almighty with your little wants, you can let the *devatas* deal with those. After all, we put the ox to the plough, not the mighty elephant!"[380]

A devotee responds: "Thank you, Maharaj-ji, for this beautiful instruction. But on another, less elevated level, are there changes we normal people can make in our everyday ways of living that will speed our progress towards this sort of enlightened awareness?"

"Food is of great importance", comes the immediate reply. "There can be exceptions, of course. When due to some calamity one's very life is threatened, then you must eat what you have to. There are examples in the Upanishads of sages who were forced by circumstances to eat indiscriminately, but generally speaking one should be very careful about what one eats and drinks".[381]

"A *sadhaka* should avoid such ingredients as salt and mustard, foods that are sour or acidic, or too bitter or dried up. Also any substances that are excessively hot and pungent; also in the beginning you should take more milk and clarified butter. Once you have attained progress these dietary restraints are not so necessary, but while you are on the path, then certainly you must observe them. And take care that the milk and clarified butter are pure, and obtained from good sources and from those people who have good intentions. In fact, impurity of food prevents many from becoming *siddhas*. With impure food, the aspirant cannot meditate well, his mind just runs away and he soon becomes dejected. All because the food was spoiled. But if your food is pure, and you do meditation, then whichever *devata* you meditate on will begin to support your wishes. We see this principle operating in the Vedic fire sacrifice too. The priests chant and meditate on what the patron wishes to be accomplished, but only if their meditations are pure enough will those benefits shower down on him like the nourishing rain".

"You mention meditation. Isn't that the preserve of reclusive types?"

"Oh no, not at all. The Veda approves all the various stations of life, householder and recluse alike, and for all of them meditation is enjoined. All that may differ is the method and the degree of success but as there are degrees in everything, so it must be with this too. Meditation is to be adopted no matter what one's particular life-stage".[382]

Everyone considers the import of the Master's words, reflecting on their own habits.

After a while he continues:

"Also, you should take care with your speech. Manu says we should speak the truth, but only speak the truth that is sweet.[383] This is not saying you should indulge in flattery, but frame your words so they are pleasant to hear. If you speak truly and pleasingly, then your aims will not be met with resistance, and because you are being truthful, some subtle power will come into your speech. But be careful to conserve that power: don't speak too much. That way your words will retain their energy. And above all, continue your spiritual practice, that is the main thing. If you do this, you will certainly meet with success. Our system of Vedanta is not something to prattle about, just keep practising with strong faith. That's all that needs to be done, keep practising sincerely".

Only in retrospect will many of those present realise the timely significance of this succinct summary of the range of the age-old teaching.

Awakening from the dream

It is now late autumn. The Master and his party are staying in a riverside ashram in Haridwar, the ancient pilgrimage town where the sacred Ganges emerges from the Himalayan foothills to begin her stately journey across the flat plains of the north to the great eastern sea. They plan to spend the winter here before beginning their journey back up into the mountains after the snows have melted the following spring.

There is a young man giving public talks each day on the riverside *ghats* after the sunset *puja*. He is a professor of philosophy who has ambitions to become a spiritual teacher. His *guru* was a householder living in the north-west who claimed to have spent time with a saint in the south, a teacher whose reputation and status are considered impeccable throughout the Land of the Veda. Informed by his own teacher that he has attained enlightenment, the young man has set out to spread his radical teaching far and wide. It is creating quite a stir amongst both locals and the many visitors who have arrived in town for the annual Durga Puja celebrations.

One morning he comes to the ashram where the Master is putting up, bringing with him a group of followers. After listening intently to what the master Vedantin has to say in answer to some questions, he begins to explain his own teaching in confident tones to the assembled company.

"As the scriptures tell us, everything is, was, and always will be the Absolute, the one eternal Self. We ourselves are that. Therefore it follows that any attempt to realise the Self by following a path of spiritual discipline, practising meditation and observing all the restraints, is a waste of time and doomed to failure because, as we are already the Self, it follows that we are already enlightened! The individual seeker who considers himself unenlightened has never really existed. This individuality is only a false imagination in the state of ignorance, so anything this deluded individual might do towards realising enlightenment is merely keeping himself in the dream of not being already liberated. All that is necessary is to awaken from the dream".

The Master says nothing.

"So, how can this happen, how do we awaken from the dream?" continues the visitor, taking the lack of comment as an invitation to expound his ideas further. "My *guru* recommended just sitting quietly without effort or striving, and simply asking oneself the question 'Who am I ?' With this enquiry revolving in the mind, when the aspirant is ripe, everything will then happen spontaneously and the dream will be shattered, revealing what has always been the case: we are the Self, already enlightened. Such a realisation can happen anywhere, at any time. Anything else is an unnecessary and tedious complication, a melodrama based on a false premise. This includes all the usual questioning and dilemmas of the spiritual seeker, as well as all the remedies offered by so-called spiritual teachers: meditation, worship, austerities, scriptures – the whole pantomime. All are equally meaningless, because they are all the expression of a point of view – the state of not being enlightened – that does not really exist! They are like questions asked in a dream, which may have appear to have meaning in the context of the dream, but are meaningless once the dreamer has woken up".

He looks expectantly towards the Master, who pauses for some time before replying softly:

"I'm sorry to have to say this, but your position is nonsensical. If anyone is dreaming here, it is you! Theoretically, it may be quite correct to say that the Self is always one and the same, and that therefore there can be no fundamental difference between an ignorant mind and an enlightened mind. But this in no way alters the undeniable and practical fact that one is enlightened and the other is ignorant. Nor does it remove the necessity of the unenlightened taking recourse to scriptures and teachers, and making whatever efforts are necessary to remove his ignorance. From the practical point of view of the man in ignorance, a path must certainly be followed if he is to do away with his confusion. How else will he be able to transcend the tenacious psychic attachment to desire, which is what propels one into passing from one body to another, life after life?[384]

"After all, if just sitting around and asking ourselves who we are was all that is needed, the whole world would have become enlightened long since, would it not? Telling yourself that there is only the one eternal Self and that you are that One, may possibly, if repeated long enough, bring about some temporary mood – a sort of self-hypnosis in the waking state – that may seem to approximate to your idea of enlightenment, but it would be quite delusory and have no lasting value whatsoever. How can you, by a mere act of will, by-pass all the *karmas* that have been accumulated over lifetimes? These *karmas* ripen into egotistic desires and those desires breed actions taken to fulfil them, and then those actions will again create more *karmas*. This whole cycle must be inspected, purified and totally transcended before the mind is clear enough to cognise the Self. Merely asking oneself waking-state questions about one's identity will not touch these unconscious activators, let alone bring about enlightenment". After another pause, the master Vedantin continues:

"I also have to tell you that your attitude is not only injurious to your own spiritual progress, but also highly irresponsible when applied to others who look to you as a teacher. How can you deny the experience of those who come to you? Whether you like it or not, they clearly experience the reality of being unenlightened, otherwise they would not come to you in the first place! For them, what you call 'the dream' is completely real, and merely telling them it is not real will only result in further confusion. As the text says very clearly, this sort of half-baked knowledge is 'like the blind leading the blind', and will soon result in everyone stumbling around not knowing where they are going.[385]

"Rest assured," the Master concludes serenely, "apart from a few very exceptional souls, the way to liberation is clearly laid out: having examined the insufficiencies of worldly life, the seeker should resolve to seek true Knowledge. Being willing to submit himself to the Holy Tradition of teaching, he should humbly approach a realised Master and under his guidance engage in sincere practice, deeply rooted in respect for spiritual authority".[386]

The young visitor sits silently, head down in thought. There is obviously no point in debating further. After some time, his group leaves the *darshan* hall, some of them evidently confused by what has just transpired.

Inequalities

There has been a violent disturbance in the bazaar over the infringement of some caste rule or other. Fighting has broken out, several men are injured, one seriously. The next day the local elders meet in the ashram grounds to discuss the incident and the Master is asked to be there to give his opinion on what should be done.

A social reformer known for his dislike of organised religion attends the meeting. He is evidently agitated, and pushing his way to the front of the gathering begins to question the Master forcibly.

Visitor:

"You are an expert in the scriptures, and the scriptures are always telling us the Supreme Reality is in each and every one of us equally. So how can there be caste distinction? It runs blatantly counter to this highest principle".

Master:

"Why do you drag in the Supreme Reality? He evidently has no complaints. Only those who do have complaints should pursue the matter".

Visitor:

"Well, you are a *mahatma*,[387] so you cannot admit to caste distinction. But I observe it in operation even in your ashram here".

Master:

"Well, it is you who say I am a *mahatma*, not I myself. Likewise, it is you, not I, who is complaining about this caste business".

Visitor:

"*Paramatman*[388] is supposed to be the same in all, isn't it?"

Master:

"Why do you bring in all these names? Let them take care of themselves; they don't need your help!"

The man will not be deterred. He continues:

"Well, what do *you* think of caste distinction?"

Master:

"How does my opinion help you? How will it be of any use to you? Surely it is your opinion that will affect you, not the opinion of others".

Visitor, slightly mollified now:

"Personally, I do not approve of the caste system, but a *mahatma's* opinion is always useful guidance. I want your blessings in the matter".

Master:

"This *mahatma's* opinion is that you direct all your efforts to finding the Self. Your search is what matters here, not my blessings".

Visitor:

"Well, I am on my own path to the Truth as best I can be, but caste distinction is just too painful to me. It must go".

Master:

"To whom, exactly, is it painful?"

Visitor:

"To members of society..."

Master:

"So you say. But we hear there are many other distant lands that have no caste system in operation. Are they free from trouble? They have their wars, their struggles between different groups and tribes, competing families and so on. Why do you not go and remedy the evils over there?"

Visitor:

"But there are the same troubles here, also".

Master:

"Yes, precisely. Differences are always here and there, and so it will always be. Not only amongst human beings, but between animals, plants and so on. This state of affairs cannot be helped".

Visitor:

"Well, let us not bother ourselves with the animals at the moment but focus on the human situation".

Master:

"Why not? I am sure that if the animals could speak they would claim equality with you and dispute your claims no less vigorously than any human being".

Visitor:

"Well, the differences between animals is beyond our control. That is just a natural state of affairs, God's work if you like".

Master:

"Aha! So the differences between animals is God's work, but those between humans is your work? Is that what you are saying?"

Visitor:

"Caste is a man-made distinction".

Master:

"Whether that is the case or not, the thing is, you don't have to notice these distinctions. There is endless diversity in the world, but that is not the whole picture: there is also a unity that runs through this diversity. The Self is the same in all; there is no difference on the level of the spirit. All differences are external and superficial, like the many varied waves of the one ocean. Find that unity and be happy, and then the pain of diversity is remedied. After all, a king may disguise himself as a servant, yet that deceptive covering makes no fundamental difference to the person himself. Rest assured, the correct measure has been given out to everyone, regardless. This cannot be altered".

The visitor thinks for a moment. Then:

"It is not so much the differences I object to; more the claims of superiority which are attached to them".

Master:

"There are differences in the limbs of one's body, yet when the hand touches the foot, the hand does not feel it has been defiled. Each limb performs its own allotted function, yet all work together for the welfare of the body. Why do you object to differences?"

Visitor:

"As I say, people feel the caste system is divisive and unjust. It must be rooted out".

Master:

"You can individually arrive at the state where such distinctions are not perceived and be happy. Anyway, how can you hope to reform the whole world? Attend first to yourself and then see what happens. On a practical level, why continue going to such places where these distinctions are observed and cause yourself pain? Why not seek out those places where they are not observed and be happy there?"

The visitor returns to the subject of inequalities in life; he is evidently not satisfied by the Master's responses. Eventually, the latter responds:

"Look, you want complete equality. Are all the people in the world equally intelligent, equally beautiful, equally pure, equally deserving? Moreover, can they ever be? To say so is to assert that all people have equal *prarabdha* [389] which is demonstrably false. Just look around you if you doubt it; there is no need of lengthy discussion on the matter".

A silence. After a pause, he continues to press the point:

"Or, if you prefer, consider this: can there be two kings in one kingdom, or indeed, one king in two kingdoms? Suppose there were. One of them could not have his way without overriding the will of the other. If the two wanted the same thing, they could not both achieve it; there would be a battle between them to attain the desired object. So the fact of equality here would be the very thing to destroy it! What is more, even if the conflict were to be undeclared, an overt superiority on one side and a hidden superiority on the other are still in opposition, are they not? Even things which may superficially seem the same actually have relative superiorities along with their apparent equality".[390]

The subtlety of the argument is lost on the visitor.

"As I said, we must work to abolish caste distinctions", comes his stubborn reply.

Master:

"Then by all means do so. If you succeed in the world, then come back and see if the distinctions still exist in this place".

The man now becomes aggressive. His face reddening, he indicates the ashram with a sweep of his hand and says in a raised tone:

"This must be the first place where I bring about my reform!"

The Master has had enough.

"Why do you exert yourself so much to bring about reform? If you are really concerned to abolish distinctions, why not just go to sleep? That is the easiest way to obliterate all differences!"

There are many smiles; after a while the man leaves. He is quieter now, but it is clear he is still not fully satisfied by what he has heard.

Later that day when the meeting is over, one of the young *brahmacharis* asks:

"Master, is Self-realisation dependent on the observance of caste rules or, as seekers after the great unity, should we ignore them?"

Master:

"No, do not ignore. Not in the beginning. Observe them to start with, while you are on the path, even if you are a *sannyasi*, who died to caste when he renounced the world. It is all to do with birth and each birth is a seed generated by countless processes operating through an unfathomable stretch of time. Each birth is the sum total of innumerable actions and their results. As Lord Krishna has taught us,[391] we cannot chart the course of this process, but rest assured all is very well set up, so we do not have to concern ourselves with it. It is in the hands of the same almighty power that determines the nature of any seed and its sprouting. Whether it is of a mango or a guava or an orange, whatever seed it is, place it in the soil and it will grow. A mango seed does not yield a guava tree – how could it? All things must follow their nature.

"And anyway, on the practical level, caste rules are useful because they serve to order society by acting as a check on the vagaries of the mind. In this way they are instrumental in its purification, which is what is needed above all. So remember, only those who are mature in *sannyasa*[392] are permitted to ignore the distinctions delineated by caste. And rest assured, there is good reason for all this, because hidden behind everything lies an appropriate order that is invisible to the uncultured eye, the vision of the typical person is just insufficiently refined to see this clearly. After all, if you do not know your very own Self, how can you reliably claim to know anything about the outside world?"

The pull of sex

Question from a young man:

'Why does sex have such a pull? Even if we are not engaging in sexual activity, we are often thinking about it, either remembering or anticipating."

Answer:

"Sex is one area of human activity in which you can forget about the little self and its boundaries. For the time being, at least for the moment, sex allows you to forget your limitations. This freedom from the restrictions of self gives some pleasure, happiness even. But it is as nothing compared to the unbounded bliss that is self-transcendence in the state of freedom."

Maya

Spring has finally come and the Master and a group of followers are travelling by stages upstream towards the great peaks that have towered over the Land of the Veda since the beginning of time, casting their divine energy and blessings down into the plains below and far beyond. From Haridwar they move up into the foothills, an area long-known as 'The Abode of the Gods'.

They reach Deoprayag, a town perched at the confluence of two sacred rivers, the Alakananda and the Bhagirathi, which combine at this spot to form what is known as the Holy Ganges. The little town has a large reputation, for it was here that the great sage Devasharma led his ascetic life and the place is also worshipped as one of the five sacred confluences. Visited by many pilgrims, the whole area bristles with temples and shrines and the Master is keen to spend time here amidst such powerful energy. In Deoprayag he stays for some time in lodgings attached to the great Raghunathji temple where Hanuman-ji, the devoted servant of Lord Rama likes to stay. He also sojourns at the Danda Nagaraja temple, where the Lord of Snakes often appears for his devotees. Other temples he enjoys visiting are those where the Great Goddess in her many forms dwells, particularly her favourite local resting place, the Durga Bhubanshvari temple in a little village upriver called Pundal. Indeed, the sublime atmosphere of the Goddess is very lively all over this part of the country, especially at this time when the hot weather begins to return. Many pilgrims are passing through Deoprayag on their way further north, where they will join the procession that takes the Goddess in her form as Ganga Mataji from her winter home downriver back up to her summer palace, the main Ganga Devi temple in Gangotri, near the source of the holiest of all rivers.

The Master seems to be in a particularly joyous mood over these weeks. By this time, a good number of South Indian *brahmins* have come north to join him, so the party is sizeable. All said, it is an impressive group, composed of intelligent, dedicated, and ritually skilled members, and it moves like a mighty wave of joyous purification through the beautiful countryside. The local maharaja is so impressed by the work of the Master's party that he grants stewardship of several of the local shrines to some of these *brahmins*, whose descendants continue to run them to this day. Temples that had fallen into disuse are re-consecrated and throughout the whole area there is a palpable stirring of religious and spiritual influence that reaches from temple officials to the simple village folk. At this time of year the rivers are full, swollen by snow melt further up the steep valleys. Alakananda Ma is coloured a muddy brown by earth brought down from the higher reaches, while her sister Bhagirathi Ma, who has had a less arduous journey to reach here, is a pristine and sparkling green, translucent in the bright sun. Together they mingle joyously and then flow on as one, sanctifying all they touch.

As evening gives way to night, the Master is sitting with many *pandits* at a spot called Ram Kunda which overlooks the confluence. Here it is said that the sacred footprints of Lord Rama are impressed into the stone, dating from when he visited the area at the time of the Great War. There has been *yajna*, Vedic recitation and *bhajan* chanting for most of the day, along with due worship of nearby images. Now all is quiet except for the sound of the waters below. A brilliant moon is overhead and the still scented atmosphere feels saturated with peace and contentedness.

Someone asks about *maya*.

"Reality is a paradox for the normal mind", begins the Master, "and this is why we have to employ the concept of *maya* if we are to understand it. This *maya* is often misunderstood, because it transcends our common-sense logic which tells us that a thing is either 'this' or 'that' and cannot be both at once. *Maya* – now what is this *maya*?"

A frisson of expectation runs around the group; people sense some important teaching is coming. Gesturing to the river below, the Master continues:

"Now, to understand this question of *maya*, let us consider the moon reflected in the water down there. If you look closely, you will see that the moon is not really immersed in the water, yet nor is it wholly outside of it. We cannot say that the moon is actually in the water, because it is a mere reflection; but on the other hand, we cannot say that it is not there, because, even though a reflection, it manifestly *is* there, right in front of us. Like that, if we are to be strictly accurate, we must say that the world of *maya* is both real and unreal at the same time. It is like a mirage, a divine mirage".

"How can this be, Maharaj?"

"Well, phenomenal appearances are very curious! On the one hand, they exist of course; no one could deny that. But at the same time they have no abiding reality: they are impermanent, utterly evanescent. There is a permanence in life, but that status belongs to the non-dual Being alone, which is unmanifest and hidden, out of sight and beyond sense perception. Because Being is hidden behind the scenes so to say, the ordinary uncultured mind is quite unaware of it, and therefore such a mind falls into the grip of the world and becomes subject to the binding power of creation. What then is the status of this *maya*? We can say it is the transitory dimension of life, superimposed upon the Divine which in itself lies forever beyond all time, space and causation. As human beings, our noble destiny is first and foremost to transcend the insufficiencies of the ever-changing realm of *maya,* and thereby live our natural inborn identity with that Divine directly. Only then shall we avoid undue entanglement in the superimpositions that obscure it. And it is only by being free of this entanglement that we shall be able to understand and enjoy the world of variety aright, which is to recognise it as the Divine made manifest".

Possessions

A wealthy merchant addresses the young sage directly.

"It seems to me, Sir, that our lives are almost exact opposites. You are still young and yet, having already renounced the world, have clearly found the eternal peace that the sacred texts tell us about. I, on the other hand am now quite advanced in years, and having devoted my life to accumulation, am very well-off and respected in society because of it. But in truth, I feel as if I am imprisoned by my possessions, weighed down by all I have worked so hard to surround myself with. And all my wealth has not given me peace".

The Master nods sympathetically.

"Yes, your intuition is correct; one must also be careful, as any degree of wealth can become a conduit of negative energies. The family lives in peace and harmony unless and until the ancestral land comes to be divided. Even dogs lick each other and sleep side by side happily until a scrap of food gets tossed amongst them...but then, watch out!

"In fact, the problem is not with possessions – after all, they are just things that have their own existence apart from us, are they not? The problem lies with our attitude to possessions, the extent to which we are attached to them. So the problem is with the mind, not the thing itself. With a strong mind, it is perfectly possible for even the most active householder to be surrounded by possessions, and yet remain free of their binding influence. All he has to do is remember that the world is not under our control anyway, but belongs to the Lord, who is more than capable of managing everything.[393] So we should just leave it up to Him! All we have to do from our side is behave as best we can and perform such life-supporting actions as are in accord with the scriptures. This way one can certainly live a long and fruitful life".

Then, after a thoughtful pause:

"Still, when all is said and done, the fact remains that most people find it very difficult to maintain such an attitude of non-attachment in the midst of their worldly lives. That is why the ancient Way recommends renunciation for all who can aspire to it. Those who take the vow of renunciation do so to devote themselves wholeheartedly to Self-realisation, and when they reach spiritual maturity, they rest forever in the contentment of the Self, free of desires".

"And how are they free of desires? Can the Self really be that satisfying?"

"Yes, it is the supreme bliss; in truth, only he who revels in *brahman* is truly happy. As *brahman* is wholly immaterial, it may seem strange to say such a thing, but do not forget that we can only desire what we think is separate from us. When we have realised the Self as our own essential nature and know directly that it is also omnipresent, we have the best of both worlds: possessing nothing, we own everything".[394]

Religion and spirituality

The old Shiva temple is built in the style found all over the mountains. Set on a rocky plateau overlooking the serpentine twists and turns of the Alakananda, it has a squat conical tower of grey granite rising over a rectangular chamber that houses the *yoni-lingam*.[395] Fronting the shrine is an assembly hall with intricately carved and painted pillars and a pitched roof made of rough slate tiles. From the top of the tower a white flag flutters, announcing to all that the deity is in residence and happy to be visited.

It is high summer now, and all around the temple plateau wild flowers and small sturdy bushes spike the rough pastures. For most of the year these meadows are dry and stony, but in recent days they have become almost a continuous marshland, due to the many gurgling streams that tumble and rush down through them, fed by the snow-melt from higher up the mountains. But despite the bright sunshine and sprinkled colour carpeting the fields, the energies of nature feel very raw up here, and the place has a wild, almost forbidding atmosphere. There are no trees, for this is well above the tree-line and rising up far behind the temple can be seen the distant lofty peaks of the high Himalaya glowing a hard, vivid white against the clear blue sky. In a month or two the long cold winter will begin and snow will once again cut the temple off from the outside world for six long months or more.

The local raja has arranged a *yajna*. A large fire-pit is constructed in the centre of the hall. Flags and streamers made of coloured cloth are hung from the pillars while the images of the gods, piled high with red and orange flowers, silently observe the preparations. All in all, the simple place has an air of unaffected festivity. Several *pandits* and dignitaries have come up by mule from the little town below and with them a group of pious locals. The Master and his disciples have also been invited to add their blessings to the proceedings.

The fire-ceremony lasted for several hours, then Ganges water was offered in the ritual lustration, and finally came the customary feast and presentation of gifts – shawls, food and money – to the officiants. And now, as half-burnt logs smoke lazily in the pit, people are sitting around in an atmosphere of relaxed contentment. Desultory questions are put to the Master. One comes from a small elderly woman with grey hair, who wears the belted tunic and bright striped apron typical of a married Tibetan. The tunic is a faded madder colour, but spotless and immaculately pressed. Though the woman's face is deeply lined from years of toil in harsh mountain conditions, her eyes are bright and she wears an expression of calm dignity. Despite her years, her voice is steady and clear.

"Maharaj-ji", she begins, "I have long been wondering about the difference between religion and spirituality. Are they one and the same or are they different things? I would be most grateful if you could shed some light on this".

Gesturing around the assembly hall, the master Vedantin answers:

"See, Ma, it is like this temple. This beautiful *mandapa*[396] where we are sitting is like religion: a nourishing and social place where the community gathers to enjoy devotional music and *bhajans*, worship, rituals and ceremonies, as well as marriages and spiritual instruction from our sacred texts such as the Gita, Puranas and Ramayana. And everything that goes on here is watched over by the gods, who look down from on high and bless the proceedings. But when you want to penetrate to the heart of the place, you have to pass through the *mandapa* and enter the *garbha griha* itself.[397] Here there is nothing of the outer, just a small, un-adorned chamber where you are quite on your own. It is only there in that uncluttered inner space that you come face-to-face with the Divine.

"Like that, the spiritual life means leaving behind all the outer trappings of life and society and taking a solitary journey deep into the silent and naked depths of your own being. It is only there that you will meet the ultimate reality. And why should this be so?"

He pauses a moment to let the point sink in:

"Because that ultimate reality you are seeking is nothing but your own inmost Self".

Techniques of devotion

Question:

"Master, what is the way of devotion for one who for some reason cannot always be in the company of his gurudev?"

Answer:

"Such a devotee should meditate whenever, and for as long as, he feels impelled to. As to his meditation, he should form in his mind a vivid image of his guru, the expression of his face and particularly of his eyes. This way, after some time, his guru's physical presence will be there with him".

Question:

"When should he do this meditation?"

Answer:

"As I say, whenever he has the natural inclination. And at special times as well, such as before coming to any important decision or when confronted by some difficult situation. Because the realised guru is unshakeably united with the Absolute that is the Self of the world, remembering him in this way will have the effect of bringing the devotee to that Self, which is the fullest expression of his own powers. By this means, the appropriate answer for his predicament will be there spontaneously. In addition, this practice has the benefit of regulating the devotee's behaviour, so that he will be saved from doing anything which he would not have done in his guru's presence".

Question:

"How much then should the devotee practice this dwelling on the guru's physical presence as you advise, Sir?"

Answer:

"As much as he can! Every second spent in this way will be good for him. So, he should practice as long as his eyes can stand the sight, and he'll get great benefit from it, no doubt at all".

After a pause:

"One more thing. He should remember his guru's voice, and his laughter also".

The real cure for illness

A gathering of eminent Vaidyas has been convened and the Master invited to bless the proceedings. After several of the medical authorities have had their say, the organiser of the event, an elderly *brahmin* much respected in the locality, turns to the young *sannyasi*:

"Maharaj-ji, you have heard our prescriptions for living a balanced life and enjoying good health, well-being and longevity. Do you have anything to add from your side on the matter?"

"As *Vaidyavidyavarenyas*, the sons of Dhanvantari, you are all the representatives of a noble and ancient tradition", begins the Master.[398]

"However, my approach is from a different angle. The holy tradition of Vedanta that I represent sees all humankind, both those the world calls 'healthy' and those it calls 'unhealthy', to be suffering from the same universal and debilitating disease. And what is this? The repeated birth and death into a life of attachment to the body. Fortunately, Vedanta does not stop with merely diagnosing the malady, but presents both the medicine and the correct diet to be followed to ensure this illness does not return".

Several of those present look rather nonplussed; the discussion is taking a radical turn that they were not expecting. For whatever reason, the young sage is in an uncompromising mood today. He continues with great force:

"What is this wonderful medicine that brings peace and happiness in the ups and downs of daily life and also secures release from repeated births? Surrender to the Lord and behaving in a spirit of service to Him. And the diet that goes along with this medicine is to undertake actions in accordance with one's nature, and to perform all the duties stipulated in the scriptures in a righteous and proper manner. Mark well, both these are necessary. If the medicine is taken but the accompanying diet is not followed, no lasting benefit will be obtained".

"But surely Master, only a few people can undertake such a discipline?"

"That may be, but without resorting to this Vedantic remedy, beings will inevitably fall into the same old trap of egotistic attachment, and from this will stem all manner of woes: the lust for power, arrogance, pride, and all the rest of it. Some rich and haughty people may perform religious rites and think that doing so is enough to save them, but such insincere activity is meaningless and amounts to mere hypocrisy. Everywhere people are driven by the craving to acquire wealth and amass things for themselves, and they rejoice in their own might and their material happiness. But in fact, to act in this way is to display hatred for the divine non-dual principle which dwells both in ourselves and in all creation. And as a result of ignoring this supreme principle, we have created a hell on earth, characterised by envy, disdain for those who are treading the right path, all the cruelty and malice readily observable everywhere. The typical human being has become a demonic creature".

The company is visibly shocked by this stark analysis.

"What is to be done, Swami-ji?" asks the senior *brahmin.*

"Well, the basis of this soul-destroying state is the typical person's subjection to passion, anger and greed. So if we are truly concerned with a heathy life, my friends, then nothing less than renunciation of these three negative attributes is needed".

"Are you saying that our regimes of Ayurveda serve no purpose then?"

"No, I am not saying that, good Sir, but one thing is certain: we shall all have to leave this world sooner or later, so we should not spend all our time and energies trying to shore up the rickety building of this life. As I say, the most useful prescription for all our ills is: perform the righteous tasks of which you are capable, so that your mind does not become tarnished, and pass your time in dedication to the Lord".

"What can help us do this?"

"The role of scripture is essential here. Without such guidance, you cannot maintain purity in your practical life, with the result that whatever you may do to worship the Lord will not bear real fruit. It's just like taking the medicine, but ignoring the proper diet. The Vedas and the Shastras have laid out very clearly what to do and what not to do; all we need is to follow their injunctions. Without this, if we just rely on the whims and fancies of the unpurified mind, there will be no happiness in this world, let alone fitness for liberation and the attainment of the supreme goal of life".

"And what is that goal, Swami-ji?"

"Realisation of the One, the bodiless in all bodies".[399]

The vendor of shawls

Three brothers from the adjacent valley have come for *darshan*. They sell woollen shawls and high-quality cloth made from a number of looms they own, which are distributed around several villages in their home region. The men will take the finished articles down to the big cities in the plains and go from door to door in the wealthiest areas to sell them. Given all the travelling, it is hard work, but profitable. The two younger brothers are energetic worldly men with plans to expand the business, but the eldest has a more settled and thoughtful disposition. Long interested in spirituality, he is especially close to one of his cousins who is a Buddhist monk based in a monastery nearby and the two of them often enjoy philosophical discussions.

The Master has been speaking in glowing terms about the omnipresence of *brahman*, the absolute Reality, emphasising that nothing whatsoever can be excluded from this essential Being. For his part, however, the shawl merchant finds no evidence of such an Absolute; he sees only the world of change around him, and so prefers the view of the Buddhists.

"Swami-ji, I have heard many times from Buddhist teachers that the world is held together by cause and effect. I believe you teach the same?"

"I do indeed, but not only that! The world is only half the story, after all. Therefore I also agree with the Upanishadic texts that celebrate the omnipresence of *brahman* as unlimited Consciousness".

"This the Buddhists deny. I have to agree with them, Sir, as I cannot see any connection between the observable truth of causality operating in the world and this abstract idea of some ultimate Consciousness behind the scenes".

"Well, let us first examine what is in front of our eyes: this question of causality. If you examine the mechanics of the affair, you will allow that nothing that is not already pre-existing in its cause could come into existence in the first place? How could it? Where would it come from, and what would the means of its manifestation?"

Receiving no answer, he continues:

"This being so, it is clearly the fact that an effect exists in latent form before its actual appearance. By the same token, all effects, however varied they may be, are non-different from their causes".

The man looks unsure, but still says nothing.

"And this being so in the world of particulars, it must also be the case for the world itself when taken as a whole. In all its infinite variety, the world emerges as the effect of its cause and nor is it different from it. You see the drift?"

The man nods, aware that he has taken on a penetrating intellect.

"So, we are now led to the question: what then is the cause of the world? The Buddhists have no answer on this point, because they deny any transcendental realm, but our tradition teaches that the cause of the manifest world is the unmanifested and absolute Consciousness. Moreover, as we have just seen, the world cannot rightly be considered as different from that Consciousness, because it conforms to the law that nothing is separable from its cause. Just so, the ever-changing world is the effect of that Consciousness which alone persists, forever unchanged".

The man counters:

"I see your logic, Swami-ji, which is faultless, but if we cannot actually locate this Absolute, how can really we say it exists?"

"Well, just because a cause is imperceptible to our senses does not mean it does not exist. Look at what happens when you are doing business. You go from door to door, with your shawls rolled up under your arm, don't you?"

The man nods, wondering what on earth this has to do with metaphysics.

"Then, someone opens the door, but he does not recognise what it is under your arm. It is only when the shawl is rolled out that its real nature is recognised and all its details become obvious. Like that, the unrolled cloth is the observable effect and the same cloth, when rolled up, is its hidden cause. In fact there is no real difference, they are one and the same, are they not? Moreover, even if the roll under your arm *is* recognised to be a shawl – let's say this client has sharper eyes than most, or perhaps he remembers you from before – nevertheless all the particulars - its shape, size, colour, pattern and texture - become clear only when it is unrolled.

"Indeed", the Master is clearly enjoying playing with the analogy now, "we can take this further! The cloth was itself unmanifest for as long as it remained latent in its own cause, which is the wool or yarn. It only became known distinctly when the activity of various causal agents – the shuttle, the loom, the weavers and so on – combined together to produce the woven material. Once this has happened, the effect is clearly present. Like that, everything in this world is an effect of, and therefore not different from, its unmanifest cause, which is *brahman*, the Absolute ".[400]

Someone else then asks:

"Does this unity of cause and effect operate in the law of *karma* also?"

"Of course, how could it not? In fact, it is the very essence of *karma*. Actions and their consequences are inseparable, because as we have just seen, effects are not different from their causes. And this is so even if long periods of time separate the two, which may happen, because for the effect to manifest there must always be the appropriate circumstance, the right conditions".

"How can this be, Sir?"

"Well, let us go back to our friend here and his shawls", replies the Master, smiling kindly at the dealer. "His cloth will only be unrolled when the appropriate situation is present: the door is open, there is a potential customer standing there, he is prepared to hear all about the shawl and so on. But if the man closes the door in our friend's face, because he has no interest in buying, then at that time no opportunity to sell exists, and so the cloth will not be unrolled. In such a case the process of manifestation will have to wait for another house, another door, another day!"

There is general laughter. For those who asked no questions, but only listened to the discussion, whatever unvoiced questions they may have had evaporate.

Desire, attachment and rebirth

A monk asks:

"What is the motivation for rebirth?"

"Desire, the tenacious mechanism of desire".

"How is this, Master?"

"Well, what is a desire? It is the awareness of a lack. Desire is wanting something we do not presently have, is it not? We feel we would like to have this thing, because having it would benefit us in some way, make our life better, more enjoyable. So, a desire arises somewhere deep in the mind, a faint impulse of feeling or thought that becomes more concrete, more manifest, as it moves into conscious awareness. The initial impulse becomes a faint longing and, if unchecked, takes a more definite shape and becomes a resolve, a determination. Then the senses take over, and the determination then motivates an action that seeks to employ whatever means are appropriate to yield the desired result. Now, the result of the action taken may or may not be what was originally envisaged, but the consequence will be there nevertheless, whatever it may be. This is how the mind works, and as our mind builds our life, this is how we live, day to day, year by year. You see the process clearly?"

The questioner nods.

"Now, what is crucial here is the fact that we are attached to the outcome of our desiring. We are not neutral towards the result of a desire; we want it to materialise in the expected manner, and we want to enjoy the fruit. And the stronger the desire, the more we want it to be realised, and the more upset and angry we become if that desire is somehow frustrated. You can see from your own experience how desire and attachment are intimately linked in the normal man, the usual mind?

"It is in this way that the self who desires becomes falsely attached to the body and the organs and the desires they generate, but by the same token, even when the desire is somehow appeased, and the mind becomes serene and peaceful, the self is still attached, because it becomes identified with this absence of desire. In other words, whether we are considering righteousness or unrighteousness, anger or lack of anger, this or that, the obvious or the hidden – the limited self becomes attached to everything it experiences".

"I don't understand how righteousness can be a source of attachment".

"Because even righteousness is attendant on desire, in that it is a benign state springing up from desire's being absent. And so this habitual way of functioning, whether towards good or evil acts, creates attachment: as the mind does and acts, so it becomes".

After a time of silence, as those present consider what has been said, he continues:

"And it is just this attachment that is the mechanism for transmigration and the passing from one life to another, time after time".

"What exactly is it that transmigrates, then?"

"The subtle body, or we can say the mind, which is anyway the principle aspect of the subtle body. Either way, the limited individual self is what is signified here. So, in short, it is our good and bad deeds that are the cause of our reincarnating, and the more attached we are to them, the stronger is the link. You will remember that beautiful verse in the scriptures on this topic:

'Whoever longs for the objects of desire and makes much of them is carried by those same desires to places in which he will be able to realise them'.[401]

"Now, if on the other hand, actions are undertaken without desire, without any attachment, then such actions do not lead to the accumulation of karmic merit or its opposite. Without attachment to desire, there is no identification with it, or with its fruits or with the disappointment that comes when the fruit is not forthcoming. In every case, without such attachment there is no such identification, and therefore there is no rebirth".

The monk speaks up again.

"What you say makes sense to me, Sir, but, on the other hand, we know that desires are without end. So how then can a man become desireless and so avoid the endless process of reincarnation?"

The Master is delighted that the young man has grasped the drift of the conversation and come up with the important question.

"This is a beautiful question! As we have just seen, only the person who is free from desire does not reincarnate. Desires and their binding power have deserted him. And why have they left? Because their objects have been attained!"

Bemusement.

"How can this be?" laughs the Master, rocking gently from side to side.

"Let us follow this carefully now, for this is the nub of the matter. The man who is without desire is he who has recognised both that all the possible objects of desire are nothing but the omnipresent Self, and also that he himself is that same omnipresent One. Being itself omnipresent, spread evenly everywhere, there is nothing outside of the Self left to be attained. It is pure intelligence, infinite, homogenous, and without parts, so when everything is recognised to be the Self, what is there left over to be desired? What could such a sage see, or hear, or think of, or know that is *not* the Self? So, with Self-realisation all possible objects of desire have already been obtained, because the Self, their essence, has itself already been attained. Such a man is without and beyond desire; for him all sense of want has dissolved and thereby he attains complete and utter liberation, impeccable".[402]

An overbearing official

Generally, the Master is very courteous and attentive to all who come to him, answering their various questions with great patience and in appropriate terms, whether simple and down-to-earth or erudite and abstract. But there are times when he is clearly immersed in his own mood of bliss and seems not to care what those who are present make of it. The higher he and his entourage travel up into the vastness of the Himalaya, the more frequent such times become.

One day while on the pilgrimage to Lord Badri's place,[403] the Master is sitting quietly by the roadside resting. A brash official rides up. Used to exercising his authority over the local people, he accosts the young *sannyasi* imperiously.

"You there! I suppose you are one of those monks that spend their time roaming around the country here and there. Well, I can see from your appearance that you are not from this area, so what is your native place? Where are you stationed now?"

"I dwell alone in the temple of emptiness".

Not understanding the answer, the official replies:

"And where is that, pray?"

"Everywhere", comes the unruffled reply.

Realising the Truth

"How can I realise the Truth?"
   "You cannot realise the truth".
   "How so?"
   "Because the 'I' cannot realise the Truth".
   "Why not?"
   "Because in Truth, there is no 'you' and no 'I'".

Spending time with Lord Badri

After perhaps an hour's climb, the party has reached a high plateau open to the enormous expanse of sky. The place is enveloped in an awesome atmosphere, and one can feel the elemental power of the forces that reign here. Above the plateau towers the outline of Mount Narayana, while just below, the river tumbles and bounces down, a frothing torrent bursting with the energy of its source, which is not far above. Next to the river a natural sulphur spring rises and the large pools it feeds form a purifying bathing place much used by locals and the pilgrims who come to visit. The main focus of attention here is a small temple located at the edge of the plateau, a brightly painted shrine dedicated to Lord Badri, one of the forms of Vishnu. After they have visited the shrine, visitors will continue past the little village and up the mountainside to pay homage to the footprints he left imprinted in an ancient slab of rock when he first visited here so long ago. Altogether it is a magical place.

But there is one thing missing. On entering the shrine, the Master is distressed to observe that instead of a proper image, in bodily form adorned with all the appropriate regalia, the priests are worshipping a sanctified *shalagrama* stone.[404] Enquiring why there is no worthy form of the Lord, he learns that when iconoclastic invaders from across the border cast their ominous shadow on this holy spot, the distressed priests hid the sacred idol by submerging it in the river below. But since then, despite repeated searches, no-one has been able to locate it. One problem is the strong currents and whirlpools in that part of the river. After many unsuccessful efforts, the priests have gloomily concluded that for whatever reason, the Lord has withdrawn his favour and there is nothing to be done. As a second best, the *shalagrama* has been substituted; no one is happy about the situation.

It is said that after a long time engrossed in thought, the Master hurried down to the river, and jumped in. A long time elapsed; everyone was worried. Then eventually he reappeared, bearing the sacred image on his shoulders. With great ceremony and all the necessary prescribed ritual, it was re-established in the sanctum sanctorum. The part of the river from where the image was retrieved, known as Narad Kund, is still worshipped by devotees today.

The local raja, overjoyed at the return of Lord Badri, has received the Master and his companions with great hospitality, taking great care personally to see to their accommodation and well-being. After a couple of days he asks what more he can do for them.

"Expand the existing shrine and endow this place with a really fine temple", says the Master, "Such a noble guest as Lord Badri needs a suitable palace to make him feel comfortable and ensure he deigns to stay here with you. If you do that, I myself will guarantee the succession of well-trained priests to look after it".

The raja agrees; work is begun immediately. And so the magnificent Badrinath Temple is built, and, to this day, it is looked after by Nambudiri priests from Kerala, ritual experts born into the Master's own caste and native place.

The founding of Jyotir Math

Some hours back down the road from Lord Badri's place, the Master finds a spot he likes particularly, and the party spends some time there. The view ranges right across the valley to the distant mountain peaks, and the sage is particularly taken with a venerable mulberry tree there, under which he sits for many hours each day. One day as he is stationed there giving *darshan*, a pilgrim on the way up to the Badri shrine asks him about the nature of *brahman*, the ultimate non-dual reality.

"The absolute *brahman* is self-luminous, and pervades the entire universe both outwardly and inwardly. This Consciousness is other than the universe, yet there exists nothing that is not within its embrace. Everything that is perceived, everything that is heard, everything without exception is nothing but *brahman*. One who rises to the knowledge of Reality sees the entire universe as the non-dual *brahman*, which is always and everywhere pure being, consciousness and bliss".[405]

Everyone present is thrilled by the simple power and clarity of this exposition. Suddenly the Master announces that this very spot would be the ideal spot for a monastery to preserve and disseminate Vedic knowledge throughout the north of the Land of the Veda. He appoints his beloved disciple, the devotional and innocent Totakacharya to be the first Shankaracharya in charge of the institution and entrusts it with the particular responsibility of safeguarding the Atharva Veda. As this text contains the recondite science of sacred sound and the knowledge of the *mantras*, it is well suited to the remote purity of these mountainous regions. Two orders of monks are to be assigned the place: the *Giri:* 'those who dwell on a hill' and the *Parvata:* 'those who dwell in the mountains'. In addition, the preceptor presiding over the institution will also be venerated as the *Rajaguru*, the most senior of the special *dandi swamis* and the pontiff with ultimate responsibility for all the orders of the 'Renunciates of the Ten Names'.

The monastery, known as Jyotir Math, 'The Monastery of Light' – or Joshimath in the local dialect – still continues its work today as the seat of the northern Shankaracharya whose responsibility now, as then, is to act as the custodian and lighthouse of Vedic knowledge.

Signs

It has been a hot day, very humid. The Master and a large crowd of followers, numbering perhaps two hundred, have climbed high above the site of the ashram, and are seated on a plateau there. As there are visiting *pandits* present, the discussion turns to an erudite Sanskrit text. At one point a passage is read out: *"If it is true that this is a Yogi, a blissful Knower, then the heavens will give a sign"*.

Some present are wondering about such a sign when, suddenly, a stormy wind blows up, as if out of nowhere, tearing at the hair and clothes of those present. Strangely, the Master, who is sitting on his usual deer skin in the midst of the group, remains quite untouched. Then lightning and thunder set in, and rain can be seen pouring down all around. However, the little plateau where the group is gathered remains dry, somehow quite protected from the storm. And then, high above, a piece of bright blue sky is clearly visible through a small round hole in the clouds.

For perhaps half an hour everyone stays seated, listening to the words of the Master. Then, with the group deeply moved by the enormity of what he has revealed to them, he gives the signal for a return to the ashram. As soon as he is seated in the palanquin, and the party begins to descend the hill, the rain finally reaches the plateau. Before long the area is flooded. One hour later a brilliant, ethereal glow envelopes the whole landscape.

Universal peace

A man arrives at the ashram who has worked many years at the court of the local maharaja.

Visitor:

"I have spent my life serving His Majesty. When I began my service as a young man, there were wars in various parts of the kingdom. Now, twenty-five years later, I am a grandfather, and there are still wars going on here, there, and everywhere. Will there ever be universal peace? "

The Master:

"The world is within you. If you are at peace within, if your awareness is established in the real Self, your world is in peace. And if you are wavering and peaceless, and you are not in tune with your own eternal state of Being, then the world around you is also without peace".

The essence of the Veda

Someone comments:

"Master, the Vedas are so complex, and they require a lifetime of study to even begin to understand. Life is so short, time is so limited.

Is there any way we can know their essence, their final import? What is that?"

"The Veda declares that the Absolute is the highest Truth and this entire universe is nothing but the Absolute alone – here, there, above, below, inside and out. Any other ideas about it are just ignorance, like mistaking a length of rope lying on the path for a snake. That is the essential meaning of the Veda and that is all you need to realise. Do that and the job is done".[406]

"And yet you have taught that the world is unreal?"

"The world is that which comes and goes, insubstantial, while the Absolute is unmoving, unshakeable, infinite Being. Together they make up one totality, which we call *brahman*. Taken by itself, the evanescent world of perishable phenomena could never stand on its own feet. In itself, what is it? A pitiable realm of insufficiency! This is why our teaching is clear: the world has no reality when considered apart from its essence, which is the Absolute".

The importance of the guru

Question:

"Some say we can achieve enlightenment through our own efforts, or by relying on our own intuition. Others assert that a *guru* is necessary. What is your opinion?"

Answer:

"The Self-realised *guru* is not only necessary, he is indispensable. Such a one is by nature magnanimous and merciful. Freed from re-birth, he is like the moon that saves the earth from being scorched by the heat of the sun or ..." here the Master pauses a moment, "he is like the Springtime that brings fresh life and energy and joy to all. And he does this spontaneously – unobserved, unasked and unsought. Truly, such a *guru* is your best friend, because he is motivated only by compassion for your suffering".[407]

"How then is our suffering destroyed?"

"Through approaching a realised sage in the correct manner, which means with sincerity, humility and the desire to serve".

"Can you give us some idea of his state of consciousness?"

"Such a one is at peace. He is like a fire that has consumed its fuel, and he is like an ocean filled to the brim with compassion. He is a friend to all, learned in the texts and possessed of spiritual insight. He does not labour under the erroneous feeling of being an active agent confined to a limited body, but experiences himself as being unborn, immortal, beyond danger and fear. Such a one is omnipresent".[408]

"And what is it that gives such a sage this extraordinary status?"

"The fact that he has realised his unfailing identity with the Absolute. He has consciously become what he really is, always was, and always will be: the Totality, *brahman*. As such, he is freed from duality, a unique and lovingly compassionate figure, transparent to the Divine. And therefore he naturally acts as the Divine in this world; his actions carry out the will of the Divine on earth. Make no mistake, in our Vedic knowledge the importance of the true *guru* is supreme". [409]

"Can you say more about the relationship between the disciple and the guru, Sir?"

"It is an entirely natural affair. The great *guru* is like the turtle, who protects her eggs from a distance without being near them. He does not need to stay always close, like the fish or the bird when they look after their young. Such a *guru* helps, protects and guides his sincere disciple by observing his behaviour from afar, just keeping a watchful eye on him. This gives the disciple room to grow and develop as he must, and from his side it is never a question of trying to mimic the *guru's* behaviour. If the disciple follows his teacher's instructions to the letter, the blessings will naturally flow from the greater to the lesser, and this way the disciple will shine in the world. So, each and every disciple should worship his *guru*".

"Given what you say, surely everything can just be left to the grace of such a *guru*?"

"Oh no! Personal effort is also indispensable. The *guru's* grace may sometimes appear to be doing the work, but in such a rare case the seeker must already have put in tremendous effort in order to deserve that grace. No one can simply enlighten another. Sons and others may be able to absolve a man from the debts he has incurred, but we are not talking about mere material things here, we are talking about a complete transformation of consciousness. Others can remove a load you are carrying on your head, but not the pain that carrying it around for so long has caused. For that, you yourself have to take healing herbs and eat nourishing food and so on. Similarly, if you want to see the moon clearly, you must use your own eyes, there is no use in hiring some scholar to do it for you!"

"How should the seeker's effort be directed then? There seem to be so many paths and different ways to achieve the goal ..."

"Actually, there is only one way. Neither yoga, nor philosophising, nor religious rituals will do the trick. Only one thing is really useful here – and that is awakening consciously to your own identity with the Absolute. The glory of the *guru* is that he is your path to that supreme awakening".

The death of the Master

Most people believe that the Master left the body at the temple he revived in Kedarnath, up in the high Himalaya. There is today a simple shrine there to mark the spot.[410] Others say he died in the precincts of the famous Vadakkunnathan Temple in Vrishachala,[411] perhaps a hundred miles from where he was born. This accounts for the four ancient monasteries situated nearby that temple, believed by those who follow this version of the story to have been founded by his four closest disciples after his death. Yet others claim he left this earth at Kanchipuram in Tamil Nadu, at the Kamakoti Peetham monastery he had founded there many years previously, and which still stands today as a spiritual lighthouse for all of South India and beyond.

But those who follow the spirit rather than the letter of the Master's teaching, say that what matters is not so much his death, but his life. And what matters even more than his short life is the Truth that he lived and taught so impeccably: the ever-abiding fact of non-duality.

NOTES TO THE INTRODUCTION

[a] These are Kedarnath in the Himalayan state of Uttarakhand and Kanchipuram in the southern state of Tamil Nadu.

[b] The five principal Shankara monasteries (*maths*) are:

Shringeri Sharada Peeth in Chickmagalur, Karnataka (regulating the centre of India);

Jyotir Math near Badrinath, Uttarakhand (regulating the north);

Kanchi Kamakoti Peetham in Kanchipuram, Tamil Nadu (regulating the south);

Govardhan Math in Jagannath Puri, Odisha (regulating the east) and

Sharadapeeth in Dwarka, Gujarat (regulating the west).

Taken together, these 'centres of knowledge' (*vidyapiths*) trace a five-pointed mandala of sacred energy that operates through the four cardinal points and the centre to unite, charge and sanctify the Land of the Veda. While both texts and tradition refer to Shankara's founding other major *maths* and their many satellite institutions, these five are considered the most important. The three holding records of a lineage going back twenty-five hundred years are the ones at Dwarka, Puri and Kanchipuram.

Alongside their sanctity and age, the great *maths* are also human institutions and so not exempt from human follies. Since their founding they have witnessed various intrigues, mainly disputes over the rightful succession of a Shankaracharya (i.e. the presiding abbot) that arise when the retiring pontiff has not appointed a clear and willing successor. Such disputes continue up to today, sometimes resulting in lengthy court battles. In addition, it is becoming increasingly difficult for a Shankaracharya to remain aloof from the political trends that are sweeping a country which likes to refer to itself as 'the world's greatest democracy'.

It should also be mentioned here that the foundation of the Kanchipuram *math* by Shankara himself has long been disputed by the other four, which are collectively known as the *amnaya peeths*. Whatever the rights or wrongs of such an argument, the fact remains that the southern seat produced in its 68th pontiff a saint who has had an extraordinarily profound influence on South India and far beyond in recent times. The life and teachings of Swami Chandrashekharananda Saraswati (1894 – 1994), known throughout the world as The Sage of Kanchi, are widely acknowledged to be an impeccable example of the wisdom of *advaita*. A highly accessible and well-illustrated collection of his discourses is: *An Introduction to Hindu Dharma* published by World Wisdom Books, USA.

[c] The head of each of the five principal monasteries is given the title Jagadguru Shankaracharya, which translates as 'Guru of the World and Teacher of Shankara's Wisdom of Liberation'. Adi Shankara is thus an abbreviation of the formal title Adi Shankaracharya i.e. 'the first or original (*adi*) Shankaracharya'.

[d] This is the Shringeri *math*.

[e] Commentary on the Brahma Sutra 1.3.33.

[f] Madhava Vidyaranya was the 12th Jagadguru of the Shringeri Sharada Peetham, reigning from 1380-1386. In response to the devastation caused by the Islamic Sultanate of Delhi, he inspired the re-creation of the Vijayanagara Empire of South India and served for a time as its prime minister. His writings on *advaita* helped re-establish Shankara's message as a rallying symbol of orthodox Hindu values at a time of great social and political instability.

[g] A further confusion here is caused by the fact it was not an uncommon practice for scriptural commentators to append their teacher's name to their own work if they felt it accurately reflected his views without distortion.

[h] There are a number of books on this perennial teaching. See for example: *The Perennial Philosophy* by Aldous Huxley; *The Common Experience* by Jack Cohen and John-Francis Phipps; *Mysticism* by F.C. Happold; *Ecstasy: a Study of Some Secular and Religious Experiences* by Marghanita Laski and *Coming Home* by Lex Hixon. An excellent recent study is *The Supreme Awakening* by Craig Pearson.

[i] The five sites of the Shankaracharya monasteries (*see note b above*) are pilgrim centres in their own right because major Hindu temples of historical importance are attached to them or nearby. Thus at Badrinath in the north, where one tradition has Shankara leaving his body, and at Puri in the east with its revered Jagannatha temple dedicated to a form of Lord Krishna, pilgrims gather in huge numbers. Dwaraka in the west is one of the seven sacred cities of Hinduism, believed to be the ancient capital where Lord Krishna lived and ruled. Kanchi in the south is another town with ancient associations, this time with venerable Buddhist, Jain and Hindu monastic institutions while Shringeri, occupying the centre of the *mandala*, also enjoys considerable popular sanctity thanks to its temple, founded by Shankara himself, which is dedicated to the goddess Sharada. (*See also note 303 below*).

[j] Commentary on the Brahma Sutra 1.1.4.

[k] Commentary on the Chandogya Upanishad 8.1.1.

[l] 'The Last Awakening' by John Donne

NOTES TO THE TEXT

Part One: The Boy

[1] The Sabhanayaka temple at Chidambaram, dedicated to Shiva Nataraja, Lord of the Cosmic Dance.

[2] Modern Trichur, the cultural capital of Kerala state.

[3] The great Guruvayurappan temple, dedicated to Krishna.

[4] Shani: the planet Saturn; often a malefic or troublesome planet in Vedic astrology.

[5] Indra: the King of the Gods.

[6] cf the South Indian saying: 'Kings, children, pregnant women, deities and gurus should never be visited empty-handed'

[7] Indra urges the life of the road upon a young man named Rohita in a passage from the Aitreya Brahmana.

[8] *Brahmachari*: 'student'; literally, 'one who moves in *brahman*'. The first of the four stages of an orthodox *brahmin's* life, followed by the stage of 'householder' (*grihasta*); 'forest dweller' (*vanaprastha*) and 'wandering mendicant' *(sannyasa)*.

[9] *Chatan*: one of a large number of spirits in Keralan folklore believed to enjoy possessing humans.

[10] A traditional *brahmin* physician, some of whom specialise in *graha*, which is healing the mental and physical ill-effects of spirit possession.

[11] *Ghee*: clarified butter.

[12] *Amalaka*: Indian gooseberry or myrobalan *(phyllanthus emblica)*, highly valued for its medicinal properties.

[13] Taken from Verse 8 of the Khanakadharastava stotra, the hymn to Lakshmi traditionally said to be Shankara's first composition.

Part Two: The Monk

[14] The temple of Omkareshvara in Madhya Pradesh.

[15] Shivaratri the 14th day of the dark fortnight in the lunar month of Phalgun (i.e. February-March) each year.

[16] Taken from Gaudapada's commentary (karika) on the Mandukya Upanishad, one of the most celebrated and perhaps the most absolutist texts of classical Advaita Vedanta.

[17] The Absolute personified as Lord Vishnu, in his form as the supreme causal energy.

[18] The lunar month of January-February.

[19] Shankara: the Redeemer, one of the epithets of Lord Shiva. The staff is known as a danda, and those Dashanami sannyasis who chose to retain it after initiation are known as Dandis, whereas those who in their extreme renunciation, chose to abandon even this stark symbol of their monastic status, are called Tyakya Dandis 'those who abandoned the danda' or more commonly, Paramahansa 'Supreme Swans'. This is one example of what can be called 'the theatre of renunciation', i.e. those outward and visible signs of an inner psychological, or even spiritual, reality. Shankara himself was a Dandi, as were his four favourite disciples, and thus Dandis have a special place in the Dashanami tradition. As these four disciples were the first in the historical line of Shankaracharyas (see note c above) it is the custom that all subsequent Shankracharyas must also be Dandis. To this day, Varanasi remains the centre of Dandi activity.

[20] Modern-day Varanasi, formerly known in British times as Benares.

[21] The Kadam (Neolamarckia cadamba) which grows up to 45 m high, is traditionally associated with the Buddha by Buddhists and with Shiva and Parvati by Hindus.

[22] Literally: 'sloping place' i.e. the long steps leading down to the river.

[23] Bhaja Govindam. The poem totals thirty-one verses, of which the first twelve are traditionally attributed to Shankara.

[24] Gestures and postures.

[25] Communal hymn singing.

[26] *Avimukta* means 'the never-forsaken', so-called because it is said that Lord Shiva never forsakes his beloved Kashi, even at the end of the worlds. Avimukta, an area between today's Marnikarnika and Pancha Ganga *ghats*, was the area of the city where the most renowned teachers lived in Shankara's time.

[27] Bhagavad Gita 2.23-24 and commentary.

[28] The Eight Virtues.

[29] Commentary on the Bhagavad Gita 4.39

[30] c.f. The well-known Sanskrit adage: *Na guror adhikam.*

[31] In Vedanta, these bodies are technically called the 'sheaths' (*koshas*) that obscure the pure light of the Self. They are known, in their ascending order from gross to subtle, as: 'the sheath made of food' (*annnamayakosha*); 'the sheath made of breath' *(pranamayakosha);* 'the sheath made of mind' *(manomayakosha);* 'the sheath made of knowledge' *(vijnanamayakosha)* and 'the sheath made of bliss' (*anandamayakosha).* For the textual source of all that follows on this subject, see the Taittiriya Upanishad 2.3.1; 2.4.1 and 2.5.1 and commentaries and also The Crown Jewel of Discernment verses 151–218.

[32] The Tamil word *khutumbay* means literally a kind of jewelled ear ornament worn by women, but is also used in South India as a colloquial term of endearment for girls.

[33] These are the three qualities *(gunas* = 'strands of a rope'*)* enumerated by the Sankhya philosophy as *rajas*: activity or motion; *tamas*: inertia or mass and *sattva*: harmony or light. They are the constituents of the matter-energy (*prakriti*) that creates the material universe and, in various combinations and proportions, are present in every aspect of material creation.

[34] Two of the *Satdarshana* or Six Right Perspectives, i.e. the six orthodox systems of philosophy.

[35] Commentary on the Bhagavad Gita 2.47-50.

[36] The magical and protective materialisation of lotuses is a popular theme in Indian myths. Another example concerns the Buddha: once a fanatical enemy of the enlightened one named Shrigupta tried to lure him into a house surrounded by hidden pits of fire. As the Buddha approached the building, however, lotuses sprang up over the pits and he was able to walk across them unharmed.

Together with Sureshvara, another of Shankara's closest followers, Padmapada developed ideas that led to the founding of the Vivarana school of Advaita commentary. His only surviving work is the Panchapadika, written as a response to Shankara's commentary on the Brahma Sutra, but unfortunately, all that survives of the text is an extended gloss on the first four verses. He also founded a monastery named Thekke Matham at Thrissur in Kerala, his native place.

[37] These four – discrimination (*viveka)*, non-attachment *(vairagya)*, right conduct *(shatsampat)* and right desire *(mumukshutva)* – are both the practical discipline on the path and also the sign that it is bearing fruit.

[38] *Shatsampat*: 'The six aspects of right conduct' according to Advaita Vedanta.

[39] *Aghori*, 'the Fearless', a type of tantric ascetic whose spiritual path lies in complete disregard for all the norms of conventional social propriety.

[40] Yama: the Vedic Lord of Death.

[41] This is a classic refrain of Shankara's, found often in his writings, in various forms and expressed in varying degrees of intensity. See among many such examples: The Thousand Teachings 10; The Crown Jewel of Discernment 85 - 93, etc.

[42] Yoga Sutra 2.40 and commentary.

[43] The Thousand Teachings 15.11-34.

[44] *Samskaras*: The seeds of the previous actions deposited deep in the mind. They serve as unconscious activators by sprouting as future desires.

[45] Commentary on the Bhagavad Gita 14. 22 – 25.

[46] Commentary on the Bhagavad Gita 14. 19 -20.

[47] Commentary on the Bhagavad Gita 4 .19-20; 37 - 42.

[48] These are all names and forms of the god Vishnu. Interestingly, although the hagiographies and popular tradition consider Shankara to have been an incarnation of Shiva, the sparse evidence we have from his life and writings point to an equal preference (apparently shared by his parents) for Vishnu as a chosen personification of the Absolute. He and his immediate followers refer positively and not infrequently to Vishnu as a theistic focus, hardly at all to Shiva. This may be partly affected by the circumstances of teaching: Vishnu and his incarnations is traditionally the focus of the householder and theistic devotion, whereas Shiva appeals more to the recluse and seeker of metaphysical knowledge. Although ascetics from the Shankara orders have consistently worshipped a variety of personal gods, in the five major Shankara monasteries today, the twenty-eight Shaiva scriptures (*agamas*) are a basis for a great deal of the regular performance of *puja*. It is also worth mentioning here that, just as the absolute Self is above and beyond sectarian partialities, so can the sage who knows the Self move freely between affiliations to various *devatas*, unlimited by any one of them and enjoying, while simultaneously transcending, all of them. This explains how Shankara composed hymns to the Goddess replete with great devotional feeling while remaining a staunch non-dualist. It also explains how a prominent later Vedantin, Vachaspatimishra, would call Badarayana, the author of the resolutely absolutist Brahma Sutra, an embodiment of Vishnu's creative intelligence (Narayana).

[49] These three types correspond to the three qualities (*gunas*) explained in note 33 above.

[50] Probably modern day Maheshwar in Madhya Pradesh. As with so much of Shankara's life story, there are several variant versions. Some local legends claim that Mahishmati is Maheshvar near the sacred pilgrimage town of Ujjain; others that it is Mahishi in Bihar. Such divergent opinions are fiercely held and attest to Shankara's continuing influence in all parts of the subcontinent. In 1970 no less than 400 scholars descended on Mahishi for a three-day function to celebrate the famous debate they believe took place there.

[51] *Shraddha*: rituals performed by a son for his deceased father to enhance the parent's evolution through the various subtle realms

after death. The ritual also opens up a channel for the departed to bless their children in return.

⁵² *Dharamshala*: pilgrim resthouse.

⁵³ *Dharma*: born duty; the Natural Law that sustains creation.

⁵⁴ *Varna*: caste. The Sanskrit word means literally 'colour'; the English word 'caste' derives from the Portuguese *casta*, meaning 'race, lineage, or breed', that British travellers in India encountered in the early 17ᵗʰ century. Each of the four *varnas* – *Brahmin*, *Kshatriya*, *Vaishya* and *Shudra* – is subdivided into numerous sub-caste groupings, known as *jatis*, literally: 'births'.

⁵⁵ Bhagavad Gita 3. 5-8.

⁵⁶ Bhagavad Gita 3. 26 and 29.

⁵⁷ Bhagavad Gita 3. 3. and commentary.

⁵⁸ Bhagavad Gita 3. 19; 26-28. and commentary. *Mahamahopadyayaji*: an honorary title for a great textual expert.

⁵⁹ *Gotra* ('clan') an unbroken line of male descent stemming originally from one of eight legendary Vedic sages. Members of the same *gotra* are believed to possess certain common characteristics by way of nature, inherent tendencies or profession. The institution is observed especially among *brahmins*, but people of the same *gotra* can be found across different castes. Traditionally, marriage between members of the same *gotra* is prohibited, whereas it is deemed best when between those of the same caste or *jati*.

⁶⁰ The Jaimini Sutras are one of the principal texts of the Karma Mimansa ('Enquiry into Action') orthodox school.

⁶¹ Brihadaranyaka Upanishad and Commentary: 3.8 & 4. 2-4. These are among Shankara's favourite scriptural passages.

⁶² Quoted verbatim from the Mundaka Upanishad 1.1.4.

⁶³ Quoted verbatim from the Bhagavad Gita: 2. 43-46.

⁶⁴ The Thousand Teachings (Verse) 1.24.

⁶⁵ *"Ram nam satya hai!:* 'The name of God is Truth!"

[66] The yogic power known as *parakayapraveshavidya*: 'the art of possessing another's body'. For details see Patanjali's Yoga Sutra 3.38 and commentary.

[67] Sureshvara was popularly known as Vartikakara, 'the Composer of Commentaries', in acknowledgement of his formidable literary output. He was charged by Shankara to write commentaries elucidating several of the Master's own works, including the commentaries on the Brihadaranyaka and Taittiriya Upanishads. But Sureshvara's most important work was his own composition 'The Perfection of Acting in Freedom' and, although less well-known than Shankara or Gaudapada, the converted exponent of Karma Mimansa became one of the most important exponents of classical Advaita Vedanta.

[68] *Gali*: the narrow alleys in Kashi/Varanasi. (Compare the *calli* of Venice).

[69] All the biographies of Shankara describe this meeting with the Untouchable as a crucial event in his life. Perhaps predictably, it is often cited as a criticism of orthodox views on caste and the social exclusivity of orthodox *brahmin* life. However, this present study sees the significance of the event as going beyond sociology, being rather a dramatic indication of a radical shift in the young teacher's awareness. This shift was a direct, unmediated and permanent cognition that 'In truth, all beings are seen in the Self, and the Self in all beings' (Bhagavad Gita 6.29 – 31) and with it Shankara entered fully and finally into the mature phase of his enlightened vision and teaching mission.

In this interpretation, the figure of the despised outcaste symbolises the 'impure' relative realms of boundaries and distinctions, the realms of matter that hedge in our native spiritual boundlessness. In other words, the young *brahmin's* embrace of the despised social inferior describes and symbolises the dramatic, irreversible and liberating transcendence of duality once and for all. To the fully enlightened, there is no 'other', all, without exception, is his own Self.

This dramatic transformation is the culmination of a profound journey in consciousness that is described in the wisdom traditions as proceeding through identifiable stages or stations. The first is the unchanging experience of the Self as separate from the ever-changing world of activity, in which category is included the sense of individual agency rooted in a separate selfhood constituted by one's own body/mind.

This, the preliminary stage of enlightenment, is known in the Advaitin teaching as *turiyatit chetana*: 'being established in the awareness of the fourth'. It is so called because 'the fourth' *(turiya)* is the transcendental awareness that lies, forever undisturbed, prior to our three habitual modes of mind: waking, dreaming and sleeping. This unbroken continuum of consciousness is the constant preoccupation of many of the major Upanishads upon which Shankara wrote his authoritative commentaries. It is most clearly described in the Mandukya Upanishad.

This initial stage of freedom is also known in the texts as *jivanmukti:* 'Liberation of the individual' or by such English phrases as 'Self-realisation' or 'Cosmic Consciousness'. It is classically described in The Yoga Sutra of Patanjali, the philosophical background of which is the dualistic system of Sankhya.

Mature realisation, however, cannot be satisfied with a freedom that is only subjective. Somehow, the outside world of change, in its entirety, must also be realised to be imbued by the unchanging 'fourth'; both Self and 'other' must be reconciled in, and as, the one unbroken Divine. This seamless Unity that underpins, informs and maintains diversity, while in no way obliterating it, is what Vedanta calls 'non-dualism' (*advaita*). The journey to full Enlightenment (*brahmi chetana*) thus proceeds through a double transformation: firstly, as a passing of the limited individual into the Divine, and then as the infusion of the Divine into everything.

Part Three: The Master

[70] The spiritual lineage (*guruparampara*) of Advaita Vedanta is taken to derive initially from deities (e.g. Narayana, a form of Lord Vishnu, who governs the continuance of the evolutionary process) then descends through Vedic seers (*rishis*) such as Vashistha and Vyasa and is maintained through a succession of fully enlightened human beings or Masters, for example, Govinda and Gaudapada.

[71] Since earliest times in India there have been orders of monks, traditionally known as the *parivrajakas*, ('travelling mendicants')

who, though loosely affiliated to a particular monastery, remain itinerant except for the annual rainy season of four months when they stay put in one place. In their outward rejection of fixed society they paradoxically act to stabilise and balance it by enacting the spiritual, rather than just the material values of life. If the cosmic principle of movement is eclipsed by that of stasis, imbalance and suffering will result.

[72] Bhagavad Gita 4.35; 6.29-31.

[73] Rig Veda 1.164.46.

[74] Vedanta accepts six valid methods of gaining knowledge: (1) direct experience or perception *(pratyaksha)*; (2) inference *(anumana)*; (3) analogy or comparison *(upamana)*; (4) scriptural authority *(shabda)*; (5) implication or inference from circumstances *(arthapatti)*; and (6) negative proof *(abhava pratyaksha)*. Of these six, Shankara consistently holds the first to be the most important as, incidentally, did the Buddha.

[75] Shankara deemed learning and familiarity with the scriptures to be essential both for a truly proficient teacher and a worthy *sannyasi*. See for example The Thousand Teachings 1.3; Commentary on the Katha Upanishad 1.2.7; Commentary on the Brahma sutra 3.4. 47-50.

[76] *Puranas*: 'old, ancient' – literary records the West would call myths; *itihasas*: 'thus it happened' –literary records the West would call epics. Both these bodies of literature would be considered to be factual history by the orthodox Hindu. *Rishis:* 'seers' who cognised the Vedic scriptures; *siddhas:* 'perfected ones' with the ability to enjoy supernormal powers.

[77] Commentary on the Brahma Sutra 2.1. 24-25. (See note 84 below).

[78] Patanjali's Yoga Sutra Chapter 4, verse 27.

[79] As in, for example, the Shvetashvatara Upanishad: 6.19.

[80] Commentary on the Chandogya Upanishad: 6.2.2.

[81] Chandogya Upanishad: 6.2.1.

[82] *Prakriti*: a term used, mainly in the Sankhya teachings of Kapila, to denote the primal energy-matter from which all manifestation springs. Sankhya enumerates and categorises the various strata of

creation and many of its terms are employed by Advaita Vedanta in its analysis of the world. The term *pra-kriti* means literally 'the coming forth of what has been done'. To speculate, there may be an equivalence here, or at least an analogy, between *prakriti* and the fields of dark energy and dark matter currently being posited in the theories of quantum physics.

[83] Shvetashvatara Upanishad: 4.10.

[84] All the foregoing is an exposition, derived largely from Shankara's commentary on the first quarter of the second book of the Brahma Sutra, on the topic of *sat karya vada*, a crucial tenet of Advaita Vedanta, both before and after Shankara. *Sat karya vada* deals with the question of causality. It argues that any observed effect is not the creation of something new, *ex nihilo*, but the emergence into manifestation of something that already necessarily exists in latent form. All that is needed for this emergence are the appropriate conditions, just as all that is needed for the emergence of an oak tree from an acorn are the appropriate conditions of sunshine, rain, nutrients in the surrounding earth, etc. Shankara argues that the entire world of time, space and causation is but a series of changes that, as they emerge into manifestation from their causal seeds, are in reality non-binding and substantial modifications of an essential constituent that itself remains unchanging. This is the absolute intelligence, realisable by an individual as their Self. The medium through which these changes are generated, the primal causative energy or *prakriti*, is essentially at one with the Self. Thus the Self retains its unbounded integrity throughout, despite and beyond whatever changes it appears to be undergoing in the limited view of the empirical mind.

[85] Hari Stotra 41.

[86] See Yoga Sutra 2.47 and commentary. *Nididhyasana:* a type of one-pointed mental absorption that leads to an immediate experience of the Absolute (see note 88 below). In all his writings Shankara mentions a total of only perhaps a dozen *asanas*, and he pays them little heed. His interpretation of the classical yogic *Ashtanga* ('Eight Limbs') as laid down by Patanjali is to internalise the entire process as various stages of inner absorption and refinement of awareness rather than treat the first half as is normally done, i.e. as a set of behavioural stipulations (*yama, niyama*) followed by a regime of

physical exercises (*asanas, pranayama*). He once commented that *hatha yoga* was 'a cart with only one wheel'.

[87] Commentary on the Bhagavad Gita 16.1; 18.52.

[88] The Direction Perception of Being (*Aparokshanubhuti*) 116. The three stages of hearing (*shravana*), reflection (*manana)* and absorption (*nididhyasana*) constitute the classic methodology of Vedanta, spelled out in the Brihadaranyaka Upanishad 2.4.5. and explained in Shankara's commentary thereon. The great Vedantin refers to this triple means more than any other as a preferred teaching methodology; see, for example his own composition called Self Knowledge (*Atmabodhi).*

[89] *Mahavakyas:* the four 'great sayings' of Vedanta, that affirm the identity of the Self (*atman*) with the Totality *(brahman).* See, among many such examples: Brihadaranyaka Upanishad 5.1.1.; Chandogya Upanishad 3.14.1. and 6.11; Katha Upanishad 2.1.11.; Mundaka Upanishad 2.3.9.; etc.

[90] Here Shankara plays on the word *rakta*, which means both 'red' and 'impassioned' in Sanskrit. Antithetically, *vairagya*, usually translated 'non-attachment' also means 'colourless', and is thus another word-play with the analogy of the 'colourless sap' in the previous discussion. The usual Sanskrit term for these latent mental impressions that are the seeds of our thoughts, desires and actions is *samskaras*. When a *samskara* becomes activated it is known as a *vasana* ('scent'). Interestingly, smell is the only one of our five senses that is located in the old brain, a reminder of the time before the human eye took over from the animal nose when our species began to walk upright. The evocative power of smell is well-known; thus 'scent' is a peculiarly apt way to describe an echo of the deep subliminal past emerging into consciousness.

[91] Yoga Sutra 2.52 and commentary and also commentary on Bhagavad Gita: Chapter 2. 61-62.

[92] Commentary on Brihadaranyaka Upanishad: 2.3.6.

[93] It would be hard to overestimate the importance that Shankara attributes to the tradition of enlightened Masters through whom the wisdom of life has been passed down over the centuries. His commentaries always begin with an acknowledgement of this

tradition and its blessings. See, for example: The Crown Jewel of Discernment 51 and onwards; Introduction to the Taittiriya Upanishad, and then 1.1.1 in the same text; Commentary on the *karika* to the Mandukya Upanishad 4.100; Introduction to the Brahma Sutra; Commentary to the Bhagavad Gita 4.1-2; The Thousand Teachings 17.2-3; 89; and 18.233. In one place (Commentary to the Brihadaranyaka Upanishad 6.5.1-4.) he even traces this blessed lineage back through the mothers of these teachers as they were the ones who gave the sages life.

[94] *Sammelan*: a gathering of the religious to debate and discuss doctrine.

[95] Brahma Sutra 1.2. 1-8 and commentary.

[96] The Thousand Teachings (Verse portion): 17.72; The Direct Experience of Being 24-28; 40.

[97] e.g., The Brihadaranyaka Upanishad 1.4.10; the Taittiriya Upansihad 3.10. 5-6, etc., and see also note 89 above.

[98] The Thousand Teachings (Verse portion) 17.35. See also the Yoga Sutra 4.19. and commentary.

[99] Introduction to the Commentary on the Brahma Sutra.

[100] The Thousand Teachings (Verse portion) 18. 24-33; 56-58.

[101] The Thousand Teachings (Verse portion) 18.37-43.

[102] The Thousand Teachings (Verse portion) 19.27-28.

[103] Vedic fire ceremonies to elicit the support of the gods. See Bhagavad Gita 3.10 - 15.

[104] Commentary on the Brahma Sutra 2.3.40.

[105] The teacher referred to here is Gaudapada. These lines come from his commentary (*karika*) on the Mandukya Upanishad 1.16. See also the Commentary on the Brahma Sutra 2.1.9.

[106] e.g. Taittiriya Upanishad 2.8.; the Brihadaranyaka Upanishad 4.3.33.

[107] These successive subjective levels are known in Vedanta as the five *koshas* or 'sheaths' that cover the Self (see note 31 above).

108 Commentary on the Taittiriya Upanishad 2. 6. The intense personal experience of this level of life is often expressed as devotion to one of its divine personifications. See in this regard Shankara's compositions 'The Wave of Bliss' (*Anandalahari*) and 'The Wave of Beauty' (*Soundaryalahari*) which are both hymns addressed to the Goddess.

109 Commentary on the Brahma Sutras 2.1.13.

110 Introduction to the Commentary on the Brahma Sutras. This doctrine of 'superimposition' (*upadhi* or *adhyasa)* is crucial in Shankara's teaching and occurs in many contexts (see, for example, notes 158 and 182 below).

111 Gaudapada's *karika* on the Mandukya Upanishad 1.9.

112 Commentary on the Brahma Sutra 2.1.32–33.

113 Bhagavad Gita Chapter 8.5-6.

114 'Mind-stuff': *chitta* in Sanskrit. In Shankara's teaching, and Indian thought generally, the mind is considered to be a subtle material entity that absorbs and holds impressions of what is presented to it. There are analogies here with the Western psychoanalytic concept of the 'unconscious'.

115 Yoga Sutra of Patanjali 3.10 and commentary.

116 Bhagavad Gita 8. 7-14 and commentary.

117 Commentary on Bhagavad Gita 18. 66.

118 Yoga Sutra 2.9 and commentary.

119 This analysis occurs frequently in Shankara's writings; see for one example among many: The Thousand Teachings (Prose) 10 – 18.

120 Bhagavad Gita: 2. 20 – 30 and commentary.

121 Commentary on the Bhagavad Gita 3.3.

122 Bhagavad Gita 3. 3-8; 18-20 and commentaries; see also Bhagavad Gita 5.5 and 11.

123 Commentary on the Brahma Sutra 2.1.34. Compare also the New Testament teaching that God 'gives his sunlight to both the evil and the good, and he sends rain on the just and the unjust alike' (Matthew 5.45).

[124] When *samskaras*, the subconscious activators or latent tendencies seeded by past actions in the deep levels of the mind, begin to stir, manifest and sprout into desires, they are known as *vasanas*.

[125] Commentary on the Bhagavad Gita 2. 47-48.

[126] Gaudapada's Karika on Mandukya Upanishad 3.10; 4. 33-37 and commentary.

[127] Commentary on the Taittiriya Upanishad 1.11.1-2.

[128] *Varna*: the Sanskrit term means 'colour' and is usually translated as 'caste'. See note 54 above.

[129] The word used is *guna*; for a definition see note 33 above.

[130] Laws of Manu 6.42.

[131] Bhagavad Gita 3.35; 18.40–48 & commentary; commentary on the Brihadaranyaka Upanishad 1.4.6; 1.4.11-15 and commentaries.

[132] The Crown Jewel of Discernment 236. Shankara here reiterates a crucial definition, common to all Indian wisdom systems, of Reality as 'that which is unchanging'.

[133] The Crown Jewel of Discernment 268.

[134] Katha Upanishad 1.3.8; 2.3.14-15.

[135] The Thousand Teachings (Verse) 10.10.

[136] The Crown Jewel of Discernment 569-574.

[137] Bhagavad Gita 2. 48-52.

[138] Ashtavakra Gita, a classic text of Advaita Vedanta that takes the form of a dialogue between the great ruler Janaka, King of Mithila, and the eponymous sage Ashtavakra.

[139] Bhagavad Gita 3. 21; 3. 25-29.

[140] Bhagavad Gita 3.1.

[141] Commentary on the Yoga Sutra 1.15.

[142] The Sanskrit word for this dispassionate non-attachment is *vairagya*, which literally means 'without colour'. Hence Shankara's use of the crystal analogy.

[143] Commentary on the Brahma Sutra 2.1.33.

[144] Mundaka Upanishad 2.1. 1-10 and commentary.

[145] Brihadaranyaka Upanishad 3.7.3-23 and commentary on the Brahma Sutra 2.1.25.

[146] To follow Shankara's argument here, we must bear in mind his unfailing adherence to the Vedic definition of Reality as 'that which does not change'.

[147] Brahma Sutra 3.2.25 - 30 and commentary.

[148] Commentaries on the Bhagavad Gita 4.37; Chandogya Upanishad 6.14.2 and Brahma Sutra 4.1.15.

[149] *Prarabdha*: the *karma* that has precipitated the present birth and is being worked out in the present life.

[150] The Crown Jewel of Discernment 451-464; 548-552 and 558-561.

[151] Commentary on the Brihadaranyaka Upanishad 3.2.12 - 3.3.1.

[152] Bhagavad Gita 5.12-14 and commentary.

[153] Commentary on the Bhagavad Gita 13.2. Shankara here plays on the word *kshetra* which means 'a field', both in a literal, agricultural sense and also as a spatial metaphor, as in 'a field of vision', 'a field of influence' etc. In yoga, the word is also used to describe the body and the world of objects, when differentiated from the subjective Knower, i.e. the Self. To judge from the unusually long commentary appended to this verse, it was evidently one that Shankara thought particularly important.

[154] Trishanku: a character in the Ramayana, who aspired for heaven but got stuck half-way there. In common parlance the phrase 'Trishanku's heaven' still describes a middle ground or compromise between one's desired goal and the current reality.

[155] Here Shankara is quoting from the eleventh book of the popular Vaishnava scripture the Shrimad Bhagavatam.

[156] The Thousand Teachings (Prose) 1.64-5.

[157] i.e. Those who subscribe to what Shankara ironically calls the philosophy of *dehatmavada*, i.e. 'the body is the real Self'.

[158] Introduction to the Commentary on the Brahma Sutra. This erroneous superimposition is technically called *adhyasa* in Vedanta and is central to Shankara's understanding of the world.

[159] Technically: 'the six stages of transformation' (*shadbhavavikara*)', i.e. latency, birth, growth, transformation, decay and destruction. The world, and anything in the world, is invariably subject to these transformations and therefore is not permanent *(nitya)* but impermanent *(anitya)*. In this specific sense, Vedanta defines the impermanent as being 'unreal' or 'untrue' (*anritam; asatyam*) because 'reality', according to Vedic thought, necessitates permanence.

[160] Bhagavad Gita 13.26-30 and commentary.

[161] Commentary on the Brahma Sutra 3.3.53. *Paan* is a popular intoxicant, made of the chopped nut of the areca palm, the leaf of the betel creeper, lime paste and various spices to taste.

[162] Commentary on the Brahma Sutra 3.3.54.

[163] Brihadaranyaka Upanishad 3.4.2 and commentary.

[164] Commentary on the Brihadaranyaka Upanishad 2.3.6.

[165] Commentary on the Brahma Sutra 2.1.11.

[166] Commentary on the Brahma Sutra 2.2.38.

[167] Commentary on the Isha Upanishad 4.

[168] These are the four *mahavakyas.* 'The Great Utterances', i.e. 'I am the Totality' *(aham brahmasmi)*; 'You are That' *(tattvamasi)*; 'This Self is the Totality' *(ayamatmabrahma)* and 'The Totality is Transcendental Knowledge' *(prajnanambrahma).* They are to be found in the Upanishads, at Brihadaranyaka Upanishad 1.4.10; Chandogya Upanishad 6.8.7; Mandukya Upanishad 1.2 and Aitareya Upanishad 3.3, respectively.

[169] See among many examples: Taittiriya Upanishad Commentary 1.3. 2-4; Bhagavad Gita Commentary 2.42-45; Brahma Sutra Commentary 1.1.4.; 3.3.10 & 59-65; 4.1.7-12 Chandogya Upanishad Commentary 1.1.1. and Brihadaranyaka Upanishad Commentary 1.3.9; 4.3.7.

[170] Commentary on the Mandukya Upanishad 4. 45.

[171] Devotional hymns.

[172] Isha Upanishad and commentary 4-5.

[173] Isha Upanishad 17-18.

[174] Shvetashvatara Upanishad 4. 8-9 (*author's translation*). In this regard it should be noted that Shankara himself does not use the term *maya* extensively, and nowhere does he describe himself as a *mayavadin*, i.e. 'a proponent of *maya*'. It is true to say that Shankara's teaching on this point has not been well served by his successors who took over the torch of Advaita after his death. They were professional metaphysicians concerned with theorising about 'illusion', whereas Shankara's primary concern was to comment on the ancient texts in such a way as to bring liberation to seekers living in the everyday world.

[175] Bhagavad Gita 3. 27-29 and commentary.

[176] Bhagavad Gita 2. 45-46 and commentary.

[177] Commentary on the Brahma Sutra 3.4.26.

[178] Shankara agrees with Upanishadic tradition on the rigorous conditions laid down to determine the eligibility (*adhikara*) of a student. These include: calmness, humility, devotion, sexual continence and knowledge of scripture and ritual. In Vedic culture there were many different types and grades of student. The period of spiritual apprenticeship, when the student lived with and served his *guru*, was never less than twelve years and could often last for at least twice that time. For the importance of the *guru-shishya* relationship and the necessary qualifications of the student see, for example: the Chandogya Upanishad: 4.4.5; 4.9.3; 4.10.2-3; 6.14.2; the Prashna Upanishad: 1.2; the Mandukya Upanishad: 1.2.3; 3.2.10; the Shvetashvatara Upanishad: 6.22.23, etc.

[179] Commentary on the Bhagavad Gita 13.2.

[180] Commentary on the Brahma Sutra 2.1.11.

[181] Kena Upanishad 1.3-4 and commentary.

[182] This concept of 'superimposition' (*upadhi*) is key in Shankara's explanation of the relationship between the innumerable relative worlds of time, space and causation, and the one Absolute that underlies, supports, interpenetrates and simultaneously transcends them all. The mysteriousness of this relationship is explained in Shankara's use of the concept *maya*, which accords well with the rapidly growing body

of scientific evidence supporting the hidden continuity of consciousness, including near-death experiences, after-death communication, reincarnation, and neurosensory information received in altered states. The young Advaitin in his teaching on the unfailing persistence of an unlocalised consciousness beyond the demise of the body – which means that, in our essence, we are immortal – preceded by centuries the current awakening of science in this area. In general, his teaching on *maya* based on the sacred Vedic tradition, correlates well with theories in cutting-edge physics which posit that things in our plane of time and space are not intrinsically real, but are manifestations of a hidden dimension where they exist in the form of superstrings, information fields, and energy matrices. Among the many books now available on this topic, see for example: 'The Philosophy of Consciousness Without an Object' by Franklin Merrell-Wolff, and 'The Immortal Mind: Science and the Continuity of Consciousness Beyond the Brain' by Ervin Lazlo and Anthony Peake.

[183] Commentary on the Brahma Sutra 4.1.7.

[184] Commentary on the Brahma Sutra 4.1.8.

[185] *Shad darshana*, often referred to as 'the six orthodox systems of philosophy'. These are: Nyaya, Vaisheshika, Sankhya, Yoga, Karma Mimansa and Vedanta.

[186] Qualities (literally: 'strands of rope'): *sattva, rajas* and *tamas*. See note 33 above.

[187] Commentary on the Bhagavad Gita 2.49-53.

[188] This is the classic Vedantic definition of the undefinable Absolute as: *sat* (Being), *chit* (Consciousness) *ananda* (Loving Bliss).

[189] It is its unbroken endurance that gives the Self its absolute status as ultimate Truth. Shankara, and his illustrious predecessor in the *guruparampara* tradition Gaudapada, often refer to this fact.

[190] Commentary on the Brahma Sutra 3.2.4-8.

[191] This is a doctrine technically known as 'Difference within non-difference' *(bhedabhedavada)*.

[192] This is the literal meaning of Vedanta; i.e. *Veda* ('knowledge') and *anta* ('end; culmination.').

193 See, among many such examples: the Mundaka Upanishad: 2.2.11; the Brihadaranyaka Upanishad: 1.4.10; 2. 4. 6; 3. 7. 23; 3. 8. 10-12; 4.4.19-20; 4.4.24-25; the Bhagavad Gita: 7. 19; 13. 2; 13. 27; the Isha Upanishad: 7; the Chandogya Upanishad 7.25.3; etc.

194 Commentary on the Brahma Sutra 1.4.21-23.

195 *Prasad*: food that has been blessed by either being offered to the deity or having received the spiritual energy of a holy being.

196 Yoga Sutra 3.37 and commentary.

197 Yoga Sutra 3.38 and commentary.

198 Bhagavad Gita 6.29-31 and commentary.

199 Commentary on the Yoga Sutra 1.25.

200 Commentary on the Brihadaranyaka Upanishad 1.5.20.

201 Commentary on the Brahma Sutra 4.4.17-21.

202 Badarayana: the author of the Brahma Sutra.

203 These are the concluding words of the Brahma Sutra.

204 Commentary on the Brihadaranyaka Upanishad 3.9.26. Yajnavalk-ya and Shakalya were two well-known characters from Vedic lore. The former was an enlightened sage, the latter an imposter whose head fell off when he lost a debate. To make matters worse, his bones were stolen by robbers as they were being carried to his home for the funeral rites.

205 Commentary on the Brahma Sutra 2.3.17.

206 Commentary on the Brihadaranyaka Upanishad 2.1.20.

207 Commentary on the Brahma Sutra 1.1.4. and 4.1.12.

208 Shvetashvatara Upanishad 2.10.

209 Commentary on the Brahma Sutra 4.1.9-11.

210 Commentary on the Brahma Sutra 1.4.14.

211 Gaudapada's *karika* to the Mandukya Upanishad 3. 15 and commentary.

212 Shvetashvatara Upanishad 3.8-21.

213 Commentary on the Brahma Sutra 1.1.11. These two aspects of *brahman* are classically known as *saguna* ('with attributes') and *nirguna* ('without attributes'). Thus both the relative and the absolute realms together constitute the one Totality (*brahman*), though in the case of the former, its transcendental substratum is obscured, giving rise to what Shankara calls 'ignorance' *(avidya)*. See also note 282 below.

214 Commentary on the Brahma Sutra 1.4.15.

215 Commentary on the Brahma Sutra 2.3.9.

216 Commentary on the Taittiriya Upanishad 2.1.1 & 3.10.5-6; Commentary on the Chandogya Upanishad 7.25.2 & 8.12.3.

217 See, for example, the Katha Upanishad 1.2.22-3; the Mundaka Upanishad 2.1.2; the Brihadaranyaka Upanishad 4.3.15-19 and the Chandogya Upanishad 8.12.1.

218 Commentary on the Chandogya Upanishad 8.10.4.

219 Isha Upanishad 6-8 and commentary.

220 Brahma Sutra 4.2.12-16 and commentary; The Thousand Teachings 10.1-14.

221 This is the Sankata Mochana ('Destroyer of Sorrow') temple dedicated to Hanuman-ji, the embodiment of devotion and loyal service.

222 Commentary on the Brihadaranyaka Upanishad 1.3.1.

223 The Thousand Teachings (Prose) 1.30-32.

224 Commentary on the Brihadaranyaka Upanishad 3.3. Introduction.

225 Commentary on the Brahma Sutra 3.1.8.

226 Commentary on the Brahma Sutra 1.1.1.

227 Commentary on the Brahma Sutra 3.1.7; the Bhagavad Gita 3.11; the Chandogya Upanishad. 3.6.1. Commentary on the Brihadaranyaka Upanishad 1. 4. 10; 2.1.20. As regards the 'debt' Shankara mentions in this section, it is traditionally said that human beings are obliged to repay three kinds: to the gods, the ancestors and the sages. The means of repayment of such debts are, respectively: sacrifices, procreation and celibate study of the Vedas.

228 Bhagavad Gita 4.18-22 and commentary.

[229] Brihadaranyaka Upanishad 4.4.7 and commentary.

[230] Bhagavad Gita 4.24 and commentary.

[231] Commentary on the Brahma Sutra 2.3.48.

[232] Brahma Sutra 3.4.50. and commentary; Brihadaranyaka Upanishad 3.5.1.

[233] Mundaka Upanishad 2.2.11. Following Gaudapada in his Mandukya Upanishad Karika 2.7 and 4.32., Shankara often describes the world as *mithya*, 'misperceived' by which he means that the normal understanding of the world as a time-space duality is a false perception that overlays an essential unity. This unity is unbounded Consciousness and in its light all material reality is only provisional. A metaphor useful in understanding this could be the concept of 'fatherhood'. If X is the father of Y who in turn is the father of Z, then we can say that the 'fatherhood' of Y is real from the standpoint of Z, but not from the standpoint of X. It is a relative term only and has no absolute, abiding reality. The technical term Shankara frequently uses to describe the relationship of the changing relative world's relationship with its unchanging absolute substratum is 'superimposition' (*adhyasa*). Nonetheless, what some proponents of Shankara's view often overlook is that he never claims the world is simply 'unreal'. It has a reality, i.e. an existence, quite obviously, only that reality is provisional and wholly contingent.

[234] Bhagavad Gita: 6.25-26 and commentary.

[235] Yoga Sutra 1.36 and commentary. The discriminating intellect is known as *buddhi*.

[236] A statement found in many places. See for example: the Chandogya Upanishad 6.16.3. 8.12.3, etc.

[237] Mundaka Upanishad 3.2.9. and commentary.

[238] Commentary on the Brahma Sutra 1.3.19.

[239] Brahma Sutra 2.3.39-40; 3.2.24 and commentaries; The Thousand Teachings 1.17.22.

[240] Bhagavad Gita 2.16-17.

[241] The Sanskrit word translated here as 'abiding existence' is '*vastubhava*', a crucial concept in Vedanta and one that is often

misunderstood. Shankara's analysis of the world of the senses is virtually synonymous with the Buddha's teaching of 'no-self' (*anatta*). Indeed, some of Shankara's critics referred to him as a 'crypto-Buddhist'.

[242] c.f. The commentary of Shankara's illustrious predecessor, Gauda-pada, on the Mandukya Upanishad 4.31: 'Whatever does not exist in the beginning or the end does not really exist in the present'. This is the essential Vedantin critique of the 'reality' of the world. It does not, of course, mean that the world does not *exist*, but that is has no ultimate, that is to say abiding, status.

[243] Commentary on the Bhagavad Gita 2.15-18.

[244] This story also occurs in the Shrimad Bhagavatam, Book 11. Alluding to the arrow, Shankara here extends the concept of 'one-pointedness' (*ekagrata*), originally a technical yogic term referring to fixity of mind in meditation (e.g. Yoga Sutra 3.12) to refer to steadiness of intent applied in daily activity outside meditation.

[245] e.g. Chandogya Upanishad 8.1.5.

[246] Katha Upanishad 1.2.22.

[247] The Thousand Teachings (Prose) 1.33-37.

[248] i.e. The Golden, Silver, Copper and Iron Ages (*Sat, Dvarapa, Treta* and *Kali Yugas*). These are the sequential, and descending, phases of each cycle of cosmic manifestation, evolution and dissolution. We are currently in the *Kali Yuga*, when humanity's possibilities are least, and its suffering greatest. This cyclical process is considered to continue without end.

[249] Subsidiary branches of Vedic knowledge, including astrology.

[250] *Jyotishis*: Vedic astrologers.

[251] Commentary on the Brahma Sutra 1.1.17.

[252] Commentary on Gaudapada's *Karika* on the Mandukya Upanishad 1.7. This must be the first recorded mention of the famous 'Indian rope trick'.

[253] It is worth mentioning here that within a hundred years of the Buddha's death, there were no less than eighteen schools claiming to have the Master's original teaching. Only one of these – the

Theravadins or 'Doctrine of the Elders' – survives in any substantial form; most of our knowledge of early Buddhism, including other early Buddhist schools, derives from its records.

Much has been made of Shankara's antagonism to Buddhism. While it is certainly true that he dismissed the Buddhism he saw around him and engaged in fierce debates with contemporary Buddhists, it is easy to place undue emphasis on this difference. Much of the confusion is semantic and centres on the concept of 'self'. Shankara championed the cosmic Self, (Sanskrit: *atman)* whereas the Buddha denied the reality of the limited empirical 'self' (Pali: *atta).* (In Indian languages, as in English, the same word can refer to both). In effect, both teachers celebrated the unicity of what transcends the limited sense of selfhood but from opposite, or complementary angles.

The Buddha, who as a member of the ruler-warrior *kshatriya* caste was debarred from performing brahminical rituals, framed his message as a timely reaction to the Brahmanism of his day, a ritualistic religion that had at that time become corrupted and overly complex. As a reforming counter-balance, his message was presented as a practical psychology addressed to what he saw to be the central problem of the human condition – suffering. In his analysis of this congenital illness and his prescription for its cure, he resolutely avoided both theology and metaphysics, mindful that these could easily degenerate into sterile theorising and be used to justify the religious exploitation he saw all around him. His focus was always directed to the problematic nature of life and the way to overcome its inherent suffering.

Shankara on the other hand, as a high caste *brahmin* and the heir of a lineage of extraordinary spiritual genius – Vyasa, Shukadeva, Gaudapada and his own master, Govinda – represented the quintessence of orthodox Hindu metaphysics firmly grounded in the sacred texts of the Upanishads. While the Buddha's starting point was to employ an analysis based on phenomenal realism, Shankara's perspective was to affirm the blissful and non-dual Consciousness of the Self that underlies, interpenetrates and transcends all relative existence, in both its apparently 'happy' and 'unhappy' modes.

In fact, both these approaches, despite their seeming divergence, end up at the same place. Buddha's way culminates in *nirvana,* the defeat of suffering that results from following the eightfold noble path of morality and meditation, while Shankara's path reaches its goal of *moksha* through the purifying disciplines of ritual (*karma*), worship *(upasana)* and finally, direct spiritual intellection *(jnana)*.

To sum up simply: the Buddha analysed the insufficiencies of the relative world (including its subtle or astral dimensions) and presented a path to transcend them all and arrive at freedom, while Shankara, as heir to the Upanishadic tradition, celebrated the plenitude of the Absolute that contains, but lies beyond, time, space and causation and outshines all worlds – gross, subtle and causal.

It should be noted that in Buddhism 'suffering' (*dukkha*) is a quasi-technical category. Originally an agricultural term denoting a wheel that is not properly fixed to the axle and so causes the cart to lurch and sway, the word refers to the intrinsically unsatisfactory nature of so much of our lived experience. At another level, the concept of *dukkha* is extrapolated to refer to all unenlightened worldly experience that is predicated on the erroneous identification with a body-self and its limitations. The Buddha called this identification 'the false idea of self', while in Shankara's terminology it is 'ignorance' (*avidya*). Both teachings agree that this egotistic self-possession is only finally destroyed by direct insight into the nature of reality.

Shankara's denial of Buddhism, therefore, was not on the basis that Buddhism was fundamentally in error, but rather that he could not accept the Buddha's teaching as it was framed and still remain true to himself and his born destiny as the guardian of Vedic orthodoxy. This orthodoxy included all sorts of regulations and observances for living in society prior to the dawning of metaphysical insight and consequent liberation. To the extent that Buddhism's monastic orientation deviated from Vedic orthodoxy, not in its ultimate goal of liberation but in its rejection of the social and ritual requirements incumbent on householders prior to liberation, Shankara was bound to oppose it.

In this context it is interesting to remember a couple of further points. Firstly, the Buddha never denied the existence of the Vedic gods; what he did deny was that their worship brought a real end to suffering. This, in fact, is precisely Shankara's view, as witness his famous debate with the celebrated exponent of *karma mimansa* ritualism, Mandana Mishra (see text above). Secondly, not only are the terms *nirvana* and *moksha* used virtually interchangeably to describe enlightenment in Buddhist and *advaitin* texts, but both are unfortunately often misunderstood, even by so called 'experts', to mean physical death, or some freedom consequent on physical death, rather than liberation in life.

[254] This is the Buddhist doctrine known as 'Momentariness', a necessary correlate of the 'no-self' *(anatta)* teaching. Several early schools – such as the Vaibhashika, Sautranika, Yogachara and Madhyamika – held this theory in various forms. In a very different cultural context, a similar theory of 'no-self' was also held by the leading philosopher of the eighteenth-century Scottish Enlightenment, David Hume.

[255] Commentary on the Yoga Sutra 1.32.

[256] Brahma Sutra 2.3.7 and commentary.

[257] Bhagavad Gita 6.28-31 and commentary.

[258] The Direct Experience of Being: 107-109. For Shankara's devotion to Dakshinamurti, see his *Shri Dakshinamurtistotra*. Among the large number of devotional prayer-poems attributed to Shankara, this is one of the few that scholars agree is his composition. However, see note 48 above for Shankara's Vaishnavite leanings.

[259] Commentary on the Kena Upanishad 2.1.

[260] Brahma Sutra: 2.3.18 and commentary; 2.3.50 and commentary.

[261] Chandogya Upanishad 6.11.3.

[262] Commentary on the Brihadaranyaka Upanishad 2.4.12.

[263] Commentary on the Chandogya Upanishad 3.14.2.

[264] Commentary on the Chandogya Upanishad 6.3.2.

[265] The Thousand Teachings (Verse) 18.28-33; 38-39.

[266] Bhagavad Gita 2. 20-29 and commentary; Brihadaranyaka Upanishad 4.4.6.

[267] The foregoing idea of different levels of truth is crucial in Shankara's teaching. Already prefigured in the Upanishads (see one example, among many, the Brihadaranyaka Upanishad 2.3.6) it was shared by some Buddhist teachers, such as Nagarjuna and the Madhyamika school. It is not merely a question of different opinions

held in the waking state but of different perspectives based on radically different levels of consciousness and, by extension, different states of physiology and brain functioning. The highest level of truth confounds all empirical experience of the usual waking state (see Gaudapada's *Karika* on the Mundakya Upanishad 2.31-32; 4.72-75 and Shankara's commentary thereon). To those who experience the non-duality (*advaita*) of the unbounded Consciousness, all common experience is seen to be an unreliable basis for true understanding, because it is predicated on the limitations of egocentricity and duality (and their corresponding physiological functioning), which are, *a priori*, states of metaphysical ignorance.

[268] An ancient order of wandering ascetics whose best-known historical guru is Gorakhnath.

[269] Commentary on Gaudapada's *Karika* on the Mandukya Upanishad 3.37-44.

[270] *Dhobi:* laundry; *dhobi wallah:* washerman.

[271] Bhagavad Gita 4.22.

[272] Chandogya Upanishad 6.8.7.

[273] Commentary on the Brahma Sutra 1.4.6.

[274] Bhagavad Gita 5.8-9 and commentary.

[275] Bhagavad Gita 5.18 and commentary.

[276] See note 33, above.

[277] Taken from Chapter 4 of the Ashtavakra Gita (see note 138 above).

[278] Commentary on the Brahma Sutra 2.1.23.

[279] Commentary on the Bhagavad Gita 2. 21; Brihadaranyaka Upanishad 4.4.19 and commentary.

[280] Literally 'the fourth' i.e. the unchanging basis of the three transient states of waking, dreaming and sleeping. 'The fourth' is the name commonly given to the transcendental Self in early literature and is most clearly described as such in the Mandukya Upanishad.

[281] Commentary on Gaudapada's *Karika* on the Mandukya Upanishad: 4.45-52.

[282] Commentary on the Brahma Sutra 1.1.11. These two aspects of *brahman* are classically known as *saguna* ('with attributes') and *nirguna* ('without attributes'). Thus both the relative and the absolute realms together constitute the one Totality, though in the case of the former, its transcendental substratum, without which it could not exist, is obscured.

[283] Commentary on the Chandogya Upanishad 8.1.1. This is the doctrine of 'skilful means' *(upaya)*, the pragmatic use of provisional truths. It is perhaps the central method of teaching non-dualism.

[284] Commentary on the Brihadaranyaka Upanishad 4.4.25. Shankara lauds this verse as summing up the entire Upanishad in a nutshell.

[285] The major annual Buddhist festival of Vesak, the Spring full moon which celebrates together the birth, enlightenment and death of the Buddha.

[286] *Bhikku*: the usual word for a monk in the early (i.e. Theravadin) schools of Buddhism.

[287] The 'Three Marks of Impermanence' by which Buddhism characterises the shortcomings of human life and, by extension, the world.

[288] This is Shankara's preferred definition of the word *nirvana*, emphasising the affective aspect of liberation. See for example the commentary on the Bhagavad Gita 2.71 and 5.24-26. It is thus a more positive interpretation of a state classically described by translations of early Buddhist texts as 'extinction'.

[289] The passage Shankara quotes here, taken from *Udana* 80, is the clearest extended description we have of *nirvana* in words reliably attributed to the Buddha himself. As a practical spiritual teacher Gautama was always unwilling to characterise the state of freedom, for fear that such a description would degenerate into just another set of theories and concepts to burden his followers. Here Shankara cleverly uses both the words and the formal debating style of the Buddha himself to present his teaching of Advaita Vedanta to these Buddhist monks.

[290] The famous teaching known as 'The Flower Sermon'. In general, however, Buddhist schools value debate as a way of sharpening the mind as a tool fit for realisation, and we know that there were many such discussions between Buddhist and non-Buddhist schools.

Great teachers such as Nagarjuna, Aryadeva, Buddhapalita, Chandrakirti, Dharmakirti and, later, Shantarakshita and Kamalashila wrote comprehensively about the ancient Hindu schools of thought.

[291] Kena Upanishad 1.3-9.

[292] Shankara here speaks in terms that mimic the seminal Mahayana text the *Lankavatara Sutra*: (see especially Chapter 2.9.122-4). In its radical non-dualism the *Lankavatara* is very close to Shankara's doctrine, and its vocabulary in places also recalls the words of Gaudapada, the teacher who Shankara seems most to cherish among his predecessors in the *guruparampara* succession of Advaita Vedanta. Gaudapada was renowned for his commentary on the Mandukya Upanishad and possibly the commentary on the Sankhya sutras, which form the philosophical basis of Yoga, early Buddhism and Jainism.

[293] Brahma Sutra 2.1.1-3 and commentary. See also Hari Stotra 41. In advocating 'the great texts of the Upanishads', Shankara is referring to the *mahavakyas* (see notes 69, 89 and 168 above). It is the direct realisation of the import of these sayings that takes the aspirant from knowledge of the Self (*atman*) which is the goal of *yoga*, to knowledge of the Totality *(brahman)* which is the goal of Vedanta. The Sanskrit terms for these discreet and successive stages of enlightenment are respectively: *turiyatit chetana* (or Cosmic Consciousness) and *brahmi chetana* (or Unity Consciousness). It is this profession of enlightenment as the state of complete non-duality which distinguishes the lineage of Shankara.

[294] Taken from Totakacharya's *Totakastakam*, the hymn composed on his reaching enlightenment.

[295] This text is The *Shrutisarasamuddharanam*, a poem of one hundred and seventy-nine verses.

Part Four: The Mission

[296] The four places where the divine nectar fell to earth are Allahabad, Nasik, Haridwar and Ujjain, each situated on a holy river. The Mela is held between the auspicious dates of Makra Sankranti and Maha Shivaratri, at each place in rotation over a twelve-year cycle. The Purna ('Full') Kumbha Mela is held at Allahabad every 12 years. After 12 Purna Melas, i.e. once every 144 years, the Maha ('Great') Kumbha Mela, is also held at Allahabad and deemed particularly auspicious due to the planetary configuration that only occurs then. Each Mela draws at least 10 million participants; at the last Maha Mela celebrated in 2013, it was reckoned 100 million people attended, including perhaps a million from outside of India. The Kumbha Mela is thus by far the largest regular gathering of people on the planet; the nearest contender probably being the Haaj to Mecca, which draws approximately 2 million pilgrims annually.

[297] Modern Allahabad, renamed as such ('The City of Allah') by the Mughal Emperor Akbar in the seventeenth century.

[298] Braj is the area around modern Vrindavan, south of Delhi. The Dark Lord is Krishna, who is always depicted as blue.

[299] Marquee-like awnings.

[300] These two groups of ascetics are ancient indeed; the Keshavins are mentioned in the Rig Veda and the Vratas in the Atharva Veda, texts going back to at least 2000 BC.

[301] 'The Eternal Law' i.e. what the West calls 'Hinduism'.

[302] The 'ten directions of space' are the four cardinal points and their mid-points making eight, with above and below added to complete the picture. In a temple these would be represented by guardian deities placed at the appropriate places of the building or circumference wall.

In each of the five monasteries Shankara is here establishing (see note b above) there is to this day an observable pattern of wholehearted theistic worship conducted within the overarching framework of pure non-dualism. Thus the goddesses Kamakshi, Sharada, Vimala, Bhadrakali and Purnagiri are the focus of devotion in Kanchi, Shringeri,

Dwaraka, Puri and Jyotirmath respectively. These five divine embodiments of the cosmic feminine energy are balanced in each case by the presence of a *lingam*, which, as the 'emblem' of Shiva, signifies the cosmic masculine principle. The *lingam* is an abstract icon; it cannot be said to have form, but nor is it quite formless; its shape has neither a clear beginning nor a well-defined end. In addition, the fact that the *lingams* in these five potent Shankara sites are made of crystal quartz accords well with the *advaitic* understanding of ultimate Reality: having no colour themselves, they take the colour of whatever object is presented before them. Thus, the crystal *lingam* is a most appropriate image of the attributeless *brahman*. While remaining infinite and devoid of form or qualities in itself, the Absolute seemingly succumbs to its own perfection, and under the influence of *maya* appears temporarily to adopt all forms and assume all limitations.

In addition, according to the present Shankaracharya of Shringeri, Adi Shankara placed the Shri Chakra, a *yantra* symbolising the supreme Goddess Tripurasundari, inscribed with various *bija* mantras, at each of the seats of learning. This is the symbol of the teaching known as Shri Vidya 'the most auspicious Knowledge' which reconciles the various strands of theistic, yogic and non-dualist perspectives into one whole.

303 This form of deity worship is known as the *panchayatana* ('five altars'). Popularised by Shankara in his travels around India, it continues to this day to be the principle ritual of orthodox *smartas, i.e.* the non-sectarian followers of Vedic Hinduism.

304 Shankara's heirs, the abbots of the monasteries he established, who are known as Shankaracharyas, i.e. 'teachers of Shankara's wisdom' (see notes b and c above).

305 Bhagavad Gita 1.40-43.

306 Taittiriya Upanishad 2.6.

307 'Name and form' *(nama-rupa)*, is the shorthand term in Vedanta for the relative reality of time, space and causation.

308 Commentary on the Taittiriya Upanishad 2.6.1.

309 The part of India where Shankara was born, known since 1956 as the state of Kerala, was until that time effectively the Western seaboard of the Tamil country that stretched right across the

south of the subcontinent. While Kerala had its own Malayalam language, its own vibrant tribal traditions and was ruled by local dynasties who were frequently at war with neighbouring royal families, it was also home to many high caste and religiously orthodox who enjoyed a great degree of cultural homogeneity with the rest of the south.

[310] This is *Soundarya Lahari* or 'Wave of Beauty'.

[311] i.e. the Vijnanavadins.

[312] Commentary on the Brahma Sutra 2.2.28.

[313] i.e. the Sarvastavadins.

[314] Commentary on the Brihadaranyaka Upanishad 4.3.7.; and The Thousand Teachings 16.23-32; & 18.141-144.

[315] Commentary on the Brahma Sutra 2.2.25 & 32.

[316] *Yama*: the Lord of Death.

[317] Commentary on the Chandogya Upanishad: 5.10.1. & 2. Traditionally, it is taught that at death the celibate who has lived a pure life leaves the body by the Northern Path associated with the sun, whereas the householder, who has been concerned more with ritual fire offerings rather than pure knowledge, leaves the body by the Southern Path of smoke and the moon. More generally, the spiritual path of the recluse is known as *Nivritti marga*, the path of turning away from activity (*nivritti* = negation), whereas the spiritual path of the householder is known as the *Pravritti marga*, the path of involvement in the world (*pravritti* = action, engagement).

[318] Vivekachudamani verses 246-64.

[319] Bhagavad Gita 3.26-29 and commentary.

[320] Gaudapada's Karika on the Mandukya Upanishad 1. 14-18.

[321] See the Brihadaranyaka Upanishad commentary 4.3.7.

[322] See above and also the Bhagavad Gita 13.33; 15. 12 and the Katha Upanishad 5.13.

[323] This state of suprasensual cognition, whose object is clearly seen without any error, is known as *Ritam bhara pragya*; see the Yoga Sutra 1.48-9 and commentary.

[324] Indian basil.

[325] A stone pillar in Kaladi's Aryadevi Samadhi Mandapam marks the spot of the cremation today. The shrine is maintained by the Shringeri Shankaracharya math.

[326] The modern town of Kollur in Karnataka. This legend is attributed to several other sites as well as Kollur.

[327] Taken from the twelve verses of the *Hastamalaka stotra.*

[328] A medicinal fruit, also known as the Indian gooseberry, much valued in Ayurveda.

[329] Modern day Dwarka.

[330] This is a favourite argument of Shankara's against those – for example Buddhist logicians such as Nagarjuna – who sought to negate the reality of the world.

[331] Self Knowledge 62-64; and Mandukya Upanishad Karika 1.17.

[332] Another meaning of the word *maya.* See the commentary on the Bhagavad Gita 15.3.

[333] Bhagavad Gita 2.24-25 and commentary.

[334] Commentary on the Bhagavad Gita 4.24.

[335] Bhagavad Gita 4.19; 27 and 37.

[336] Brihadaranyaka Upanishad 3.9.28.7 and 4.5.13; Taittiriya Upanishad 2.1.1.

[337] Commentary on the Brahma Sutra 2.3.18.

[338] Modern day Kashmir; part of the Pir Panchal range of the middle Himalaya.

[339] This concept of layered meaning, known as *paroksha,* is an important device in orthodox exegesis.

[340] Yajurveda Taittiriya Samhita 1.8.6.1.

[341] Yajurveda Taittiriya Samhita 4.5.11.1.

[342] Brihadaranyaka Upanishad 3.9.1.

[343] Mahabharata 12.110.62.

[344] All the above discussion is taken from the commentary on the Brahma Sutra 1.3.27.

[345] Yajurveda Taittiriya Samhita 1.2.1.1 & 1.3.13.1.

[346] Shatapatha Brahmana 6.1.3.2 & 4; Chandogya Upanishad 6.2.3 & 4.

[347] This doctrine of the presiding deities (*abhimani devata*) is spelled out in the commentary on the Brahma Sutra 2.1.5.

[348] Yajurveda Taittiriya Samhita 1.2.1.

[349] Commentary on the Bhagavad Gita 4.38.

[350] Bhagavad Gita 4.18-20 and 5.7-9 and commentaries.

[351] Commentary on the Brahma Sutra 4.1.13.

[352] Mundaka Upanishad 3.2.2. and commentary.

[353] Bhagavad Gita 4.20 & 5.13 and commentary.

[354] Brihadaranyaka Upanishad 4.4. 5-7 and commentaries.

[355] This view is one of the main subsidiary versions of Advaita, known technically as *bhedabheda vada*.

[356] There are, as Shankara says, innumerable textual references to this unicity. See for some examples: Mundaka Upanishad 2. 2. 11; Brihadaranyaka Upanishad I. 4. 10; 2.4. 6; 3. 7. 23; 3. 8.11; 4. 4. 19; 4. 24; Bhagavad Gita 7. 19; 13. 2; 13. 27; Isha Upanishad 7; Kaushitaki Upanishad 6. 2. 1; 7.25. 2; etc.

[357] Commentary on the Brahma Sutra 1.4. 20-23.

[358] Commentary on the Brahma Sutra 2.1. 32-33.

[359] In Vedanta, the concept of *vada* ('discussion') is an essential element in the process of enlightening the student. The popular pedagogic axiom to which Shankara refers here runs: *vade vade jayate tattvabodhah'*.

[360] *Sadhaka*: someone on the spiritual path; a seeker.

[361] Commentary on the Brahma Sutra 1.4.18. The text Shankara refers to here is the Kaushitaki Upanishad 4.19.

[362] The five elements: earth, water, fire, air and space. According to Vedanta, in various combinations these elements, collectively known as the *pancha mahabhutas*, compose the entire universe, gross and subtle.

[363] Brihadaranyaka Upanishad 4.4.4 - 6.

[364] Patanjali Yoga Sutra 2.20 and commentary; The Thousand Teachings 1.18.43 & 83-85.

[365] *Mauna*: a vow of silence. The common word for a sage – *muni* – is derived from this, but refers not so much to an external vow, but to the inner silence of such a being.

[366] Practitioner of traditional Ayurvedic medicine.

[367] The Direct Experience of Being 143; Hari Stotra, 41.

[368] *Nididhyasana:* a level of mental expansion that transcends thinking and leads to an immediate experience of the real Self beyond the mind. This praxis is central to Shankara's teaching as the culmination of the triple process of hearing (*shravana*), reflection *(manana)* and deep meditation (*nididhyasana).* The great Upanishadic sage Yajnyavalkya defines *nididhyasana* as 'right knowledge' *(vijnana)*, by which he means an immediate and direct experience of unbounded consciousness, and Shankara himself often uses the two terms synonymously. See the Brihadaranyaka Upanishad 2.4.5 and commentary, and 4.5.6. and commentary.

In all his voluminous writings, Shankara hardly ever mentions the physical side of Yoga. In his lack of interest in physical practice, he follows the most authoritative commentator on Patanjali's Yoga Sutra, the sage Vyasa (c. late 4th century AD) who mentions just five *asanas*. The one place Shankara does discuss the subject is in his own commentary on the Yoga Sutra (2.46), where he refers specifically to twelve postures, adding 'and others' after this list, which clearly indicates knowledge of more. He also refers to: 'asanas mentioned in other scriptures', but whatever these may have been, he did not consider any of them important enough to spend time explaining.

Instead, Shankara's genius led him to internalise the whole of the Patanjali's *Ashtanga Yoga* sequence, treating the eight limbs not so much as a means to realisation, but as the expression of true insight into reality. Thus *yama* is the natural restraint over the senses due to the awareness 'All is *brahman*'; *niyama* is the oneness of consciousness with *brahman* as separate from the physical universe; *asana* is that state in which *brahman* is unceasingly contemplated with bliss; *pranayama* is the spontaneous control of the life force that comes from seeing all creation as *brahman* (Shankara adds that 'painful breathing exercises are for the ignorant'); *pratyahara* is to consider the sense objects as the Self ('seekers of liberation should practise this rather than its physical counterpart') ; *dharana* is the blissful steadiness of mind that sees *brahman* everywhere; *dhyana* is the thought-free awareness 'I am *brahman*'; *samadhi* is the blissful identification of consciousness with *brahman*.

This radical perspective also informs his treatment of specific Yoga poses. In general, he tells us that 'the inner state which permits the uninterrupted contemplation of *brahman* is to be considered the best posture' *(asana)*. Specifically, Shankara sees the *mulabandhasana*, for example, as 'the origin of all existence in which the mind can rest fixed' and the *siddhasana* as 'the immutable substratum of the universe in which the true yogi abides'. See The Direct Experience of Being 102-126.

[369] The Direct Experience of Being 116. For the full list of yogic qualities, see the Bhagavad Gita 16.1-3; 18.51-54. and commentary.

[370] Vyasa, believed by the orthodox to be the compiler of the Vedas, the author of the Mahabharata and commentator on several important texts, including the Brahma Sutra.

[371] Bhagavad Gita 8.6. and commentary.

[372] Brihadaranyaka Upanishad 4.4.2-3 and commentary.

[373] For the correct approach to a realised teacher, see, for example, Shankara's The Crown Jewel of Discernment v. 34-36.

[374] See, for example, Patanjali's Yoga Sutra 4:1.

[375] *Prarabdha*: the *karma* from our actions in previous incarnations that has already begun to fructify in this lifetime. The sum total of our individual *karmas*, by contrast, is known as *sanchita* ('the piled up') *karma*.

[376] The Kantakari fruit (Botanical Name: *Solanum Xanthocarpum*) is still widely used in Ayurvedic medicine for its good effects on the blood and internal organs.

[377] *Devatas*: subtle energetic beings, gods and goddesses. For the fact that all these *devatas* are ultimately reducible to the one prior Self, see for example the Brihadaranyaka Upanishad (3.9.1-9) where the sage Yajnavalkya presents the same argument as Shankara does here. In his

commentary on these famous verses, Shankara makes the point that the *devatas* are in fact infinite in number, while adding that the Self as *brahman* infuses and transcends them all. Thus being both one and infinite, the Self is the empty set that includes all possible numbers between these two limits. To signify such an abstract nature, the Self is often described as 'That' *(tat)*, which, Shankara says, is 'a word denoting remoteness'.

[378] On the *gunas*, see note 33 above.

[379] *Klesha*, literally an 'affliction'. The five *kleshas* are: ignorance *(avidya)*, egotism *(asmita)*, attraction *(raga)*, aversion *(dvesha)* and fear *(abhinivesha)*.

[380] See the Brihadaranyaka Upanishad 4.4.6 and commentary. See also the Bhagavad Gita 7. 19-25 and commentary. In these latter verses, it is significant that Lord Krishna, the personification of the Absolute, refers to himself as Vasudeva, i.e. 'that in which the *devatas* dwell'. Another way to understand this Sanskrit term is: 'the God that dwells within'.

[381] Brahma Sutra 3.4.28-31 and commentary.

[382] Brahma Sutra 3.4.47-49 and commentary.

[383] "One should speak the truth, one should say that which is pleasing; one should not say the truth that is not pleasing". *(Satyam bruyata priyam bruyata na bruyata satyamapriyam)* Manu Smirti 4.138

[384] Commentary on the Brihadaranyaka Upanishad 4.4.5. and the Mundaka Upanishad 3.2.2.

[385] Mundaka Upanishad 1.2.8.

[386] Mundaka Upanishad 1.2.12-13 and commentary.

[387] Literally: 'great soul'; saint.

[388] The supreme Self; the Absolute.

[389] *Prarabdha karma*, see note 375 above.

[390] Commentary on the Yoga Sutra 1.24. The same point, framed in the case of the clash of desires between two so-called omnipotent beings, occurs in Brahma Sutra 4.4. 17 and commentary.

[391] 'Unfathomable is the course of action' (Bhagavad Gita 4.17 and commentary).

[392] The formal vow of renunciation.

[393] The word translated as 'The Lord' is *isha*, which comes from the verbal root *ish*, meaning to rule, control or have power'. In Shankara's teaching this refers to the ultimate causal level of material manifestation. This personified causative power is still subordinate to the unqualified Absolute *(nirguna brahman)*.

[394] Isha Upanishad 1-2 and commentary.

[395] The abstract image of Shiva *(lingam)* and Shakti *(yoni)* that is the main conjoined image in the holy of holies of Shiva temples. The *yoni-lingam* symbolises the complementary masculine and feminine principles, which together create the universe.

[396] Temple meeting-hall

[397] Holy of holies (literally: 'womb-house').

[398] *Vaidyavidyavarenya*: an honorary term for an eminent physician. Dhanvantari: the celestial physician who is the father of Ayurveda.

[399] Bhagavad Gita 16.6 - 24 and commentary.

While it was not Shankara's sole approach, devotion to the Lord became the path for a number of later schools of *advaita*, most significantly the Vaishnavite Pushti Marg of Shuddha Advaita founded by the hugely influential fifteenth century saint, Vallabhacharya.

[400] Brahma Sutra 2.1.18-19 and commentary. See also note 84 above. In this teaching Shankara throws a new light on the standard analysis of phenomenal existence presented by early Buddhist schools, the theory known as the 'Chain of Dependent Origination' *(pratityasamutpada)*. This states that everything without exception depends on something else for its existence. Shankara accepts this dependent necessity to be operating in the entirety of the relative worlds of time, space and causation, but follows the Upanishadic position in locating and identifying an unborn, uncaused, and totally independent Absolute – i.e. *brahman* as pure Consciousness without an object – to be the transcendental essence of causality. Many later Buddhist schools of the Mahayana would come to agree with him, positing similar absolutes, such as 'emptiness' or 'Pure Mind' 'Original Nature', etc., as the uncreated and acausal context in which the realms of time, space and causation arise. Moreover, they would agree with the master Vedantin that both the unlimited Absolute and limited relative exist together, inseparably. This mutuality is described through such

common Mahayana phrases as: 'Form and emptiness exist together' or 'Samsara and nirvana are one', and it explains how Padmasambhava, the founder of the influential Dzogchen school of Tibetan Buddhism, could write: "Though my view is as spacious as the sky, my actions and respect for cause and effect are as fine as grains of flour".

[401] Mundaka Upanishad 3.2.2.

[402] Brihadaranyaka Upanishad 4.4.5-6 and commentary. See also the Mundaka Upanishad 3.2.2. as above, and commentary.

[403] Badrinath, one of the four dhams or major sacred mountain pilgrimage sites.

[404] Ammonite fossil, worshipped as a symbol of Vishnu. Shankara mentions the shalagrama principally in discussions on the subtle body, as for example his commentary on the Brahma Sutra 1.3.14 and on the Taittiriya Upanishad 1.6.1.

[405] Self Knowledge, verses 62-64.

[406] Commentary on Mundaka Upanishad 2.2.11.

[407] The Crown Jewel of Discernment 39,40.

[408] The Crown Jewel of Discernment 33-38; The Thousand Teachings 17.52, 59; 87-89. Also, see Dakshinamurti stotra for Shankara's fulsome praise of the enlightened guru.

[409] The Crown Jewel of Discernment 54-58.

[410] Revived by Shankara, the Kedarnath mandir is one of the twelve jyotirlingas, 'lingams of light', the holiest of the shrines dedicated to Shiva. Interestingly, the temple was left virtually undamaged in the catastrophic flooding that engulfed the area in 2013. While the walled complex, surrounding areas, and Kedarnath town all suffered extensively, with many buildings collapsing into the Mandikini river below, the shrine itself did not suffer any real damage, apart from a few cracks on one of the four walls, caused by the debris flowing down from higher up the mountain. A large rock among this debris acted as a barrier, protecting the temple from the flood.

[411] Modern Trichur, the cultural capital of Kerala state.

APPENDIX

A chronological list of the principle teachings in the order they occur throughout the text:

Paperbacks also available from
White Crow Books

Jesus of Nazareth with Simon Parke—
Conversations with Jesus of Nazareth
ISBN 978-1-907661-41-9

Thomas à Kempis with Simon
Parke—*The Imitation of Christ*
ISBN 978-1-907661-58-7

Julian of Norwich with Simon
Parke—*Revelations of Divine Love*
ISBN 978-1-907661-88-4

Allan Kardec—*The Spirits Book*
ISBN 978-1-907355-98-1

Allan Kardec—*The Book on Mediums*
ISBN 978-1-907661-75-4

Emanuel Swedenborg—*Heaven and Hell*
ISBN 978-1-907661-55-6

P.D. Ouspensky—*Tertium Organum:
The Third Canon of Thought*
ISBN 978-1-907661-47-1

Dwight Goddard—*A Buddhist Bible*
ISBN 978-1-907661-44-0

Michael Tymn—*The Afterlife Revealed*
ISBN 978-1-970661-90-7

Michael Tymn—*Transcending the
Titanic: Beyond Death's Door*
ISBN 978-1-908733-02-3

Guy L. Playfair—*If This Be Magic*
ISBN 978-1-907661-84-6

Guy L. Playfair—*The Flying Cow*
ISBN 978-1-907661-94-5

Guy L. Playfair —*This House is Haunted*
ISBN 978-1-907661-78-5

Carl Wickland, M.D.—
Thirty Years Among the Dead
ISBN 978-1-907661-72-3

John E. Mack—*Passport to the Cosmos*
ISBN 978-1-907661-81-5

Peter & Elizabeth Fenwick—
The Truth in the Light
ISBN 978-1-908733-08-5

Erlendur Haraldsson—
Modern Miracles
ISBN 978-1-908733-25-2

Erlendur Haraldsson—
At the Hour of Death
ISBN 978-1-908733-27-6

Erlendur Haraldsson—
The Departed Among the Living
ISBN 978-1-908733-29-0

Brian Inglis—*Science and Parascience*
ISBN 978-1-908733-18-4

Brian Inglis—*Natural and Supernatural:
A History of the Paranormal*
ISBN 978-1-908733-20-7

Ernest Holmes—*The Science of Mind*
ISBN 978-1-908733-10-8

Victor & Wendy Zammit —*A Lawyer
Presents the Evidence For the Afterlife*
ISBN 978-1-908733-22-1

Casper S. Yost—*Patience
Worth: A Psychic Mystery*
ISBN 978-1-908733-06-1

William Usborne Moore—
Glimpses of the Next State
ISBN 978-1-907661-01-3

William Usborne Moore—
The Voices
ISBN 978-1-908733-04-7

John W. White—
The Highest State of Consciousness
ISBN 978-1-908733-31-3

Stafford Betty—
The Imprisoned Splendor
ISBN 978-1-907661-98-3

Paul Pearsall, Ph.D. —
Super Joy
ISBN 978-1-908733-16-0

**All titles available as eBooks, and selected titles available in Hardback and
Audiobook formats from www.whitecrowbooks.com**

Lightning Source UK Ltd.
Milton Keynes UK
UKHW011804020819
347296UK00001B/134/P